FIT, FIRM & 50

JAY LEHR & KEN SWANSON

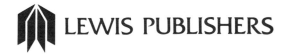

LEWIS PUBLISHERS

Library of Congress Cataloging-in-Publication Data

Lehr, Jay H., 1936–
    Fit, firm & 50 : a fitness guide for men and women over 40 /
Jay Lehr, Ken Swanson.
        p.   cm.
    Includes bibliographical references (p.).
    ISBN 0-87371-399-0
    1. Physical fitness.   I. Swanson, Ken.   II. Title.   III. Title:
Fit, firm, and fifty.
    GV481.L55   1991
    613.7--dc20   90-44553
                                                                        CIP

LEWIS PUBLISHERS, INC.
121 South Main Street, Chelsea, Michigan 48118

PRINTED IN THE UNITED STATES OF AMERICA

ACKNOWLEDGMENTS

Jay Lehr has attracted frequent media and public attention with his physical accomplishments as a middle-aged athlete. Whenever he has been asked to share his views on fitness, he has obliged, partly because he is an educator who enjoys lecturing and teaching. Thus, due to public interest in his fitness regimen, he decided to write a book to present the knowledge and findings he has acquired by training hard and by experimenting on his aging body. His idea was to write for older readers and to put the book in the form of an encyclopedia with topics ranging from "A to Z."

Jay's wife, Pat, liked the book idea, but she thought it should be broadened to include profiles of other older athletes who are in excellent physical condition. Pat suggested that I should write the profiles, and Jay agreed.

Thanks to Pat's suggestion, I've had the opportunity to acquire immense rewards from the athletes interviewed for this book. Talking with these athletes was a delightful experience as they discussed their athletic history. The accomplishments of these athletes are included in a large number of books, magazine articles, and newspaper articles. Although they have had previous media exposure, these athletes provided time and photographs to help with this exciting project. Many, many thanks to every athlete, including those who responded but were not included in the book.

Athletes were selected based on a combination of fitness, age, and athletic accomplishments that were predetermined through research, observations, and/or third-party recommendations. It would have been nice to have all men's and women's sports included, but that consideration was secondary to the people. Our goal was to interview the first ten athletes who satisfied the criteria established for each chapter, and we added an 11th "younger generation" athlete when a favorable response was submitted before the 10th interview was completed.

Recommendations on potential role models were sought from a variety of league, team, and event offices. The following people were especially helpful in providing information:

— Susan Hahn of the United States Tennis Association

— Barbara McQuitty of the United States National Senior Olympics

— Jim Ricca, President NFL Alumni, Washington Redskins Chapter

— Anthony "Don" Tall of the United States Orienteering Federation

Talking with the athletes was an exhilarating experience because they are enthusiastic people with a positive outlook toward life. Many spoke about the need to give something of themselves to help others. Their willingness to share personal information may be a significant help to the readers of this book.

Anita Stanley deserves special recognition and many thanks for editing this book and for lending moral support along the way. Special thanks also to friends and family members for their support and tolerance during the time required for this writing. This is especially true of our wives, Pat and Gloria, for putting up with their husbands' enthusiastic pursuit of fitness, athletics, and life in general.

Ken Swanson
Columbus, Ohio

CONTENTS

FIT, FIRM & 50

1

IMAGINE YOURSELF FIT

PHYSICAL FITNESS IS A STATE OF MIND

It's not too late for you to acquire a level of fitness that will allow you to live a healthier life. It doesn't matter whether you are 40, 50, or over 60; whether you are a current, former, or would-be athlete; whether you are exercising or vegetating. Nothing matters if you set your mind to developing your body to the best fitness level possible within your physical limitations. Your state of mind is your only real obstacle or, conversely, your primary mechanism to achieving physical fitness.

Unfortunately, our minds and bodies are typically weak links in our travel toward achieving personal goals. Only a small percentage of people develop the mental toughness needed to overcome human tendencies toward laziness. Often this toughness results from a compelling reason such as the desire to overcome an ailment. For example, co-author Jay Lehr conquered severe knee problems, including four operations and arthritis, to complete nine Ironman Triathlon events in Hawaii.

Mental toughness is a characteristic needed to maintain a daily regimen for improving skills. Successful athletes perfect winning skills because their physical attributes would be meaningless if swings, throws, and moves were not honed to perfection. As any athlete or serious spectator knows, outstanding athletes like Jack Nicklaus, John

Havlicek, Walter Payton, Chris Evert, and Edwin Moses spent thousands of hours practicing and training to achieve success. The individuals featured in this book have also worked hard to achieve their goals. Since mental, emotional, and physical attributes are inexorably linked, great athletes have had to acquire mental and emotional strength in order to fine-tune physical skills over a period of many years.

Individual accomplishments are usually the result of hard work coupled with a determined and positive state of mind. Achievers set goals and expect to reach them; their mission in life is purposeful. But for each person who achieves a desired level of physical fitness, there are thousands who don't. The long winding road to personal fitness is lined with quitters who emitted feeble excuses: "I don't have enough time." "I'm too tired." "I'm too old." Too often these people began their journey with too little understanding of where they were going and what it would take to get there. They were ill-prepared mentally to sustain their journey.

The road to fitness is an uphill journey; the route is steep and treacherous, culminating in a narrow frigid perch buffeted by strong winds. Strong mental discipline is required to reach this pinnacle of fitness and to remain there. Personal sacrifices of time and ingrained habits are required, but the rewards are great.

Mental preparation is necessary before beginning a fitness program. You should begin by seeking medical advice from your doctor so you won't worry about harming yourself. You should understand that the process is long, but that you can expect miraculous results over a period of time if you put forth your best effort to make the miracle happen.

To avoid boredom and disappointments, you must develop an enjoyable program with realistic objectives. Since athletics is a means for accomplishing this, older athletic-oriented persons who would like to be physically fit should find considerable mental stimulation within the covers of this book. Some already active readers will learn to improve their current performance levels, while others will learn how to begin or resume sporting activities in their advancing years. Others who simply enjoy spectator sports can focus entirely on improving their physical appearance and condition.

Many physical fitness books focus on exercise and nutrition, and some of these are cited in the bibliography included in this book. But *Fit, Firm & 50* differs from exercise and nutrition books because it focuses on the mental state necessary for beginning and maintaining an effective fitness program for men and women over 40. This book addresses the reality of applying oneself to a conditioning program that will culminate in a desired level of physical fitness.

The principle ingredient in a physical fitness program is the mind, which must think positively to overcome obstacles such as pain, chronic ailments, excuses, demands for time, tiredness, and laziness. To help cope with many reasons for quitting or not starting a program, athletes of the past and present are offered as role models for positive imagery and a simple program is suggested as a way to develop good fitness habits.

Role model athletes can help change your life if you initiate the action. The authors feel certain that you will relate to at least one of these role models if you are over 40. The key to role model support is the powerful factor of self-suggestion. Since we become what we are due to dominating thoughts and desires, our purpose is to impress our subconscious mind with the specific characteristics we want to acquire.

Choose your role model advisors and hold imaginary councils with them. Close your eyes and imagine yourself talking with them and getting instructions. Ask them for their knowledge and guidance in helping you achieve your desired level of fitness. Work with as many advisors as you need to build the composite fitness person you dream of being. With perseverance, you can reshape yourself by imitating the people who most impress you.

The role models in this book are older athletes who have maintained excellent health and fitness. An effort was made to choose men and women from different sports, including those who were at least 40 by 1968, when Dr. Kenneth Cooper's book on aerobics marked the beginning of the modern fitness era. Before 1968, the general feeling was that people over 40 should not indulge in endurance activities. Those who did developed personal fitness routines without the benefit of the medical and scientific advances that exploded subsequent to Cooper's book.

The authors, who are neither first-class athletes nor health professionals, are in the "over 50" age group, and they subject their bodies to the continuing rigors of exercise and sport. With self-motivated, enthusiastic, and positive personalities, the authors refuse to succumb easily to the passages of time, and they drive themselves daily to achieve objectives despite human frailties and the inevitable process of aging. Through different paths they have achieved victories and gained wisdom to share with others who have similar dreams of youthful vigor and vitality. The authors have no secret formula for achieving fitness and do not pretend to be substitutes for medical professionals. Their message is simple: it's not too late to achieve your desired level of physical fitness if you work daily to do so. Success depends on your state of mind — not your age.

If It's Not Fun, Don't Do It

No one wants to grow old and die. We often fear death, illness, poor health, and not being able to care for ourselves. On the other hand, recent polls indicate that about sixty percent of Americans avoid exercise which could improve the quality of their lives.

Exercise daily at a level that your body finds comfortable. If your body feels like going fast, let it go; if it does not, don't push it. Your objective is to develop good exercise and nutrition habits which, in turn, will develop good fitness. You will be less inclined to develop a habit when you associate pain with the activity, so allow your body to set a comfortable pace or rate.

Instead of pushing yourself through a painful program to achieve excellent conditioning in a few weeks, we advise you to proceed with medical guidance in a long-term program designed for gradual improvement and lifetime maintenance.

Physical fitness has progressed from obscurity to center court, with many fitness enthusiasts believing that pain is necessary and most beginners dropping their programs due to discomfort and frustration. Now the "no pain" fitness philosophy is recommended by an increasing number of specialists and leaders in physical conditioning. This is a recent change in thinking as more has been learned from athletic injuries and fitness studies. Pushing exercise to the extreme is usually not the best way for most people to achieve their desired level of physical conditioning.

This turnabout is revolutionary to those of us who remember being pushed to the limit in school and military athletic programs. The group workouts during the first week or two of each school athletic program were painful despite our youth and our good fitness. Coaches drove us through rigorous calisthenics and running for several days before settling down to teach sports fundamentals. Each morning after those first few workouts would be agony, as aching muscles were called upon to get us through the school day and another physical workout. Physical training in the military was similarly painful, especially since it was not done for sport and therefore lacked an enjoyable incentive.

Before exercise became a popular subject, older people were not expected to be involved in sports. These activities were more common among the wealthy, who had time and money for leisure sports, but few members of the middle class pursued fitness.

Middle-aged working-class men never seemed to exercise or play sports during the 1940s and 1950s. Perhaps the work ethic, memories of the Depression years, and the need to provide a good living played a part in not allowing time for such frivolous activities. But the economic improvement of the middle class has given more people the opportunity to enjoy prosperity and athletics.

One of the significant changes in our society since the 1940s has been an aging population. As a result, the number of people over 40, 50, and 65 is increasing. Physicians and scientists have been increasing their knowledge of bodily changes, destructive lifestyles, and treatable diseases. With better knowledge and improved medical help, we are being given opportunities to live longer and healthier lives. The opportunities are there for our choosing. With medicine reducing our risks for premature deaths, we can enjoy our potential extra years if we are physically and mentally able.

A small percentage of our "over 40" population is fit and ready to enjoy every year of their remaining lives. The Hawaiian Ironman triathletes show how people are improving their physical conditioning, and they reflect the potential fitness capabilities that can be achieved at all ages. For example, the winner of the men's 50–54 age group in the 1987 Hawaiian Ironman completed the event in less than 11 hours. His time was 51 minutes faster than the winner's time in the 1978 Ironman.

Dr. Bill Malarkey, who is profiled in this book as a role model athlete, conducted research on triathletes at the 1989 Ironman. Since data analysis is still in progress, Dr. Malarkey doesn't have results to report other than a dramatic change observed in hormones, but he offered some observations.

"These people were quite a bit into themselves," Malarkey said. "However, their actions were appropriate for what they put out that week and for what they were trying to accomplish. They displayed a real enthusiasm for living. Basically, these men and women were very optimistic, and many looked a lot younger than their chronological age. Their physical accomplishments spilled over into all areas of their lives, including relationships with their families and their peers at work. These triathletes are the missionaries in terms of what people can accomplish physically."

"I think the people who will really take hold of an exercise program are the same people who have taken effective hold of other areas in their lives," Malarkey said. "Everyone I have seen who is competitive and who has an excellent exercise regimen also seems to be doing well in other areas."

"The body hates inactivity," Malarkey explained. "For example, when our astronauts were weightless and without movement in space, their skeletons began to dissolve and they experienced other difficulties. The same is true with bed-ridden people who develop complications in a very short time. A study done three years ago by our cardiology group at The Ohio State University discovered a rapid rate of decay among well-conditioned athletes who were kept inactive for three weeks."

"I lecture most of my patients on exercise," Malarkey added. "It's hard to convince people to change behavior, but we can influence people who are leaning toward our position and need only a small push to be convinced. This fringe group has an important number of people, and our efforts are worthwhile if we can help convince them."

"Alcohol and cigarettes can damage almost any organ in the body," Malarkey said. "There is a proven increase in incidence of cancer in most organs of heavy smokers, and about the same thing has been proven for heavy drinkers. The same thing is true for obesity. The story I tell my obese patients is this: 'I look at obesity as a malignancy, and it has five- and ten-year survivals. To lose weight is relevant, but you're a survivor if you lose weight and keep it off five or ten years. I take care of cancers, like thyroid cancer, and their survival curves are almost the same as in the entire population. I can guarantee that you won't have a normal survival curve if you keep all that weight. Have you ever been to a nursing home?' They say, 'Yes.' 'How many 90-years-olds do you see who are overweight like you?' They say, 'None.' 'How many 80-year-olds?' They say, 'None.' 'How many 70-year-olds?' Usually they say none, but someone occasionally says, 'One.' 'Is the message coming across?' I get a little rough with them and I say, 'You know where all those overweight people are, don't you?' I'm not going to say that this little talk changes their behavior, but for a moment I have their attention. People often have to be shocked before they change their behavior."

"Obese people have the same struggle that smokers and drinkers have," Malarkey explained. "They have the same kind of addictive behavior. There's a gene for obesity, but there also seems to be a gene for inactivity. These people just don't walk as much, and they watch TV 7–8 hours a day. Their eating behavior is not always bad."

"This book's focus on older people has important implications for an aging population," Malarkey said. "I believe this is a critical area because its ramifications are economic as well as emotional, spiritual and physical. A bed-ridden nursing home patient is a big liability to their family and to society. We don't traditionally think of the economic savings of exercise, but they are enormous. Life expectancies have increased six years, but quality years have increased by only two, leaving an additional four years of poor health which can cost a fortune."

GETTING STARTED

Today people of all ages participate in some form of exercise. Some push themselves through levels of pain as they seek the highest threshold of physical fitness. A few punish their bodies in endurance events such as marathons and triathlons, and runners, who carelessly compete with cars for space on city streets, are often the brunt of quips by the non-runners who drive past them. "Have you ever seen a smiling runner?" is a frequent comment.

On the other hand, walkers of all ages never seem to be in pain and they usually appear to be enjoying themselves. Often they walk in pairs, husband and wife or friends. They talk and sightsee and exercise the dog while improving their mental and physical fitness.

Walking is being touted as one of the best exercises, especially for the elderly and non-athlete. It takes longer to cover a mile, burn calories, and improve physical fitness, but the fewer injuries sustained during walking may overcome these minor disadvantages by providing better consistency and quality exercise in the long term.

Consulting your physician and walking is a good way to start physical conditioning while developing a long-term fitness program such as the one we recommend. We believe everyone should use the following simple methodology to get started, regardless of age and current level of physical fitness:

- **Mental preparation** — You must want to improve your physical fitness, you must have the right attitude, you must set a goal, and you must find an enjoyable way to exercise. Choosing an activity you like is important because you must stay motivated. Another way to stay involved is to join a group or form your own group.
- **Habit** — You must develop good high-priority habits to

negate a myriad of reasons for improper eating and not exercising.

- **Exercise and nutrition programs** — You should develop a simple low-cost lifetime program with small milestones that will achieve your long-term goal. Do what your body feels like doing, but do something every day. Strive for specific results, because that will do much to keep your program going.

This approach to achieve physical fitness will not necessarily help you live longer, although it may, but it should make you feel better and improve your productivity. We advocate a simple and enjoyable conditioning program that will endure through the aging process. Conversely, some people who are overly anxious to acquire good fitness take off like a shot from a cannon, only to have their program fizzle and die when the momentum from the initial propulsion is gone. The better approach can be found in a Frank Sinatra song: "Just take it nice and easy."

Everyone has to get started at some time if they want to reach their goal. Remember the age-old saying that "even a journey of a thousand miles must begin with a single step." This truth pertains to everyone regardless of their current level of fitness. Advancing to the next highest level requires modification of habit, and a beginner advancing to level one is really no different in this sense from someone in good condition seeking improved fitness. Both require modification of habits because continuation of current habits will not achieve improvement.

Our immediate objective is to change your attitude and your habits and to encourage self motivation, leading to greater successes. However, habits are not easily changed because they are ingrained through repetition. You must decide which current habits are negative relevant to your long-range fitness goals and you must replace them with positive habits developed through repetition.

In order to replace negative habits with positive ones, you must have goals that you want very much to achieve. Every goal-related thought must create within you a desire to reach the level of fitness that you have targeted. These thoughts must be with you at all times, thereby establishing priorities as you weigh your daily options and visualize your happiness after reaching your goals. You must envision your well-conditioned body, fit and trim, playing your favorite sports with ease, never having to give in to fatigue, and being admired by others for your youthful appearance.

Mental preparation can be strengthened and maintained through imagery. By thinking of others and how they accomplished similar goals, you can be more confident that you can succeed. If your role model athlete did it, so can you.

In addition to fixing your mind on a specific goal and reinforcing your confidence with positive imagery, you must avoid boredom. Many people begin a program with great enthusiasm and high ideals, but soon boredom sets in as they see little or no improvement in their physical conditioning after a short burst of energetic exercise. Boredom kills more individual fitness programs than any other factor. Therefore, it is essential to perform a variety of enjoyable exercises on a regular basis without worrying about speed and repetition. Competitive sports are a wonderful addition to a fitness program because they add enjoyment and prevent boredom.

Doubles tennis is a sport that can be played by many older citizens. Two couples who are in their mid-sixties often play doubles at a local park in mid-morning, regardless of the summer heat and humidity. They have developed a habit of playing on a regular basis and their enjoyment is obvious. Also, because they form a special group of four, they lend each other encouragement and they need each other to participate. One person could not skip tennis without impacting the others' enjoyment, and that factor helps continue regular participation by minimizing the number of acceptable excuses for not participating.

Thus, when developing a personal fitness program, involvement with a group is beneficial to habit-forming exercise. Join a league or enroll in a class and involve others in your program. Then, schedule your individual aerobic, strength, and stretching exercises accordingly. Warm up before sporting activities and perform your individual exercises each day at a regular time if possible. Perform a lighter routine on days when you schedule a sporting activity.

Individual fitness programs must include good nutrition in order to be complete. There are many good nutrition books available for guidance; this book is limited to the listing of some fitness books in the bibliography and to a key dietary recommendation. We strongly recommend that you minimize your intake of saturated fats.

Fitness programs can be simple and low-cost. There is no need to join an expensive health club or to buy costly equipment for a home gym. It's fine if you can afford it, but not essential for the program to be effective. Good walking shoes may be all that you need to buy. A set of lightweight dumbbells would be a helpful addition, and an indoor exercycle or bicycle with a stand can easily accommodate a well-rounded program.

The comfortable "nice and easy" program we recommend is a lifetime plan for good health. It must be viewed at all times as a long-term effort to achieve your goal. But since your goal is long term, you need to establish a series of small graduated milestones that will give you short-term and intermediate satisfaction when they are achieved.

Getting started is simple, but continuance is a challenge. An ongoing fitness program certainly benefits from a good start which includes the effective mental preparation needed to develop good habits. The replacement of negative habits with those more positively aligned with goals will help ensure success in the long term.

Progress up the ladder of fitness requires tightening of the screws at each level. The mix of positive and negative habits that allowed you to move up one level are apt to be insufficient to raise you one more. Thus, your habits will probably need adjusting so that progress may continue. Whereas negative habits may still linger at the initial levels of the fitness ladder, they may be intolerable as you climb higher. Getting started or moving from one level of fitness to the next requires similar dedication, habit modification, and additional effort to achieve success.

Making Your Way Along the Long Road to Feeling Great

America's modern interest in fitness can be traced to 1968 and the first book, *Aerobics,* written by Dr. Kenneth Cooper, who captured the American public's attention with his caloric evaluation of various exercises. An interest in physical fitness thus began tormenting the minds of a large percentage of the population, but the impact on the nation's overall health was limited, with only a small percentage of the population really doing something about fitness.

Health clubs have proliferated throughout the nation and they attract a number of exercise devotees. But three things are evident from an analysis of the population:

1. The fitness scene is mostly an upper middle-class phenomenon related somewhat to social status.
2. The number of participants remains steady rather than increasing because the migration in and out of the field is balanced.

3. Most participants are youthful and have a less critical need for a fitness program.

These factors reflect a problem in the way fitness has been approached, described, promoted, and taught within our society.

Interest in Jane Fonda's exercise routine picked up when interest in Dr. Cooper's aerobic exercise values dwindled. This brought about an ardent group of followers whose participation in aerobic activity led to a large growth in similar classes, particularly Jazzercize. Following the Jane Fonda bandwagon were other celebrities and self-styled fitness advocates who created videotapes, books, and manuals for the purpose of converting our sedentary population into an active, enthusiastic, and fit society. Unfortunately, many individuals who endorsed or created these products were more interested in personal profit or self-aggrandizement rather than truly swaying America's mind.

Few people have stopped to analyze the impediments along the road to fitness for those who are willing to invest considerable time to achieve the small rewards that are recognizable each day. Newspapers, magazines, and television shows have capitalized on the fitness craze but have not adequately analyzed the dilemma which has made it difficult for a significant percentage of our population to convert their desires into deeds. Fitness in America is more of a perception than an accomplishment.

This book deals with the reality of fitness improvement for people who have passed the mid-point in their lives. The intent of the book is to energize the "over 40" group, which is more in need of fitness achievements than any other group. Their genetic codes are naturally unwinding in a normal decline, with a resulting decrease in physical capacity. We desperately need to slow this unwinding, to slow the decline, and to enhance the quality of everyday living for the people in the afternoon of their lives. This is not just a plea to those who can afford health clubs, health spas, videotapes, and equipment apparatus; this is a plea to anyone who can achieve a dramatic quality improvement in life at a time when a vast majority of people believe that decline is inevitable and that the best part of life is likely to have been left behind them.

The purpose of this book is to get the growing army of gray panthers and its new recruits marching on the long road to feeling great. There is no need to hurry; the race does not always belong to the swift, but more commonly to those who simply keep on running.

This book adds a mixture of information which should serve as a motivational guide to those who want to look and feel better. To think better is another possible objective because scientific studies show a positive correlation between good physical condition and good mental capabilities for members of the older generation.

It is our goal to deal with every subject, concern, and detail that could cross the minds of mature individuals who may have misconceptions about fitness, a totally negative outlook regarding their capabilities, or uncertainties regarding the path they should take. Many of us have admired older athletes, particularly those like hockey great Gordie Howe, football star George Blanda, and basketball champion Wilt Chamberlain, who played their sports at high levels of excellence well into their 40s. We want to help clarify the role of fitness in the lives of older athletes, and first-hand information sources are helpful in reducing misinformation.

Outstanding athletes who have remained physically fit throughout their lifetimes are presented for consideration as role models and also for enjoyment in learning about the fitness in their lives. Perhaps you can learn from them how to develop and maintain an enjoyable physical conditioning program. Whatever program you choose, these role models will be a source of encouragement as you embark on a similar path.

In Chapter 2 on "The Older Generation Role Models," we have sought to establish credibility among our readers of advanced years by profiling a significant number of prominent individuals who have achieved and maintained fitness in a manner that has contributed positively to their lives. Our purpose is to present role models from a period in time when physical fitness was not a household word. Although fitness was not then a high-profile issue, these role models, who were born before 1928, understood the benefits of fitness and pursued lifestyles which achieved for them significantly higher quality lives than were commonly encountered.

In Chapter 3, featuring "The Younger Generation Role Models," we describe men and women born in the 1928–1948 timeframe and who are living a fit life among us. Some achieved national fame. All have been featured by various media and are well-recognized locally or nationally within their athletic associations. We are interested in athletes who have trod the common path of life and have maintained excellent fitness through perseverance and good old-fashioned hard work and sweat. Our focus is not on cosmetic fitness but on fitness that translates into enthusiasm and a zest for life too few of us have.

When we speak of enthusiasm and active participation in a fitness program, many readers may feel a bit skeptical because they have known enthusiastic people who relish life despite never having embarked on a fitness program. Some people live healthy, productive lives while doing little that can be described as planned exercise. A brief explanation of this situation may disarm the skeptics.

It is a safe guess that 10% of the "over 40" age group are leading healthy lives while not exercising. An examination of their ancestry will show them to be products of excellent genes. In other words, they come from a healthy stock of long-lived people. They had the luck of the draw in life's lottery. Their good genes enable them to experience the highest quality of life with little or no additional input or effort.

Another 10% of the older population is equally fit, enthusiastic, and ambitious without an apparent exercise program, but this is the result of an excellent mature lifestyle that has worked for them without conscious effort on their part. They happen to eat properly, have sound mental attitudes, and get sufficient exercise from their work and personal activities.

An additional 10 to 20% of the "over 40" population falls into the third and last group that is classified as fit. The people in this group have acquired and maintained their excellent physical condition by dedicating themselves to an ongoing fitness program.

There is no scientific study to back up these statistics. Still, if you should take a statistical sample of the population, we contend you would probably find that 60 to 70% of this "over 40" age group are not physically fit or satisfied with their health and outlook on life. Thus, this latter group could benefit from a fitness program if they could find or devise a program focusing on their stage in life.

Fitness needs and capabilities vary among people over 40. What's right or best for one person is not necessarily right or best for another person. Improved health and appearance is a significant motivator. Other needs pertain to improved competence and capacity for physical performance in sports and an improved state of readiness for action. Our simple program can help any older adult regardless of fitness goals, because each participant must begin with a positive and purposeful state of mind to develop effective nutritional and exercise habits.

Make no mistake about the intended reader of this book. The focus is on men and women over 40 because their concern for physical fitness is more serious, practical, and warranted than is the younger generation's concern. In addition, those over 40 question whether or not it is too late to act on their concern.

Our intent with the book is to be realistic in all things. We recognize the common mental attitudes toward developing an active lifestyle held by individuals who have done little or no exercising as adults and attitudes toward health held by individuals who have suffered with illnesses. Our intention is to be honest, simple, understanding, and entertaining. We discuss the long hard road which leads you through levels of fitness and ultimately to your goal. We tell you that this road can be followed to its end if you have the right mental attitude and if you develop a habitual long-term fitness program. It's easy to do because this is not a quick fix program aimed at accomplishing a great deal in a short time, but rather a long-term program aimed at accomplishing a great deal over time but with discernible progress during the next week, month, and year. We focus on mental attitude toward your body, health, and general fitness rather than on any specific regimen of exercise and diet. What eventually defeats most people along the road to fitness is the inability to conquer the mental objections, including boredom, rather than the physical difficulties.

People who recognize these problems have often asked Jay Lehr to address their groups. One of the best lectures on this subject, "Let's Talk About Fitness" by Jay Lehr, is included as a chapter in this book.

Another section, "An Encyclopedic Discourse on Physical Fitness," is the A to Z approach to various subjects relating to the mental barriers to fitness. Thumb through the words in this "encyclopedia" and you will quickly recognize the comprehensive effort to address questions and concerns that could arise in the mind of an individual who is concerned with physical health.

The "A to Z" fitness encyclopedia presents information in a way that allows the reader's mental and intellectual obstacles to be eliminated and that builds a positive attitude from page to page as the simplicity of our approach toward fitness becomes more obvious. We strive continuously to obtain the positive state of mind rather than create a how-to by-the-numbers approach to fitness without explaining the essence of each subject. Our goal is to allow the reader to internalize every aspect of the subject such that little memorization of technique is required. Instead, a positive approach is attained through mental programming.

Positive imagery is nothing new. For example, it is reflected in many cliches: "You are only as old as you feel" and "It's never too late." The state of one's mind is the critical difference between success and failure. Potential candidates for fitness can control their minds, but will they? Since few people can exercise complete mental control, the concept of daily exercise without pain, discomfort, counting reps, or timing cycles reduces the sources of possible negative information. It is also best to work out at the same time each day because this removes the aspect of decision making and therefore another possible point of negative input. Using this approach, daily exercise can become an enjoyable habit.

After launching a "no fat, light exercise" program and developing good daily habits, personal programs can be developed to acquire specialized results.

It's your life and your body; what you do with them is up to you. We recommend that you seek advice from your doctor, set your goals, and begin a gradual program to achieve short-range objectives. With each accomplishment, strive for a higher level objective. As you progress, read books on nutrition and exercise to learn more about physical and mental fitness, and think about your role models as needed to help you progress toward your goal.

Enjoy your program. You must enjoy what you are doing because you will then have a better chance for success. And remember, it's never too late to begin marching with the gray panthers along the long road to feeling great!

2
THE OLDER GENERATION
ROLE MODELS

The role model athletes featured in this chapter were born prior to 1928, thereby differentiating them from athletes profiled in later chapters and classifying them as the "older generation." These athletes grew up at a time when little was known about the benefits of exercise, when few people were active in athletics during their middle and later years, and when there were few competitive opportunities for athletes beyond the college level. Television had not yet brought sports into everyone's living room, and the "big money" of professional sports was unheard of when these athletes were in their prime.

Despite their limited opportunities, the "older generation" athletes found ways to become champions during their prime or later years. Evelyne Adams, Bill Dudley, and Vic Seixas achieved fame and enjoyed recognition as champion athletes while they were in their 20s and 30s. The others earned recognition by winning national and international titles in senior-level age-group events.

These role models have traits in common such as enthusiasm, motivation, and a positive view of their lives. They have worked hard and persevered to achieve goals, and their futures are bright with hope as they look forward to continued success. To give themselves opportunities for enjoying their lives as long as possible, they are maintaining their best weight, staying active, eating balanced meals, and exercising regularly. The octogenarians (Evelyne Adams, Ken Beer, Ron Drummond, and Jack Staton) are in better physical condition than many adults of any age. Pearl Mehl, who is in her mid-70s, began running at age 63 and runs a mile in nine minutes, which is a good pace for any adult, and she maintains this rate over long distances. How many adults of any age can run faster or longer than Pearl?

There is commonality among the "older generation's" fitness programs, but each program reflects an individualistic approach to achieve and maintain a desired fitness level for life. The common elements of their programs are doing some physical activity on a regular basis, choosing enjoyable activities, and employing moderation. In summarizing their philosophies, these older generation role models don't overdo, overeat, or worry; they live each day as best they can, help others, and look forward to satisfying future goals.

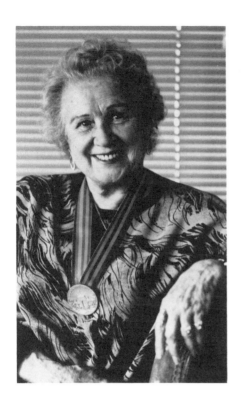

Evelyne Hall Adams

born: September 10, 1909

height: 5′ 3″

weight: 128

home: Oceanside, California

athletic highlights:

- awarded silver medal in 1932 Olympics after she and "Babe" Didriksen ran the 80-meter hurdles in the same world record time of 11.7 seconds
- elected to The Athletics Congress Hall of Fame
- elected to the National Track and Field Hall of Fame
- three-time national indoor hurdles champion
- coached the women's track team in the 1951 U.S. Pan American Games

Evelyne Hall Adams has cherished her Olympic experience all her life, and she hopes the Olympics will always mean an exchange of good will. "All Olympians are lovely," she said.

Evelyne's beliefs are idealistic, paralleling those of Frenchman Pierre de Coubertin, who was instrumental in founding the modern Olympics and who sought better international understanding through the universal love of athletics. Evelyne believes Olympians live in a separate world where they learn fair play and where they learn give and take. Since they can't always win, the athletes learn to keep going, thereby molding their character. "I think most Olympians have a set of rules they live by," she said.

Evelyne believes the Olympics are a test of individuals and not of nations. "During the 1932 Olympics, I was voted the friendliest girl in the village and the Japanese women's team chose me as their adopted daughter," she said. "I traded jewelry and clothing with Japanese and German women athletes, and you realize, after meeting athletes from other countries, that all people want to love and be loved. They're not enemies and they're not different from us. After the war broke out, I felt badly because people spoke hatefully about the Japanese and Germans. These women athletes were my friends, and I could not hate them because I could see how good and nice they were. I think this shows the spirit of the Olympic games."

"I don't know any strangers," Evelyne adds. "Whether people are homeless or governors doesn't mean anything to me. I'm not affected by color, religion, nationality, or politics. What's important to me is how they are personally."

"If you have clean habits when you're young, you will keep them for life," stated Evelyne. "I want to help the boys and girls today. One good person can spread good as well as a bad apple can spoil the bunch, and we can give youths an example of clean living and something to accomplish."

ATHLETIC HISTORY

Evelyne was born in Minnesota and her family moved to Chicago when she was a child. She attended Bowen High School and later the American College of Physical Education, which was merged into De Paul University.

"I was a premature, scrawny, and lonely child," Evelyne said. "During my early years, I had a lot of illness, including double pneumonia and scarlet fever together. When I was 10 or 11, I got started in athletics, partly out of necessity. I used to go to picnics, and they would have races with nice prizes. Since my folks didn't have much money, I would run and race bicycles for these prizes."

While Evelyne grew up in Chicago, roller skating was popular and she said she did a lot of that. She also began swimming, which she later taught along with water safety. "I did other things, too," she said. "You name it and I did it — to a degree. I earned awards in swimming, volleyball, roller skating, bicycling, and miniature golf."

Evelyne's activities included a parachute jump in 1929. Her husband was a pilot and belonged to an air club which needed a woman parachutist for an air show. The club paid her $25, a lot of money at that time, and she loved the jump, but her track teammates convinced her not to jump again for fear of injuring her ankles.

In 1928, Evelyne helped collect money for the United States Olympic team, thereby sparking her interest in becoming an Olympic athlete. She began training for a track career which proved successful and led her into the world of the Olympians. Unfortunately, two specters blocked her path to the ultimate fulfillment of her dream to be an Olympic gold medalist.

Evelyne's first specter was money. Her family had little money and had moved back to Minnesota. Then, in 1927, a week after her 18th birthday, she married Leonard Hall, her childhood sweetheart, and moved back to Chicago, where she started hurdling and ran her first competitive race at a relatively late age. Money was still a problem, but training for track was inexpensive. She ran on the school track and in parks, spending a little money for gasoline to drive to Ogden, Jackson, and Lake Shore parks, which had hurdles.

Because of her short frame, Evelyne developed a unique hurdling style. Her progression into hurdling was not difficult due to youthful experience in running and jumping. "I played a lot of jump rope," she said, "and they had maypoles in the parks. Around the maypole were rope and wood ladders for use in swinging around the poles. There were high jump standards there, and we would put them near the maypoles so that we could run and swing over the top. This exercise strengthened my arms and legs. Also, because there wasn't much else to do, we used to run around the park."

Evelyne was introduced to competition by a girlfriend in the Illinois Athletic Club in Chicago. "When this girl asked me to jump forward over the hurdles, it didn't bother me because I had experience jumping rope and swinging on the maypole. I was used to going forward over hurdles whereas most fellows at that time would go over sideways."

Evelyne's training program led to the Olympic trials, where she ran against Mildred "Babe" Didriksen, the second specter to haunt Evelyne's running career. In the trials, they had a confused finish that resulted in a split decision, but the judges gave first place to Babe. Both women qualified for the Olympics that July weekend in Evanston, Illinois, and the following Monday the women's track team was on a train for Los Angeles. According to Evelyne, she was on her way to becoming the first married woman to participate in the Olympics.

The worst year of the Depression was 1932, and women's track team members felt its hardships. Evelyne said, "I spent my lunch money for transportation to a distant practice field, and the United States Olympics Committee gave me new shoes, otherwise, I would have had to compete in ones worn down to nothing. Several of us came to Los Angeles with five dollars in our purses. Our room and board were provided, and if we did our own laundry, we were given seventy-five cents a week."

The 1932 Olympics was held in Los Angeles from July 30 through August 14. There were 1408 athletes from 37 countries, and women's track and field events, which were added to the Olympics in 1928, featured the 80-meter hurdles for the first time. Babe Didriksen, who had qualified for all five events, was allowed to compete in only three, including the 80-meter hurdles, which became one of the most controversial races in Olympic history.

On August 4, the fifth day of the Games, Babe Didriksen and Evelyne Hall raced in adjacent lanes to a dead heat finish in the 80-meter hurdles. Evelyne said many of her teammates congratulated her for winning, and she thought she had won, especially since her neck bled from the half-circle cut made by the finish line thread. Ties were not recognized in 1932 and the on-site judges from different countries huddled to decide the winner.

Several factors made it difficult to determine the winner: finish line photography was in its experimental stages, photographers stood at different angles, and there were no precision timing devices. A thread was used to mark the finish line, and Babe, the larger woman and a highly publicized athlete, was between Evelyne and the judges. Both hurdlers were timed at 11.7 seconds, which held as a world record for several years and a national record for 17 years. When the judges broke their huddle and awarded the gold medal to Babe and the silver medal to Evelyne, she could not believe they had decided in Babe's favor. She said one judge later examined the film and told her there was no way to determine a winner and she would also get a gold medal, but that never happened. Photographs showed both women with the thread against their necks and Evelyne's one foot clearly out front, but this evidence was found to be inconclusive.

Evelyne continued running hurdles until 1936 when the money specter foiled another attempt to win Olympic gold. "My husband and I got some money to go to Providence, Rhode Island, for the Olympic Trials, but I was still captain of Illinois track club and I used that money to take our team. When we got to Providence, I was exhausted and sick to my stomach and did not run as well as I could. Four of us finished the 80-meter hurdles within one foot of each other, and I could have gone to the Berlin Olympics if I could have raised $1000. But I could not raise the money and the limited national support went to higher priorities. Some girls who went to Berlin came from small towns that supported their athletes. Three or four of us from Chicago could not get sponsors, so we didn't get to go." As it turned out, the top four finishers in the 80-meter hurdles in Berlin were timed at 11.7, the same time Evelyne ran in 1932 and was still running in 1936.

Evelyne stopped running competitively after the 1936 Olympic trials and focused her efforts on coaching and teaching athletics. She became a "professional" when she began teaching physical education and coaching track for the Chicago Park District. "It was difficult to earn a living then," she said. "We would work, go home to bed, and then get up to go work again. In 1947 I left Chicago for California where I supervised the women's and girl's programs in Glendale's recreation department, and from 1957 to 1965 I was recreation director at Mira Loma Hospital in Lancaster, California. All the time I was teaching, I was also coaching. I coached pee wees, teenagers, and national track teams. I coached the women's track and field teams from 1936 to 1951, concluding with the first U.S. Pan American Games track team in Buenos Aires. In the 1930s, I served as chairman of the women's track and field team for the U.S. Olympic Committee and the Amateur Athletic Union."

In addition to coaching, Evelyne has volunteered to help others in many ways. By helping her friends' cerebral palsy children into the water, a program for special children was developed. She inaugurated the first Easter Seal Society Swim Program for crippled children in 1953 and was its first swimming instructor. She also helped with the Special Olympics and Jesse Owens programs.

Evelyne helped found the Southern California Chapter of U.S. Olympians and served as its president for 3 years (1968—70) and secretary for 12. Prior to the 1984 Olympics in Los Angeles, she worked as a voluntary member of the Olympic Spirit Team, which included former Olympians serving as goodwill ambassadors, to promote fund-raisers and to speak throughout Southern California to community organizations, civic groups, and schools. Prior to the games she carried the Olympic torch through the streets of Carlsbad, New Mexico, fulfilling a dream to carry the Olympic flame.

During her track career, Evelyne won five national hurdles titles and was a member of three national champion relay teams. In 1932, her Illinois Women's Athletic Club tied the world record for the 440-yard relay.

Several honors have also been bestowed on Evelyne. She was elected to the National Track and Field Hall of Fame and The Athletics Congress Hall of Fame. The California Assembly passed a resolution commending her as an Olympic medalist and a civic leader, especially for her efforts as a volunteer on the Olympic Spirit Team. Recently, the California State Games, an amateur sports festival for California athletes, awarded her the first gold medal of the games for her contributions to amateur athletics.

Evelyne has kept athletics as an important part of her life, although she and her husband have been retired in Oceanside, California, which is north of San Diego, since 1981. Evelyne first visited Oceanside because she had wanted to put her feet in the ocean some place while on a sightseeing trip to Tijuana. This trip was part of her Olympic visit to California in 1932.

FITNESS REGIMEN

"I belong to a Jazzercize class," Evelyne said as she began describing her fitness regimen. "I go a couple times a week. The stretching and jogging are great. It pumps my blood up and it makes me feel like life is worth living. I ride my bicycle around the trailer park where I live, I do some pushups at home, and sometimes I jog in the house. I don't follow a regular routine, but my husband does."

Evelyne married her husband, Brad, in 1964. A retired geologist and a member of Stanford's boxing team, Brad does mostly stretching exercises and still did backward somersaults at age 84. "He's in marvelous shape," she said. "He exercises daily and is as strong as an ox. He works like someone who is 50, and no one believes he's 87."

Describing her eating habits, Evelyne said, "I weighed 122 when competing, and the most I weighed was 140 during pregnancy [Evelyne has two children]. I watch my diet but am not fanatic about it. I'm not a health food nut, I have never liked greasy or oily foods, I limit my intake of sugar, and I don't use salt, butter or cream. I use non-fat milk and always fix vegetables with dinner, and I eat beef when I feel like it. Moderation is the key word. I believe in moderation, and I have always had a moderate diet."

Petite and energetic, Evelyne said she is never idle, although she thinks an afternoon nap is a great idea. "I'm busy from morning to night. Would you believe that after all these years I get at least two requests a week from Europe asking for autographs? It keeps me busy answering these, and I collect Olympic pins for a hobby. Another thing I do is make 'jokers.' I cut out cute cartoons, jokes, or anything that's amusing, paste them on paper, make copies, and mail or hand-deliver them to people everywhere."

MENTAL ATTITUDE ABOUT HEALTH AND FITNESS

Evelyne believes in the "use it or lose it" theory and "An Olympian's Creed":

> Today I am better than I was yesterday;
>
> Tomorrow I will be better than I am today!

Evelyne's enthusiastic and active lifestyle leads to happiness and good health. Asked to describe a typical day, she responded, "Since we are retired, we can get up when we feel like it, but we usually get up about 7:00 a.m. We keep busy all day, but we have no set routine; every day is different, thank goodness. We have lots of lovely people in our mobile trailer park, and I try to help those who are ill, need to go somewhere, and need companionship or food. I don't like to see lonely people. Our days get shorter and shorter as we age.

PERSONAL FITNESS GOALS

"Fitness is one of my pet programs and I'm still keeping up my end of it," Evelyne said. "I want to exercise, eat well, and stay active."

RECOMMENDATIONS FOR IMPROVED FITNESS OF PEOPLE OVER 40

"First, consult a doctor," Evelyne advises, "to be sure you are physically able to do exercises such as walking, swimming and biking."

"Second, stay active and do as your body feels. For example, if my foot hurts and I forego something because of my foot, I will do something else. I couldn't sit and wait until my foot felt better. This includes handicapped people who should also be active. If they can't use their legs, they should exercise their arms; if they can't use their arms, they should exercise their legs. A person can still exercise even if they have to sit on a chair. It's important to keep moving every day, and doing a little every day is better than doing long workouts on alternating days."

"Third, take aging as it is; fighting it is useless. It's a natural and I hope, slow process. Enjoy every day and never get bored; there are too many things to do."

In conclusion, Evelyne said, "Live right, eat right, and exercise. That's a good trio."

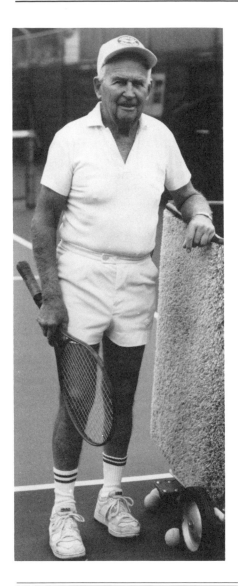

Ken Beer

born: December 9, 1903
height: 5′ 8″
weight: 150
home: Hillsborough,
California

athletic highlights:

- began playing tennis to alleviate flying fatigue
- began playing masters tennis at age 60
- has won 56 national tennis titles through 1989
- won all 1988 national singles and doubles titles in M85s (men's age 85-and-over) and repeated these wins in 1989 except for the indoor championship, which he didn't play
- ranked first nationally in 85-and-over singles and doubles

When asked about his health, Kenneth V. Beer said, "How has my health been? All I can say is I never pay any attention to it. So I guess it must be all right." When asked if he has had problems with his joints, especially his knees and elbows, while playing tennis, he replied, "Not to my knowledge, I haven't. If I have had any trouble, I'm too indifferent to pay any attention to it. I think I'm ungodly lucky. I don't have anything that I can claim to be troubles. I don't have any pains or aches or arthritis or incapacities or anything that I know of. As far as I know, I'm in perfect health. I think some of my good health is due to the fact that I don't pay any attention to it. I tore my Achilles tendon when I was skiing, but they sewed it up and now I don't know which leg it was."

Ken's attitude has been a significant factor in his life. "I've never thought of anything as being special," he said. "I've just had a lot of fun." Perhaps if his attitude had been less positive, he would not have achieved success in his various endeavors. A noteworthy achievement is his claim to having brought every aircraft home safely since he became a pilot in the late 1920s.

After completing his graduate work at Stanford, Ken joined the Army Air Corps in 1927 and went to Brooks Field, Texas, for primary and Kelly Field, Texas, for secondary training. "Flying looked as though it would be an interesting new industry," he said, "and I thought that would be the place for me."

Ken graduated from Kelly Field and completed his one-year military commitment, leaving the Air Corps to fly for Pan American Airlines from 1929 through 1963. He said he flew everything that Pan Am had from the early days right up through the jets, including the Fords, Fokkers, Sikorskys, Consolidateds, and Boeings. "That was a very interesting time because I was flying during the pioneering stages. I was involved in some of the first flights. I took some of the first seaplanes down to South America and flew throughout the South Pacific. I flew some of the first equipment down through Central America and to the Yucatan Peninsula where I had the opportunity to view from the air what looked like many pyramids. These were later excavated by archaeological societies and proven to be pyramids of the Mayan culture. I saw many of those long before they were widely known by the archaeological societies. When I went to the Pacific, I was the first to go to New Zealand and I had the pleasure of being one of the first to fly into Hong Kong and Macao, flying into those places early in the second year after they opened to air travel. I have flown across the North Atlantic to London and Paris, and I have flown across the Pacific as far as India."

"In flying, I have had everything happen to me up in the air," Ken said. "I have lost engines, I've had to return, and I have had fuel problems, but I have never injured an aircraft." He added, "An emergency is only an emergency if you are not prepared. If you are prepared, then it simply becomes a routine incident."

ATHLETIC HISTORY

Ken Beer played baseball in grade school and intramural handball at Stanford, and he did a lot of downhill and cross-country skiing in the Salt Lake City area, where he was born and raised. That was the extent of his involvement with sports until he began playing tennis.

A few years after starting with Pan Am, Ken said he discovered that exercise is one of the best antidotes for flying fatigue, so he took up tennis and found that he enjoyed the sport. He has played tennis regularly since then, initially for recreation to offset flying fatigue and later for competitive enjoyment.

Ken's competitive career in masters tennis began when he was 60 and retired from Pan Am. Ken said, "A friend came back from Florida and told me about a tournament they have for 60-year-olds. 'I think you can play,' he said, 'why don't you try it?' So, I went down and I not only tried it, I won it. And so I thought, 'Well, this is a lot of fun.' I've been playing tournaments ever since."

According to Ken, he plays about 15 tournaments a year and has won 56 national tournaments through 1989. In 1988, he won all four singles and all four doubles titles for his age group in the national indoor, clay, hardcourt, and grass championships. For this achievement, the United States Tennis Association awarded him a plaque for outstanding performance. In 1989, Ken nearly repeated his previous year's performance as he won the singles and doubles in all but the indoor championship, which he did not play.

About 12 to 16 players from all over the U.S. play in the 85s group at the national level, Ken said, and he has been playing with them for many years. Sometimes he plays down in the 75s and 80s groups and does well, but he said he doesn't win.

FITNESS REGIMEN

When asked to describe a typical day for him, Ken said he tries to be on the court at 7:00 in the morning, where he practices one-and-a-half or two hours with his ball machine. His goal is to hit 1000 practice shots five days a week. After practice he has breakfast with his wife. In the afternoon, he likes to play two or three sets of singles or doubles with friends. After returning home, he putters around his shop, as he loves to work with tools, doing all kinds of things including all the painting, plumbing, and electrical maintenance needed on his house. His evening activities include playing bridge, going out for dinner, and socializing.

Ken's daily routine is occasionally broken by rain or by other events. Occasionally he runs or rides a bike, and he does some stretching and calisthenics, usually for five to ten minutes before playing tennis. During the winter, he often goes skiing near his ski cottage in Squaw Valley. He said he's been skiing all his life and was so young he doesn't remember getting his first pair of skis.

Another thing Ken does for exercise is work with wood. He said he loves to cut wood, partly for work in his shop and also to supply wood for his cabin. "I just love to cut wood. I move those big heavy logs around, I pick them up, I pile them up, and I say to myself, 'This is the best exercise for tennis.'"

Ken's exercise regimen keeps him in good shape for tennis. As an example, he played a fellow this last year in Providence, Rhode Island. This man was younger, in the 80s age group, and Ken was playing down because the tournament didn't have an 85s category. Ken said, "It took me four hours and 15 minutes to beat him. Now a lot of people said, 'Ye, Gods, four hours and 15 minutes on the court! Weren't you dead?' And I told them, 'No, I was having too much fun.'"

When asked about his diet, Ken responded in much the same way he did when asked about his health. "How about my diet? I like everything and I eat everything. In my travels, and I've been pretty much all over the world, I haven't found a food I didn't like." When pressed for anything in particular that he does in regard to diet, he stated, "Not a thing." When asked if he tries to avoid any foods, he repeated, "Not a thing."

"My weight hasn't changed in years," Ken said. "I don't have any trouble with my weight. If it starts creeping up a little, I give up my evening meal."

Ken has an effective program to maintain his excellent health and fitness. Furthermore, he has never smoked, he said, which is remarkable considering the popularity of tobacco during the time period when he was flying for Pan American and the Army Air Corps. Instead of tobacco to alleviate fatigue and stress, he chose tennis.

MENTAL ATTITUDE ABOUT HEALTH AND FITNESS

With strength and clarity in his voice, Ken described his mental attitude as though he was reciting a memorized rule. "I'm convinced that the body is dependent on the mind. If the mind has a good healthy attitude, the body will respond."

Ken told a story to explain his beliefs. "I played tennis with a neurologist. He beat me in Nevada and I got even when I beat him in San Francisco. Later, during the course of conversation, we were discussing pills and I said, 'I never take one except when the need is specific. When I have something where a specific chemical will take care of it, I will take a pill. Otherwise, I never take anything.' I told the neurologist, 'I've got the best immune system that nature supplied and I'm not going to foul it up.' "

Ken said he sees doctors all the time, but seldom for anything except a shot or a physical, which he needs to keep his flying license. "Otherwise," he said, "I don't see any doctors except when I play tennis with them."

"I think a lot of people don't understand that the mind has such a strong influence on the body," Ken continued. "This influence of the mind is just a conclusion I came to. I don't know if I came to it on any good evidence or not."

Concerning his attitude, Ken chuckled as he remarked, "I don't know if I have a positive attitude or if I'm positive about my conclusions."

PERSONAL FITNESS GOALS

Ken's goal is to stay active and be successful in tennis and other activities. He said, "I like to succeed in anything I do no matter what it is. For the last six months I've been puttering around with electronics and a computer. I'm fascinated by the darn things and I want to succeed at it."

RECOMMENDATIONS FOR IMPROVED FITNESS OF PEOPLE OVER 40

If you are playing tennis or another sport, Ken recommends, "Keep playing regardless of age."

Staying active is important, he preaches. "The human mind needs challenge! It needs work. You don't get anywhere by sitting on your butt and doing nothing. You've got to get out and do something. It doesn't make too much difference what it is as long as you enter it with enthusiasm and the desire to accomplish. And you've got to have challenge. Without challenge you disintegrate."

Ron Drummond

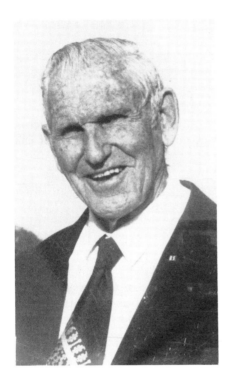

born: March 3, 1907

height: 6′ 6.5″

weight: 220

home: Capistrano Beach,
California

athletic highlights:

- placed second in a 10-mile ocean kayak race at age 81
- won dozens of swimming races in masters and senior olympic meets in Southern California
- demonstrated the emptying of a swamped canoe, jumping out to empty it and returning to the seat in 5.5 seconds
- paddled his canoe in waves more than 30′ high
- made a life-saving rescue in surf pounded by 50′ waves
- won shot put and discus events
- won handball and racquetball championships
- bar vaulted as high as the bar would go — 7′ 6″
- did 30 deep knee bends on one leg and 130 one-armed push-ups

Ronald B. Drummond is an explorer, world traveler, and all-round athlete who has challenged nature's forces for more than 80 years. As a youth, he purposefully began to develop the strength and agility needed to support his tall frame and to endure the encounters he has sought with nature. Having become a physical fitness advocate at an early age, he has found innumerable opportunities to test and prove his physical prowess in a variety of interesting ways. Except for a surprise engagement in 1943 with a powerful bolt of lightning, which knocked him about 15 feet and damaged his hearing, he has survived his active lifestyle unscathed.

One of Ron's formidable foes through the years has been the sea, with its mighty waves and unrelenting force. Understanding its potential danger but unintimidated by its ferocity, Ron learned as a youth to harness the sea for the pleasure of swimming, body surfing, canoeing, and kayaking. He sought and found huge waves for sport, riding them for enjoyment while avoiding foolhardy acts that would endanger his life.

ATHLETIC HISTORY

"When I was in Hollywood High School, I was so slim that I participated in athletics that would develop my muscles," Ron explained. "With my 6' 6.5" height, I should have played basketball, but I didn't." Ron wrestled, boxed, played handball and racquetball, and trained himself to perform feats of strength and agility such as walking on his hands. His significant sporting accomplishments related to water sports and the ocean.

BODY SURFING

Ron's family lived in Hollywood, California and spent summers at Hermosa Beach where Ron learned to bodysurf at age 6. Seventeen years later, in 1930, he was proficient with the sport and an occasional attraction on the beach. For example, the chief of Los Angeles beach lifeguards saw him bodysurfing and asked him to become a lifeguard, which he agreed to do for about six months.

The same year, Ron said he wanted to impress his future wife, Doris, on their second date, so he bodysurfed a 25-foot high wave created by an earthquake in Long Beach. "When I skidded up on the sand and nonchalantly walked up and sat beside Doris, a dozen people came over and talked with me," Ron said. Three years later they married, and in November 1989 celebrated their 56th anniversary.

Ron's bodysurfing highlights for 1930 include a book, *The Art of Wave Riding,* which he wrote and had published the next year. He said this was the first book written on bodysurfing.

Ron continued bodysurfing and, at age 70, entered a contest at Oceanside, California. In recognition of his achievements, the city awarded him a trophy inscribed, "Mr. Bodysurfer."

SWIMMING

Ron learned to swim about the same time he learned to bodysurf, and he became interested in the sport when his older brother swam for Hollywood High School in 1921. He remembers swimming, at age 14, from the Hermosa Pier to the Manhatten Pier and back, a distance of 4 miles. Ron also remembers being irked when he learned that a 17-year-old beat him out of first place in the Pacific Coast American Athletic Union Rough Water Championships for boys 16 and under.

Ron swam on the Hollywood High School and UCLA swimming teams, and in 1930 he won an ocean swimming race for lifeguards when he caught a wave and passed two national champions — Phil Daubenspeck and Reggie Harrison, who had both set records for short-distance swims.

In later years, Ron said he swam in senior olympic events held in Southern California and won about 50 gold medals a year until the number of senior meets dwindled. In 1982, he was listed in the top ten nationally for his age group in 12 swimming events. He added another five gold medals to his collection in 1989 when he entered and won five swimming events in a senior meet held in San Diego. In winning these events, he had to compete against younger men because the oldest age group was 75-and-over.

HANDBALL AND RACQUETBALL

When he was about 10 years old and in the 4th grade, Ron began playing handball. "I got Johnny Negus, the fastest runner in our class, to run and get the number one court for us to play on at recess, lunch time, and after school. As a result, Johnny and I played more than the other boys, and we went on to win doubles tournaments in grammar school, high school, and college. I had settled down at Capistrano Beach in 1946, and, in 1950, my brother helped me build a handball court, which became the only handball court between Los Angeles and San Diego; I sold it a few years ago. In later years, I entered senior olympic competition in handball and racquetball, and I won the singles and doubles titles in both sports."

Shot and Discus

George Drummond was going to work when he saw the folded front page of the Los Angeles Times sports page lying in the street. According to Ron, George saw a pair of unusually skinny legs which appeared in the lower half of a picture on the front page, and he said to himself that "nobody could have legs as skinny as that but Ron." George turned the paper over and saw a photo of Ron, who was featured because he had won the discus in all of his high school meets.

Ron threw the shot and discus at Hollywood High and in 1926 at UCLA. He won both events in the Southern California College Conference track meet, making him "high point man" for the meet.

He continued throwing the discus for fun and should have tried out for the 1932 Olympics because he was throwing over 159 feet, which would have been far enough to win a silver medal. In winning the shot put in the 1977 Pan American Masters track meet, he set a world record for the M70 age group.

Canoeing and Kayaking

"My favorite sport is surfing in a canoe or kayak," Ron said. "My first experience in a canoe was at age 13 when George rented one at a Sunday school picnic. I became so enthusiastic that I saved my lunch money for the next year and bought an old canoe. Our family was spending the summer at Hermosa Beach, and my older brother, Tom, and I took the canoe down to launch it. Big waves were breaking and I wanted to wait for calmer water, but Tommy said, 'Aw, you're chicken.' I couldn't take that so Tommy and I started out and a big, thick curling wave landed in the canoe and broke it. Tommy said, 'Aw, you're dumb anyway to try to use a canoe in the ocean.' Tommy's remark made me determined to do it. I repaired the canoe in two weeks, and I have been enjoying canoeing ever since."

Big waves have been challenging and thrilling for Ron to ride. Three times he found waves 30 feet high or more and rode them in his canoe. The largest waves he caught were in 1955 off Tijuana Sloughs on the outer reef at the California-Mexico border. When the head lifeguard phoned and told him about the "largest waves we have seen," Ron and two friends hurriedly drove down. At first they rode 20-foot waves near shore. "Then I looked out about two miles and saw enormous waves breaking on a reef," Ron said. "No one would go out with their surfboards, so I went out alone in my canoe. I took careful sights of land in Mexico and the United States to be sure to be in the exact spot to catch the waves. If I missed and a wave broke on me, it would smash my canoe to matchwood. The waves fit the description that 'You could drive a freight train through the thick heavy curl.' I had to be at the exact end of the reef to catch the wave, otherwise, I would either miss it or the ponderous curl would fall on me. I caught the waves and eventually rode my canoe safely back to shore. I remember feeling lonesome when I was at the bottom of the deep troughs, but it was thrilling to be on the crest and start sliding down the monsters."

For pleasure, Ron has made several 25-mile canoe and kayak trips between Catalina Island and the mainland. "About 1948," he said, "I paddled about 4–5 miles-per-hour from Avalon on Catalina Island to Newport Beach. Before leaving Avalon, the assistant harbor master told me that two-thirds of the large yachts had turned back to Avalon because of the rough sea. Because I left Avalon before dawn and my eyes were accustomed to my compass light, I couldn't see the breaking waves and one finally swamped me. I emptied my canoe quickly with the Capistrano Flip (see bottom of page) and turned my compass light out so I could see the waves about to break. From then on I dodged the big waves like when I'm surfing, and I never shipped another drop of water for the rest of the trip."

Ron said that he has raced and won against national champions George Sipos, Tom Johnson, and Bill Bragg. He beat George in a 500-meter kayak race at Newport Beach, and he beat Tom Johnson in a 500-meter canoe race at Marina Del Rey. He and his partners have beaten Bill Bragg in many races, Ron said. The win he is most proud of is the 50-mile race with 211 entrants down the Colorado River to the

---

CAPISTRANO FLIP

The Capistano Flip, so dubbed by Ron Drummond's friends, is a method Ron perfected for emptying a swamped canoe, and he demonstrated it some years ago in the remodeled San Clemente swimming pool. From a sitting position in a swamped canoe, Ron jumped out, emptied the canoe, and sat on the seat again in 5.5 seconds. Ron said the Red Cross and Boy Scouts have canoe emptying contests with winning times of about 20 seconds.

Imperial Dam, about 15 miles up river from Yuma, Arizona. Ron was nearly 69 years old, and his partner, John Vowels, was 33.

On February 20, 1988, two weeks before his 81st birthday, Ron finished second in a strenuous 10-mile ocean kayak race off Dana Point, California. About 30 surf skis and touring kayaks competed against a strong wind as well as each other. Ron said that white caps were breaking over the front of his kayak.

FITNESS EXERCISE

Throughout his life Ron has trained hard to improve his strength and abilities. For example, while skin-diving for four years in the West Indies, he developed the ability to hold his breath a long time, and he said that he could still hold it more than five minutes when he was in his 70s.

As a young boy, Ron learned about sports and fitness from his older brothers, especially George who was four years his senior. Like typical boys, they admired their developing muscles and wanted to hasten their growth. George bought barbells when he was 16 so that he and Ron could add one-half inch to their biceps. At an earlier age, George taught Ron how to train so that he could do one-arm chin-ups. As instructed, Ron added a stone each day to a box which was attached to a rope pulley on the grape arbor. Each day Ron would pull on the rope until finally he was pulled into the air instead of the rocks. By the time he was 23, Ron had developed the strength to do 30 deep knee bends on one leg and 130 floor dips on one arm. According to a book of records that he saw recently, his 30/130 numbers were greater than the world record.

Ron said he learned to walk on his hands when he was 12 and he got pretty good at it. In a high school show, he danced on his hands, waltzing to music — step, slide, close...step, slide, close — from one wing of the stage to the center, where he did a one-hand stand before waltzing off at the other wing. In 1930, when training for the Olympics and working as a lifeguard, he and another lifeguard used to race on their hands as fast as they could for about 200 feet along the beach. Ron said, "That's really a tiring race."

MEDALS AND TROPHIES

Ron has many hundreds of medals and trophies stored in boxes and shopping bags, and he has entered so many athletic events that he can't remember them all. During the '70s and early '80s, he said he was winning over 50 a year. He keeps three plaques on his library wall. One is from the Dana Point Athletic Club, and it reads, "DPAC 1977. Most Remarkable Athlete." Another plaque is from the 1977 Pan American Masters Games, and printed on the metal plate is, "Shot Put, World Record, Ron Drummond." The third plaque is from the American Canoe Association, and the metal plate beneath the medallion reads, "1975, Colorado River 50 Mile Canoe Race, First Place, Marathon Class, Ron Drummond."

Ron said, "According to my wife, Doris, I have a disease called medalitis! But I think that is a healthy disease. There is nothing more important to our happiness than good health, and our bodies adapt to our environment. Regular exercise is important, and competitive athletics keep you in shape."

FITNESS REGIMEN

"A typical day's exercise would be kayaking or swimming, a brisk walk and exercising with a rubber exerciser," Ron said. "I generally kayak 2.5 miles or swim for half an hour. I also exercise most of my muscles by stretching a rubber exerciser. I often take a brisk half-hour walk up and down a steep hill. I used to play handball or racquetball every day until I sold my box court."

Ron has never smoked, and, in regard to his diet, he said, "I don't eat pork and I eat little fat beef. I try to eat a well-balanced diet with fish or chicken and plenty of fruit and vegetables. If I eat ice cream, it is 97% fat-free ice milk. The most I weighed was 240 pounds when I fattened up before one of my Arctic expeditions. After returning home, I took off my excess weight quickly by playing handball every day."

MENTAL ATTITUDE ABOUT HEALTH AND FITNESS

Ron said he has always had a confident, positive, and enthusiastic attitude with no weaknesses, and he's a firm believer in exercise. "Your body adapts itself to its environment," he emphasized. "If you take strenuous exercise, you will have a body capable of strenuous exercise, and exercising regularly prevents heart trouble."

PERSONAL FITNESS GOALS

"I exercise regularly to maintain good health," Ron said in regard to his primary fitness goal. Second, he would like the opportunity to compete in more senior events in Southern California because, he said, "I would like to break the world swimming and shot put records for my age group."

Recommendations for Improved Fitness of People over 40

"Plan a regular schedule for exercise, eat sensibly, and don't smoke, drink, or overeat," Ron advises. "Choose an enjoyable activity like handball, racquetball, surfing, canoeing, kayaking, or brisk walking that provides good exercise. Otherwise, most people won't continue to exercise regularly."

"Nothing is more important to your personal happiness than your good health. Pick an exercise program that you enjoy."

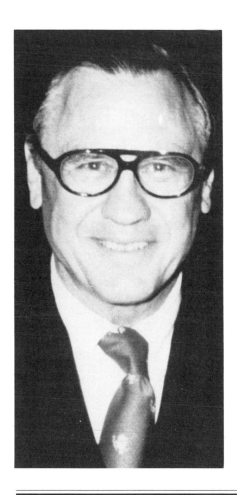

Bill Dudley

born: December 24, 1921

height: 5' 10.5"

weight: 180

home: Lynchburg, Virginia

athletic highlights:

- All-American running back at University of Virginia in 1942
- played professional football with Pittsburgh, Detroit, and Washington from 1942 to 1953
- leading NFL rusher, with 696 yards on 162 carries in 1942 and 604 yards on 146 carries in 1946
- chosen NFL Rookie of the Year in 1942 and Most Valuable Player in 1946
- elected to NFL All Star Teams
- elected to the College Football Hall of Fame in 1956
- elected to the Professional Football Hall of Fame in 1966

William M. Dudley was a football player who earned collegiate and professional hall-of-fame recognition, even though he lacked speed and size. Bill's philosophy explains his character traits and beliefs. "When I was in the 1942 All Star game in Chicago, the backs ran an 80-yard race and I finished next to last. Never fleet of foot, I've always believed that timing and positioning can be as important as speed. Reaction refers to quickness, and an athlete must be able to react. Of course, there's nothing like speed, but everyone doesn't have it and you have to do your best with what you have. Some ballplayers have made it with desire and commitment."

Explaining his thoughts about self-accomplishments and athletes who put all their expectancies into a typically short-lived sport, Bill said his father used to tell him, "Son, I want you to have an education so you can think for yourself."

Bill pursued goals based on his belief that many things don't work out in life and you have no one to blame but yourself if you have not done your best, worked hard, and prepared yourself. He believes we have responsibilities in life and we have to give rather than take. The more we give, he reasons, the less we can think about taking, and that includes giving yourself and your time to your family and society. "I think that working is giving," he concludes.

Bill said he would have enjoyed playing baseball in college, but he couldn't because it would have conflicted with spring football practice. "I felt obligated about spring practice," he said. "I was responsibile to do my best in football because the University was paying for my education, and it had been drilled into me that an education was more important than football."

NFL Commissioner Bert Bell, who shared ownership of the Pittsburgh Steelers with Art Rooney before becoming commissioner, offered Bill advice. "Commissioner Bell, who helped sign me to my first professonal contract, told me, 'Bill, you know you are only going to play pro football a short while if you play at all, and then you are still going to have to earn a living.' I think today's ballplayers will have to take a big pay cut like I did, and they should prepare themselves for it by saving their money."

ATHLETIC HISTORY

Bill spent his early years in Bluefield, Virginia, and he remembers playing football in a church lot when he was three or four. In later years, he played sandlot ball and was encouraged by his family, who gave him a football for Christmas whenever he asked for one, which was usually each year.

Bill said he was small and young for his high school class and would have graduated when he was 15, but he chose to stay in school one more year because his small size limited his opportunity to play football until his senior year. Weighing 111 pounds his first year in high school, he went out for football but did not get a uniform. He tried the next year and got a pair of shoes, but one was a size 7 and the other was a 9. Finally, as a 15-year-old senior, he got to play, and then he stayed on to play a second senior year when his weight was 138.

In high school, Bill played basketball, football, and baseball. During the summer, he swam and played baseball. He did not expect to have the opportunity to go to college, but he wanted a chance to play football because he thought it was a great game.

Football players were less specialized when Bill played than they are today. Bill said he was a running back, kicker, defensive back, punt returner, and kickoff returner all through high school, college, and the pros. He also played quarterback in high school. Playing both offense and defense was the thing to do, he said, and he played both ways until he retired in 1953. During his two-year high school career, he played every game and was never substituted.

When Bill began playing college football, he remembers being at or near the bottom of the players' list. He played wingback in the single wing and switched to tailback during spring practice his freshman year. As a left halfback in the T-formation his senior year, Bill made All-American and thinks he led the nation in scoring. Virginia won eight games and lost one.

Although World War II was in progress when Bill finished school in 1942, he said the Pittsburgh Steelers had drafted him number one and gave him an opportunity to play football for three months before he reported for military service. He played the 1942 season and performed well, leading the National Football League in rushing with 696 yards on 162 carries, being named to the All Pro Team, being elected Rookie of the Year, and finishing second to Don Hutson as Player of the Year.

Bill gave credit to his teammates for their help in his football achievements. "My teammates made me both in college and in the pros," he said. "Everybody talks about blockers and it's true. A runner is supposed to get by one man now and then but he needs a lot of help to get to the single man."

After his brilliant rookie year, Bill joined the Air Force and flew B-25s and B-29's. In 1944, when he taught future B-25 instructor pilots, he played football at Randolph Field in Texas. The following year, when the war was nearly over, he went to the Pacific Theater. On his way back to the States, he played three in-service games for the Army Air Force in Hawaii.

Bill said he got out of the service in November and joined the Steelers for the last three games of the season. "The next year, 1946, I was the MVP (Most Valuable Player), and I led the league in rushing (604 yards on 146 attempts), punt returns, and pass interceptions. I also kicked off, kicked extra points, and played defense. Coach Steve

Owens thought I was the best defensive back around and cautioned his quarterback not to throw in my direction."

Pittsburgh traded Bill to the Detroit Lions in 1947, and another trade brought him to the Washington Redskins for the 1950 and 1951 seasons. He was a backfield coach at Yale for one season and returned to the 'Skins in 1953 to play one year and to coach the running backs. For the next two years, he coached part time at the University of Virginia, and in 1956 he returned to the Steelers as a backfield coach.

Bill was elected to the College Football Hall of Fame in 1956 and the Pro Football Hall of Fame in 1966. Thinking about his outstanding football career, he said, "Probably the man who had the most effect on my life in the pros was Mr. Art Rooney. He was well respected by everyone in football and I was fortunate to get to know him."

FITNESS REGIMEN

When asked about his fitness regimen, Bill said, "I watch what I eat. I never had a strict physical program, but I have always watched what I eat, walked fast, and played golf. I stopped playing tennis about 20 years ago because I have bad knees. I think I became a fast walker when I carried papers as a kid. Although I had an angioplasty in 1985, it was successful and my health is good. I play golf in spurts most of the year, and I walk when the courses allow it, but I don't carry my bag. I don't do stretching or other exercises."

"I weigh myself every morning," Bill continued. "If I weigh over 185, I won't eat much that day. I have had to stop eating eggs and a lot of ice cream, which I love, because my cholesterol is high."

Bill described his current eating habits. "I enjoy steaks, but I don't eat them the way I used to. For the last five or six years, I have usually had fish, turkey, or chicken for my main meal, but at least three times a week I have only a bowl of soup and a salad. I have cereal for breakfast, and I was eating bran and oatmeal long before it became popular. When I was a kid, my father would heat oatmeal and put bran on it. I seldom snack before bed. Sometimes I skip lunch, typically when I play golf."

MENTAL ATTITUDE

"I try to avoid doing anything in excess, and I don't want to be fat," Bill said in explaining his mental attitude about fitness. "I got up to 195 pounds when I was in Saipan and physically inactive. In later years, I decided I would be most comfortable at my pre-training camp weight of 181 to 185 pounds. I played pro ball at 174 to 178."

"It becomes easy to maintain your weight after you develop the right eating habits," Bill continued. "Your stomach cooperates because you learn to put moderate amounts into it. As far as I'm concerned, the only way you get fat is by overeating and overdrinking, and the only way you lose weight is by consuming less. Running and other exercises burn up some calories, but this is insignificant in losing weight. Most people eat too much, and the calories we consume have to be burned up. I love to eat and I like candy, but I try to eat less than I used to. It's a matter of getting into the habit of adjusting consumption by telling yourself something like, 'I'm not going to eat any more today or tomorrow.' Once this habit is developed, it becomes easy to do because habits like smoking, drinking, eating and working are tough to break. The thing that's different about these habits is that I never heard of anybody dying from working too hard. I don't think you can work too hard."

"I've always believed that excess in anything is not good for anyone, but what is excessive for one person may be moderation for another. I've got a friend who eats like a horse. He's not as tall as me, but he eats twice as much and never gains a pound. He's been this way for 30 years and hasn't gone up or down five pounds as he just burns it off. I've seen him eat two steaks, so moderation for him would be excessive for most people. Each individual has to find their own niche in life that works for weight control."

"In regard to fitness," Bill said, "I have no doubt that pride and vanity or just a desire for good health are factors. It can also get expensive when buying clothes to fit at every weight level. I have worn the same size clothes for forty years."

"Although religion isn't fitness," Bill adds, "I think it plays a part in everyone's health. I try to go to church every Sunday. I'm also a family man. My wife and I, who have been married 42 years, have four kids and four grandchildren."

Personal Fitness Goals

Bill's longtime goal has been to maintain his weight, which he has done. Elaborating on his goal, Bill said, "I try to look decent within the framework of the body God gave me. One of our responsibilities in life is to maintain our body as best as we can, and it behooves us to accept our responsibilities. We are here for a short time and we belong to Him."

RECOMMENDATIONS FOR MATURE INDIVIDUALS

Bill recommends that mature individuals seeking improved fitness should know their comfortable weight and should weigh themselves every morning. "If you exceed your comfortable weight by two or three pounds, do not eat lunch that day," he advises. "Continue your exercise program and eat a light meal in the evening. This methodology will allow you to enjoy food and beverages while maintaining your weight. As the years go by, this method of weight control becomes a way of life and leads to happiness."

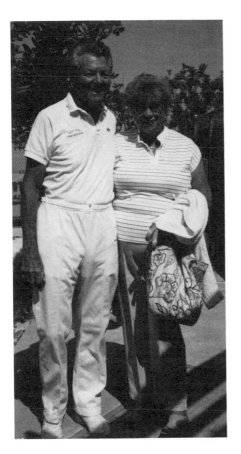

Verne Hughes

born: July 30, 1913

height: 6' 1"

weight: 168

home: Laguna Hills,
             California

athletic highlights:

- won 55 national senior tennis titles through 1989
- played international tennis for four years as a member of the United States Crawford Cup team for men over 70
- earned 1989 national tennis ranking of No. 1 in M75 (men's over 75) singles and doubles

As a young tennis player, Verne L. Hughes won many tournaments and was highly ranked nationally in doubles and singles. But after graduating from college and getting married in 1939, he did not have time for tournament tennis because he had to support his family. (Verne and his wife, Millie, who have two children, celebrated their 50th wedding anniversary in March 1989.)

When asked recently if he ever considered professional tennis, Verne replied, "When I was good enough and young enough to play at the professional level, there wasn't any money in it. I did consider teaching tennis, but I don't have the temperament to teach tennis every day. I have helped some kids on the junior program, and I've given individual lessons to a couple of them."

For nearly 20 years Verne's tennis was limited to social play on weekends while he developed his career in banking. At age 45, he resumed competitive tennis at the senior level and has earned national recognition while winning tournaments at all age levels for more than 30 years.

Senior tennis has been growing in popularity, especially in Florida and Southern California, since the over-45 parameter was divided into five-year age divisions in 1973. "Prior to these age divisions," Verne said, "the average tennis player was through with competitive tennis at age 23. Now with the increasing number of senior players in Southern California, I think you can play in a different senior tournament every week of the year."

ATHLETIC HISTORY

Born in Filer, Idaho, and raised in Long Beach, California, Verne has devoted a large part of his life to athletics. He first swung a tennis racquet at age 13 and started playing a lot of tennis at age 16. During his first year in high school, he lettered in tennis. He also played basketball, ran track, and lettered in football. The next year he concentrated on tennis and dropped the other sports. As a high school junior playing in the 18 and under age group, he won Long Beach City titles in men's and junior's singles, doubles, and mixed doubles. He once played in five finals in one day.

After high school, Verne attended Long Beach Junior College, where he played singles and never lost a league match. He completed junior college and worked until 1936 when he enrolled at the University of Southern California, attending from 1936 to 1938 on a tennis scholarship.

Verne reached the peak of his youthful tennis career in 1938–39, when he won the California men's doubles championship and earned high national rankings — No. 7 in men's doubles and No. 17 in men's singles. For eight years he was one of the top-ranked tennis players in the country, and he played with or against many of the great players such as Don Budge, Jack Kramer, and Ellsworth Vines. While touring the East in 1938, he and Mort Ballagh of Los Angeles had the national championship team of Budge and Gene Mako down to match point, but they could not put them away.

Although Verne was classified 1-A for military service, he served his country during World War II by working for Lockheed Aircraft in a critical wartime industry. In 1946, he began his banking career. He soon became active in the Lakewood Tennis Club and the Long Beach

Tennis Patrons Association, becoming president of the latter in 1961. The Patrons were dedicated to helping young people interested in tennis, and, during Verne's presidency, they were instrumental in sending a local player, Billie Jean (Moffit) King, to her first Wimbledon tournament.

After becoming eligible for senior tournaments at age 45, Verne began competing locally and was soon playing 20 to 30 tournaments a year in Southern California. In 1968, he played in his first national seniors tournament and won the hardcourt doubles title for men 55 and over. Since then, he has added 54 titles to his collection, including every senior division from the M45s through the M75s. He loves to play in national tournaments, and his titles include three grand slams, e.g., winning all four national doubles championships (hardcourt, indoor, grass, and clay) in the same year.

By January 1971, Verne estimated that he had 300 to 400 trophies packed away in boxes. At that time, he said, "I'm playing for the fun of it. I just try to get out [and play] every week and stay in shape. Enjoyment of the game rather than competition keeps me interested in tennis."

In 1985, Verne played singles tournaments for the first time in 45 years and earned No. 3 national and No. 4 international rankings to go with his No. 1 ranking in M70 doubles. His renewed involvement in singles competition resulted from an invitation to play international tennis on the United States Crawford Cup team.

Crawford Cup tennis is similar to Davis Cup tennis except it's for men 70 and over. A team consists of four players who play four singles matches and one doubles match against another team. Although Verne was chosen to play doubles, he had to be ready to play singles if one of the two singles players was injured, and so he resumed play in singles competition. As a member of the Crawford Cup team from 1984 through 1987, Verne played once in Finland and three times in Austria and helped the United States win each year against teams from 6 to 11 other countries.

Verne's recent triumphs include:

- World Cup doubles: M65 in 1986 and M70 in 1987
- M75 singles and doubles in the 1988 national hardcourt and indoors tournaments
- national titles in 1989: M75 indoors singles and doubles, M75 hardcourt doubles, M75 grass singles, and M70 grass doubles

Verne has won these doubles titles with partners Gardnar Mulloy and John Shelton. Beginning in 1983, Verne has teamed with Gardnar, who was a national champion in the 1930s and the all-time leader in national championships, to win in Austria and the U.S., and they formed the top-ranked M75 doubles pair in 1989.

Verne was recently recognized by the Southern California Tennis Association when it presented to him its first special achievement award. This annual award honored Verne for achievements, best sportsmanship, and high esprit d'corps.

Commenting on his love for tennis, Verne said, "I enjoy doubles more than singles. Doubles is a different game and it requires more skill as opposed to the stamina needed in singles. I think doubles is exciting because it has more volleying and faster play, and it suits my style as I am considered to have fast reflexes for my age."

Verne takes his wife, Millie, to tournaments with him, and they have traveled a lot since Verne retired from the bank. During their travels, they have enjoyed friendships with others on the senior circuit. Millie said the game has been good for them and has kept them healthy.

FITNESS REGIMEN

A non-smoker, Verne said his weight has been stable, increasing only 4 to 5 pounds since college. Tennis has been his primary conditioning activity 12 months a year for most of his life, and for 70 years he had no other purposeful fitness regimen. "When we were younger," he said, "they didn't know as much about exercise and nutrition as they do now. Consequently, when I was young I didn't pay much attention to it, but the older I got the more important it became to me."

In regard to a conditioning regimen, Verne said, "I have in the past been lax about it, but I'm very careful now. I practice tennis an average of three days a week, and I play tennis four to seven consecutive days in each of the 12 to 15 tournaments I enter annually. I'm diligent about doing stretching and strengthening exercises daily, principally for my back and legs. I tried running a couple times, but it bores me. On hot days when I'm not playing tennis I get exercise in some manner such as walking, riding a stationary bike, or working in the yard."

Until a physical examination in 1987 diagnosed his cholesterol to be a little high, Verne said he ate three balanced meals daily, including eggs every day for breakfast. Since his doctor recommended a low cholesterol diet, Verne has reduced his consumption of animal fats, especially red meat and dairy products, and he has cut down to one or two eggs a week. For the first time in his life he was watching his diet and eating mostly fish and chicken, vegetables, cereal, and fruit. As a result, he lowered his cholesterol from 255 to 200 in eight months.

Sweets have always been a limited part of his diet, Verne said. "As an adolescent, my doctor suggested I cut out sweets, which I did, so from high school on I have avoided them, although not 100 percent."

MENTAL ATTITUDE ABOUT HEALTH AND FITNESS

Verne's attitude about conditioning began to change about 1984 when he decided he had to do more than just play tennis. He said, "I trained sporadically for a couple years but religiously for the last two-and-a-half. I think daily exercises have been effective in my feeling better and in strengthening my back, which is the one vulnerable point I have. I have been fortunate in having good health, but my back is one place that's needed work. I have never had knee or joint problems. I had one sore elbow about 40 years ago, but that went away by itself."

Being in good health, Verne neglected to have a physical examination for about 25 years. In 1987, after insistence from his cardiologist nephew, he finally went to a doctor who diagnosed a little arthritis and elevated cholesterol.

PERSONAL FITNESS GOALS

"My goal," Verne said, "is to get my cholesterol down a little more and to continue my current conditioning program with maybe additional exercising on days I don't play tennis. If I continue this program, I should have no problem maintaining my physical well being."

In regard to tennis, Verne said he will continue playing tennis and competing in tournaments. He may reduce his singles, but he expects to continue playing doubles as long as he's physically able. By exercising daily and watching his diet, he expects to stay in excellent physical condition.

RECOMMENDATIONS FOR IMPROVED FITNESS OF PEOPLE OVER 40

It took more than 70 years for Verne to learn the importance of the following items that he recommends for improved physical fitness:

1. Maintain a regular fitness program
2. Maintain a diet program
3. Get periodic medical checkups

"I think good nutrition is more important than we realize," Verne said, "and you should have a definite conditioning program to go with it. You should set certain times for exercise because otherwise it's too easy to gloss over, which I have found with my minimum of exercises. I have to exercise first thing in the morning when I get up or else I don't do it. So, decide what you will do and schedule your activity on a regular basis. You have to really use willpower to adhere to that basis and not let inconsequential things interfere, although there is bound to be occasional interference. Anyone who follows this program will have good physical condition."

"A periodic medical checkup is also important," Verne adds, "because some life threatening developments are curable if caught in time. I changed my thinking in respect to periodic checkups. My nephew convinced me of that."

Pearl Mehl

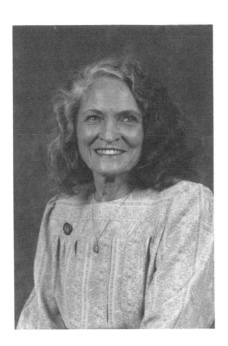

born: March 8, 1914

height: 5' 6.5"

weight: 120

home: Boulder, Colorado

athletic highlights:

- began running in 1977 at age 63 and loves to compete
- ran first marathon in 4:37.4 at age 67 in Denver
- averages about 50 races a year
- has won about 400 medals, including four golds and one silver in the 1989 U.S. National Senior Olympics and four silvers in the 1989 World Veterans Track and Field Championships
- all-round athlete who competes in running events with distances from 60m through marathon

Pearl Elizabeth (Hall) Mehl said she is often asked, especially by friends who are her age, "How do you find time to run 4 to 6 miles a day and do calisthenics 30 to 40 minutes each day with your many business and organizational commitments?" Pearl answers, "I run for my health; I have set a goal of being the best possible runner in my age group; I feel good about myself, enjoy the activity, and actually accomplish more in a day than I otherwise would."

Pearl leads an active life. Having been president of six statewide organizations and having taken courses in parliamentary law, she became a registered professional parliamentarian and now provides expertise on rules and usages for about 20 local and international organizations. Pearl also serves on two standing committees for the Associated Country Women of the World, instructs parliamentarian law in workshops and 15-hour courses, gives running clinics to women, and speaks to school and senior citizen groups on nutrition, health, and physical fitness. "Fitness for a Lifetime" has been a frequent topic of her talks.

Pearl is a qualified pilot and has been since World War II, when she and her husband, Reinhardt, joined the Air Force Auxiliary to fly search missions for lost aircraft in the Kansas area. The Mehls also supported the war effort by growing crops on their farm near Leoti, Kansas.

Pearl is not typical of a woman with two sons, a daughter, ten grandchildren, and five great-grandchildren. Sounding and looking younger than her age, she pursues her business involvements and prefers collecting running records to watching television and doing other, more typical senior citizen activities.

Pearl began running when she was 63 because she needed a re-placement activity for tennis and swimming, which she was forced to abandon because of arthritic knees and sinusitis. Her running was not hampered by the arthritis throughout her body or by the back pain emanating from a slipped disc that had nagged her for over 15 years. After six years of running, her arthritis and back pains faded away as she developed increased muscular support. As a fit woman of 69, Pearl knew she had decided correctly 22 years earlier when she chose to forego a spinal fusion.

By age 67, the thrill of competitive racing had hooked Pearl for life. She began setting running records in her age group, and she has continued her relentless pursuit of new records. During 12 years of competitive running, she has captured 24 world records and over 35 national records. When someone asked her late husband, Reinhardt, how long his wife would continue running, he replied, "She will proba-bly run until she's 100 years old unless she gets run over by a freight train."

Reinhardt's prophecy about his wife's running may become reality. Pearl has the good fortune to come from an athletic family with longev-ity. Her mother and father lived to the respective ages of 91 and 81. With good genes, an excellent attitude, and a keen eye for trains, Pearl will probably set running records for many more years.

ATHLETIC HISTORY

Pearl Mehl grew up in the Oklahoma panhandle with her athletic family of seven brothers and sisters and has been active in sports throughout her life. She ran races while in elementary school and participated in all intramural sports, including acrobatics, tumbling, gymnastics, and archery. She also ran some track, played softball, and played a lot of basketball. Later she coached and participated in many sports while she was a high school teacher.

After getting a bachelor's degree in home economics from Kansas State, Pearl taught home economics and the sciences for five years (1934–39) at high schools in western Kansas. During these years, she coached girls' athletics and played for the town's basketball team. She also played in Boulder's tennis town team tournaments during the summers of 1935–38 while working on a masters degree in home economics at the University of Colorado.

Supplementing Pearl's athletic interests was extensive knowledge of good nutrition gained from studying and teaching home economics. In addition to teaching high school for five years, she moved to Boulder in 1952 and got some college-level experience teaching chemistry of food and nutrition in the Home Economics Department at Colorado University in the mid-'50s.

Pearl remained active in sports by playing tennis and swimming through her middle years. Although she quit tennis due to arthritic knees, Pearl thinks she could play again due to her improved physical fitness. With wisdom gained from competitive running, she has learned the importance of training for casual as well as competitive sport. Whereas she did not train for tennis, she now works out daily and has recently attended exercise physiology and 10K courses at Colorado. Although consumed almost totally by her passion for running, Pearl takes time to participate in basketball events in the Rocky Mountain Senior Olympics and says she is still good at push shots.

Pearl ran her first competitve race, a 10K event, in 1979 when Boulder Memorial Hospital sponsored a marathon, half-marathon, and 10K. Her son Lanny ran the marathon and her 13-year-old grandson Shad ran the half-marathon.

In addition to her first race, Pearl has run other competitive races with family members. Two races were in 1984. Pearl, Lanny, and Shad set a record for families with their combined times in a 10-mile race in Atwood, Kansas. Later that year in West Germany, Pearl ran with

Shad and his older brother, Steele, a U.S. Air Force pilot stationed at Zimbach AFB. The trio ran a half-marathon in Kaiserslautern, and 70-year-old Pearl, the only woman older than 46, was satisfied with a 2:16.32 finish on a muddy course with rolling timbered terrain.

Pearl's running was particularly good in 1982. After only three years of competitive running, she set the following national records at age 68:

half-marathon	1:58.47
10 miles	1:30:49
15K	1:24:35
10K	54:45
5 miles	44:02
5K	25:06

Reminiscing over these outstanding results which averaged about nine minutes per mile regardless of the distance, Pearl said, "I must have been running without pain that year." Although her 4:56.52 time in the Denver Marathon was not a record, this spry 68-year-old finished first among women 55 and over.

One year earlier Pearl ran her first marathon and was paced by her son Lanny. This was the mile-high Denver Marathon, and Pearl's 4:37.4 finish is her best marathon time. She ran the Denver Marathon three more times and then ran a good London Marathon in 1985. Despite leg cramps coming off the cobblestones at the 20-mile mark, Pearl finished first among the nine women competitors over 60.

By 1987, Pearl was receiving national recognition for her running. After participating in the 1987 United States National Senior Olympics (USNSO), she was selected to represent athletes in the 70–74 age group at the closing ceremonies, where she appeared on stage with Bob Hope. She was also selected to help promote the 1989 Senior Olympics in St. Louis, where she added four golds and one silver to her growing collection of medals. Selected again as one of the five athletes to represent 3500 others during the closing ceremonies, Pearl appeared on stage with Steve Allen.

Following the USNSO, Pearl won six gold medals at the Athletics Congress U.S.A. National Masters' Track and Field Championships in San Diego, setting two more records for 75-year-old women. Pearl said that this meet was excellent training for the VIII Biennial World Veterans Championships in Eugene, Oregon, July 27 to August 7.

While the San Diego meet had 1500 participants, with 400 from 28 other countries, the World meet drew 4950 participants, making it the largest track-and-field meet in history. Twenty-two women were in Pearl's W75 age group. There were also two women over 80 and several men over 90; the oldest was 96. In one of the most exciting races, Pearl said 94-year-old Wang of Taiwan won the 200m race in 52.21, beating 90-year-old Kirk of Bozeman, Montana. In her events, Pearl said several older women and world record holders from West Germany provided tough competition, but she won four silver medals and one bronze.

Pearl said, "It was thrilling to compete with track and field athletes from 58 nations before crowds of 7500. I will remember this meet as a highlight in my career, and I'm looking forward to 1991 and the ninth (IX) World Veterans Championships in Turku, Finland."

1989 RESULTS

In March 1989, Pearl celebrated her 75th birthday. Within a month she began a remarkable racing schedule. Beginning in April with the National Master Indoor Championships in Columbus, Ohio, where she set six world records, Pearl pursued a heavier than usual schedule that netted more national and world records. An understanding of her accomplishments can be gained by viewing the table of events and times at the end of this profile. The consistency and improvement in her times are significant. Most men and women of any age should be pleased with runs as fast and far as Pearl's.

FITNESS REGIMEN

Pearl tries to run 4 to 6 miles a day wherever she is, and she logs about 2000 miles a year. When her business meetings break up in the afternoon and other participants socialize, Pearl said she runs.

When at home in Boulder, Pearl runs at the warmest time of the day during the winter and the coolest time of the day during the summer. She doesn't like to run early in the morning, and, if it's bitterly cold, she runs fewer miles or she chooses to ride an exercycle. She prefers blacktop surfaces to concrete because blacktop is easier on her feet.

Still fairly limber, Pearl works out about two hours a day, mixing distance running with sprints and exercises. She usually stretches and does calisthenics for 20 minutes before running and then does stretching exercises afterwards to relax her muscles. Pearl says her excellent mental and physical fitness enable her to accomplish more than enough each day to compensate for the two hours spent working out.

Pearl supplements her daily workout with lawn and garden work during warm weather, and she eats a balanced diet. Having studied and taught good nutrition, she knows that she needs plenty of complex carbohydrates and lots of water. She limits her consumption of sweets, fats, and fried foods, and she consumes little red meat, although she does not avoid it.

Daily workouts, a moderate diet, and strong willpower enable Pearl to maintain her weight at 120, until race time when she gets down to 116. The most she has weighed was about 130 to 135 in the mid-1930s when she was teaching high school and girls' athletics.

MENTAL ATTITUDE ABOUT HEALTH AND FITNESS

According to Pearl, her attitude toward health and fitness has been positive and unchanged since early in her career. She believes that fitness should be pursued as a lifetime occupation because physical activity makes it possible to maintain mental, spiritual, and emotional health as well as physical.

PERSONAL FITNESS GOALS

"I want to maintain my total health for as long as I am able," Pearl said, "running as fast as I can and competing in all events from 60 meters to marathons." Although she runs to win and always does her best, Pearl said she also runs for her health. She expects to run faster than last year and will continue her assault on national and world age-category records.

RECOMMENDATIONS FOR IMPROVED FITNESS OF PEOPLE OVER 40

When giving fitness talks to senior citizens, Pearl stresses that everyone needs some kind of activity like running, and the best activities are usually the ones enjoyed in earlier years. "There's no particular age to stop an activity," she suggests, "and it's never too late to start." For those who have been inactive and are now determined to develop a fitness program, Pearl advises, "Begin as soon as possible so you can improve your health and happiness. Get physical checkups regularly, exercise along with your sport, have fun, and accept the challenge to compete in a chosen activity for the rest of your life."

Senior citizens often ask what she eats, Pearl said, and she tells them, "balanced food." She then explains the balanced diet she follows.

Pearl encourages people to keep up with an activity that differs mentally and physically from their usual daily activity or work. She said this activity should help you relax, stay fit and limber, improve your muscle tone, and maintain your desired weight.

A positive mental attitude really makes the difference, Pearl believes. Goal setting is important, she adds, and people should enjoy participating in activities and eating well-balanced meals. By feeling positive and good about themselves, Pearl says they will feel better about others.

By getting out and participating in activities, Pearl believes people can develop good friendships because they are among others who have similar interests, and these people are often the up-and-comers or high achievers who have great enthusiasm for life.

PEARL MEHL'S RUNNING EVENTS AND TIMES FOR 1989
(rounded to nearest tenths or seconds)

Mo.	Race or meet	60m/ 100m	200m	400m	800m	1500m	3K/5K	10K	Medals won Gold	Silver
Apr	Natl.Indoor	13.3*	46.6*	1:46*	4:07*	7:43*	15:54*		6	
May	Bolder Boulder							1:09.56	1	
Jun	Sr. Olympics	22.4	48.3	1:49	3.55	8:19	29:53	1:07.58*	4	1
Jul	San Diego	21.9	45.9	1:43	3:57*	7:57	29:47	1:04.00*	6	
J/A	World Veterans	22.1	46.5	1:41	3:59	8:00	31:33	1:05:53		4
Aug	Rocky Mtn. Seniors	21.4	45.4	1:41	3:37*	7:44	31:10		7	
Sep	Rocky Mtn. Masters	20.9	42.9	1:38	3:37	7:48	28:12*		6	
Sep	Great Harvest						28.25		1	
Sep	Governors Cup							57.52*	1	
Oct	Cliffhangers							1:02.38*	1	
Oct	World Seniors	21.1	44.9	1:41	4:17	8:11	30:04	1:04.00*	7	
Nov	Courage Run						30.04 (3.25 miles)		1	
									41	5

* denotes national and world records.

Note: Pearl Mehl also won a bronze medal at the World Veterans Games.

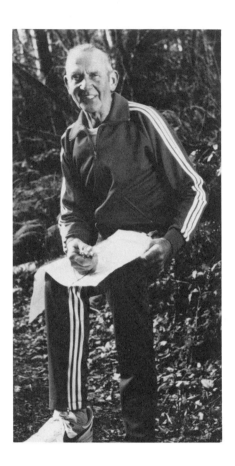

Knut Olson

born: November 9, 1922

height: 5′ 8″

weight: 150–155

home: Seattle, Washington

athletic highlights:

• won the Washington State Orienteering Championship in 1985

• won the Western States Championship in 1986 and 1987

• won the United States Orienteering Championship in 1986

Note: Each win has been in Knut's "over 60" age group.

In 1949, Knut A. Olson emigrated from Goteborg, Sweden, to the United States and began a 35-year hiatus from orienteering, his favorite sport, while working as a logger, farmer, and fisherman. Orienteering is one of the more popular sports in Europe, especially in Scandinavia, but it is unknown to most Americans and there are only a few thousand dedicated participants in the United States. Thus, at age 62 and after a long absence, Knut became excited when he read in a newspaper that a local orienteering club was sponsoring a meet.

Knut called immediately and did not get any encouragement when he explained that he had not participated in orienteering for 35 years. Undeterred, he went to the meet in Seattle's Woodland Park, where he discovered how his sport had changed. The maps he had used in Sweden were large-scaled black and white; in 1984, he was given a small-scaled color map showing detailed features such as cliffs and ravines.

"I took this colored map and couldn't understand anything," Knut said. "I didn't even understand the clue card. The terrain in the park was easy for running as it was almost flat with little vegetation. I could see everywhere, but I couldn't get going as I didn't know what to do. I looked around and everyone was gone. There wasn't a soul left. Somebody had given me a compass and I didn't know what to do with that, either. Eventually somebody showed me one control or checkpoint and then I figured out another. But everybody was back in about 15–20 minutes and I wandered around out there looking for controls for over an hour. The other orienteering participants finished eating and then went to look for me as they thought I might have broken a leg."

"This first orienteering meet was terrible; I didn't even finish," Knut said. "But after three or four meets I started getting used to it. First-time orienteers often give up. Many people look into orienteering, run in a meet, and then quit because they feel it's too much effort to use their heads. Running in an orienteering meet is not as easy as running on a road."

"Competitive orienteering is an interesting challenge," Knut said. "For example, experienced adult orienteers will run 10K, sometimes when our clothes are so soaked we have to hold them so they don't fall down. We sometimes crawl and wade through mushy growth where there are no trails. At a tough 1989 meet on Vancouver Island, British Columbia, I went through underbrush that was knee high and sometimes up to my hips or over my head. Courses are usually hilly and many have ravines. A course in Colorado Springs is one of the worst I've seen because it is so rocky."

"Anybody can learn orienteering more or less," Knut continued. "Some become good at it, some inbetween, and some never learn. But at least a small percentage stick to it. A nice aspect of orienteering is that everyone can participate any way they choose. They don't have to run in the rain, they don't have to compete, and they don't have to run. Participants can set their own pace and treat orienteering as a recreational sport by walking with others."

ATHLETIC HISTORY

Knut started orienteering in 1940 and participated for nine years, part of the time while in the military. "I did pretty well back in the old country," he said, "even though I never won in Sweden. The competition was very tough. But I did win a meet in Norway one year."

Like many Scandinavians, Knut is a runner and a skier. In Sweden, he ran the 1500, 3K, 5K, and 10K. He said he never had good national times due to lack of training, but he did well locally.

Knut did not give up after his terrible reacquaintance with orienteering in 1984. He went to meets regularly and improved his map-reading skills as well as his physical conditioning. A year later he won the state orienteering championship for his age group, and in 1986 he became a national champion with wins in the Western States Championship and the United States Championship for men 60 and over. In 1987, Knut defended his Western States title in San Diego, but he finished a close second in the national competition in Rhode Island.

Knut said he usually participates in 5K meets with 8 to 12 controls or checkpoints, and he often has to run in M55 (men over 55) because there are few participants in his M65 age group. He frequently performs better than younger competitors because orienteering requires a combination of problem-solving skills, speed, and endurance. Knut said, "It's not just a matter of running; it's how you get there."

A variety of orienteering meets are organized every year, and they can focus on any mode of human-powered transportation such as canoeing and skiing. Knut has participated in three rugged endurance events such as a 24-hour Canadian event in May 1989. "It included a 1500-foot climb," he said, "the worst I have seen. The other member of my two-man team was a 20-year-old Marine who could run away from me on the trails, but I was better on the climbs and in the woods. I was a few steps ahead of him on the big climb."

FITNESS REGIMEN

Knut said he usually runs 10K about three times a week. "It's not good when you are my age and you force yourself to do too much," he said. "I like to combine some running with real fast speedwalking. About once a week when I don't feel like running, I swim for an hour at a nearby athletic club. I used to swim more and use an exercycle at the club. Sometimes I run on the indoor track, but I never use weights because the arthritis in my shoulders is too bad. I ski a half a dozen times every winter, and I compete in many local orienteering meets, which is a form of training."

Knut, who has never smoked, gets additional exercise walking all day at his rainbow trout fish hatchery, which he has owned since 1977. The hatchery also provides him with one of his main sources of food.

Knut eats fish and a lot of green vegetables every day. The fish is mostly his own, but someone will occasionally give him halibut or salmon. He has fruit or fruit juice once in a while.

MENTAL ATTITUDE ABOUT HEALTH AND FITNESS

Knut was operated on successfully for prostate cancer in 1983. He said his blood pressure was high for a time after that, but it's down to 120/80. He recovered completely from the cancer. His attitude afterwards was not to worry about it. He decided not to let it get him down, and he took the positive approach to move forward in life.

PERSONAL FITNESS GOALS

"My goal is to stay alive, to keep going the way I am so as to live to 90 or more," Knut said. "My intention is to stick to what I'm doing for exercise and health."

Does that mean you want to keep participating in orienteering as long as you can, Knut was asked. "Absolutely," he replied, "with proper training and not overdoing it, because overdoing it doesn't help you one bit. But I may sell my fish hatchery so that I can spend time orienteering on the East Coast and in Europe."

RECOMMENDATIONS FOR IMPROVED FITNESS OF PEOPLE OVER 40

Knut has two recommendations for others:

1. Maintain a low cholesterol diet.
2. Exercise on a regular schedule by either speed walking, running, or swimming. Feel guilty if you don't keep your schedule.

"If you can get a bad feeling whenever you miss your schedule, you'll be all right," Knut suggests.

Knut calls himself an old man, but he feels good about himself, especially when he outperforms much younger people in orienteering meets. "Younger people hate to see me beat them," he said. "They don't like to see an old man run them down."

"You have to keep at it," Knut states. "Look around at people of all ages and see how many have difficulty moving and getting around. Many of them are heavy. Exercise makes me feel like a kid. It's unbelievable what it can do. It helps you walk straight, sit straight, and walk with determination. Out-of-shape people walk slowly, one step at a time, instead of purposefully."

Jacqueline Piatigorsky

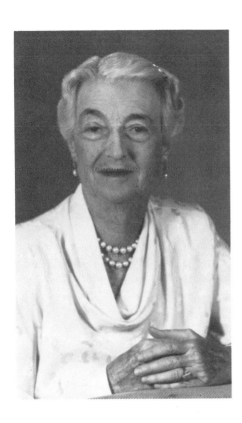

born: November 6, 1911
height: 5′ 6″
weight: 127
home: Los Angeles,
California

athletic highlights:

• played golf, went horseback riding, and rode bicycles as a youth

• learned to play tennis at age 42 and soon won Mother-Son tournament in Coronado

• ranked first nationally in 75-and-over doubles and ranked fourth in singles

• won eight or nine national senior doubles titles

• finished second a number of times as a singles player in national senior tournaments

Born into the Rothschild family and a life of luxury with her father the head of the family bank in Paris, Jacqueline Rothschild lived in a sheltered and privileged world. As a child, her home was the nursery in Talleyrand's Palace, which, she said, had so many art pieces it could have been taken for a museum. Isolated from her parents, whose quarters were far from the nursery, she was raised by a nanny who instilled fear in her life.

"Yes, I was a Rothschild, but I was a woman, an outsider, an outcast," Jacqueline explained. "Little was expected of the Rothschild women who bore the family name only until they married."

Jacqueline yearned for affection and success. Wanting to do well in something that would give her a sense of achievement, she tried the arts, chess, and sports. Finally, she found love and happiness with the renowned cellist Gregor Piatigorsky, whom she married in Ann Arbor, Michigan, between concerts. She had left the Rothschild's world and become a Piatigorsky.

When war broke out in 1939, Jacqueline and Gregor fled France with their daughter and began a new life in the United States. After the war the Piatigorskys moved to Los Angeles, where Jacqueline became well known as a tournament chess player, became a tennis champion, and learned to express herself in stone, sculpting birds and infinities for the last 20 years. Of most importance, she had found peace within herself through the love of her husband and children.

In her autobiography, *Jump in the Waves,* Jacqueline wrote that she grew up with her children. "Through them, and with them, I was reliving my childhood; this time a happy one."

At a dinner party sometime after her husband died in 1976, Jacqueline was embarrassed by a compliment from an old friend of her late husband. "She flew a plane, she is a chess champion, a tennis champion, a sculptor...," he stated in his toast to her while she shriveled inside. "I had never won the United States chess championship," she thought. "I had never won a gold ball in singles. I got involved in a variety of things, and I was a success in other people's eyes, not in my own."

"But what would it mean to me to be a success?" Jacqueline asked herself. "Getting an extra title and the adulation strewn upon winners? Would that make up for the love I didn't get when I was very young? Was any success of mine still searching for my mother's admiration? Or did it mean being at peace with myself, accepting myself as I really was? Maybe success is the physical satisfaction of striving, or the joy one helps to spread to one's surroundings.... What really matters is one's inner feelings."

ATHLETIC HISTORY

"One is athletic because it's part of one's makeup," Jacqueline stated. "When I was young, I played golf, went horseback riding, and rode bicycles."

According to Jacqueline, she was athletically gifted and loved all exercise as a youth. "Riding was my first sport, a noncompetitive activity," she wrote in her book. "We rode only for enjoyment, and I really did enjoy it. Riding seemed to be inherent to the Rothschild family."

Jacqueline said she became a good golfer, hitting the ball long and straight in practice, but she choked in competition. When she played golf on the family's course in France, her golfing instructor was her companion.

As a young adult, Jacqueline said she didn't participate much in sports. This hiatus ended in 1953 when she talked her 13-year-old son into trying tennis and began driving him to the public courts for practice. Within a few weeks she was bored sitting and waiting, so she began hitting some balls.

"I had played a few times in my childhood," Jacqueline said in her book, "so after a few weeks I became restless and wanted to try to hit the ball, but I was recovering from abdominal surgery. I was so weak at first that I stayed barely five minutes on the court, but it was fun. Little by little my strength returned and I found myself waiting and looking forward to the weekly hour. My lessons continued for several years, but with my competitive and compulsive nature tennis went beyond being only fun. I was starting to improve; I wanted to be good. I wanted to win."

"When you start at age 42, it takes a little while before you start improving," Jacqueline explained. "I started slowly; it took me at least a year to be able to play half decently. After a few years, I built up to tournament play. I had a coach and I practiced a lot with my son who became a good player. We won the Mother-Son tournament in Coronado when he was young, and that was my first tournament win. I have been playing national senior tournaments since I was 55 or 60."

After her husband's death in 1976, Jacqueline wrote, "I continued sculpting and played tennis regularly twice a week. Eventually I entered senior tournaments, often reaching the finals in the nationals, which meant getting a silver ball. Winning and getting a gold ball seemed out of reach. But as I kept improving, a top player asked me to play doubles with her, and we won. My first gold ball was a thrill."

"There are four national senior tournaments a year and I've played in all of them — the grass courts in Cedarhurst, Long Island; the indoor courts in Kansas City; the clay courts in Baton Rouge, Louisiana; and the hard courts in California. I only went twice to the grass courts because I didn't like it there. The grass is difficult to play on and the tournament is not as pleasant for me as others. The Kansas City tournament has nice people and is well arranged, and I play there every year. The tournament in Baton Rouge, Louisiana, is also nice. I enjoy meeting people at the nationals, and it's fun when it's competitive."

"I have eight or nine gold balls, which represent national titles, and I have a number of silver balls for runner-up finishes in singles. My national titles are all in doubles. It takes tournament practice to become a winner, and it took awhile before I got a good doubles partner because good players don't want you as a partner unless you are good. As I started to improve, the better players started asking me to play, and when I got a good partner, we started to win. I might have won in the 60s age group; I won several in each of the subsequent groups – the 65s, the 70s, and the 75s. In 1989, I lost in the Los Angeles finals in a close doubles match (lost 7–5 in the third set), won in Kansas City and Louisiana, and lost in the singles semi-finals in all three nationals."

Jacqueline has also played tournament chess, which is so intense and competitive in major events that participants need good health and fitness to play well. Having taught herself chess when she was a child, Jacqueline played her first tournament in Los Angeles, where she studied with 1948 U.S. Champion Herman Steiner. As her game improved, she played in the Women's U.S. Invitational National Championship, and in 1954 she and U.S. Champion Gisella Gresser represented the United States in the first women's Chess Olympics. A few years later, she quit tournament chess to focus her energy on tennis and sculpting.

FITNESS REGIMEN

Jacqueline said she tries to follow a balanced and reasonable diet of poultry, fish, vegetables, and fruit. She eats little red meat and tries to avoid animal fats. She admits to having a sweet tooth and sometimes goes off her diet with things like chocolate.

Tennis is the principal exercise in Jacqueline's fitness regimen. "I play tennis for up to three hours about three times a week," she said. "This includes weekly practice with a coach — Gordon Davis, father of Scott Davis, the tennis player. It's hard work and it's fun. I play a lot with people who are ten or more years younger than myself. One friend I often play with is 38 years younger, and that is good hard exercise because he can outrun anything. Some people use tennis as their social life, but that's not the case with me," she added. "I like the competition."

In addition to tennis, Jacqueline said she gets exercise from household chores, errands, gardening, and, in particular, working with stone in her studio. She does not do calisthenics or stretching exercises, not even before a match. "They tell me I should, but I don't," she said. "I warm up for tennis by hitting balls."

Jacqueline mentioned her studio work because it provides a significant amount of physical activity. She said, "I've been sculpturing in marble for about 20–25 years, so that's a fair amount of physical work, too. My last exhibition was in October, 1988."

MENTAL ATTITUDE ABOUT HEALTH AND FITNESS

"My mental attitude about health and fitness hasn't changed," Jacqueline said. "At this point I don't feel my age. Being interested in something keeps one alive, and a lot of it, even the physical fitness part, is mental. If one really likes what one is doing, and one is interested or stimulated, one forgets or ignores the little aches and pains that everybody has."

Jacqueline has had many strong interests, and her work with stone sculpturing best depicts her philosophy about living for something. In her autobiography, she described her feelings when she started working with stone, and she quoted her late husband as saying, "One does not choose the cello, it chooses one." So it was with stone and me, Jacqueline remarked. "I looked at my first stone. I didn't hesitate. I knew it had to become a bird. My childhood torments were tied in with birds: pheasants, pink ibises, ducks, swans. My emotions were linked with their movements."

"I knew my work had my own signature," Jacqueline continued, "and for the first time in my life I was able to express myself by letting my inner feelings flow into the stone. I was working and improving. I was starting to achieve."

In recent years, Jacqueline's analysis of her feelings resulted in a better understanding of her attitude, which she described in her book. "For many years I mistook winning for success. Of course winning is part of success. Success is achieving one's goal. But if one's goal is criminal, success is a tragedy. The inner feeling of achievement is a major part of success. The inner feeling of achievement can be reached in a variety of ways. The way I found came through love."

The last sentence in Jacqueline's book is appropriate in summarizing her mental attitude: "I may have lost many times, but I am a winner."

PERSONAL FITNESS GOALS

"I will play tennis as long as I can — as long as my body holds out," Jacqueline said, "and there are many marble pieces I want to work on in the studio. I enjoy competitive tennis and sculpturing very much."

RECOMMENDATIONS FOR IMPROVED FITNESS OF PEOPLE OVER 40

"Find an activity which is fascinating and do it because you love it," Jacqueline recommends. "Get out and have fun. Get out and try. Participate in an activity like swimming, running, or skiing and really enjoy what you are doing. I think few people will hold themselves down to artificial decisions of building up; only the professionals will do that."

In commenting on her book, Jacqueline wrote, "Most biographers relate facts and describe events; to me feelings and inner reactions to the events are more important than the events themselves. But the most important message I want to convey is that people should use their feelings to become productive."

Vic Seixas

born: August 30, 1923

height: 6′ 1″

weight: 180–83

home: Tiburon, California

athletic highlights:

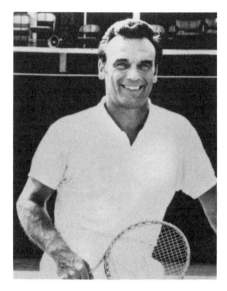

- won U.S. Open men's doubles in 1952
- won Wimbledon singles in 1953
- won French mixed doubles in 1953
- won U.S. Open singles and men's doubles in 1954
- won French men's doubles in 1954 and 1955
- won Australian men's doubles in 1955
- won Wimbledon mixed doubles from 1953 through 1956
- won U.S. Open mixed doubles from 1953 through 1955
- played 23 matches as member of U.S. Davis Cup team from 1951 through 1957
- ranked in America from 1942 to 1966, a longer span than any other tennis player

E. Victor Seixas admitted his prejudice when he said, "Playing tennis is the best form of exercise. The beautiful thing about it is that you exercise almost every part of your body while you are having fun. After retiring in 1958 from full-time competitive tennis, I kept playing for fun and exercise. I found that tennis nearly satisfied my fitness requirements if I played regularly and often. When I was playing full time, we [tennis players] thought little about aerobics, stretching and other fitness exercises. Now there's a variety of new fitness equipment and techniques available."

Vic, whose warm personality and hearty laugh make you think you have been friends for years, wrote a book, *Prime Time Tennis,* to appeal to tennis players over 40. Published in 1982, the book was written for the players from the 1960s tennis boom who had reached middle-age. Vic blended anecdotes and personal history with tennis and fitness advice for the mature player.

Prior to the publishing in 1968 of Dr. Kenneth Cooper's book, *Aerobics,* and the new age of running and fitness, the common belief was that people should not or could not run much past age 40. "I paid no attention to that whatsoever," Vic said. "In my book, I told a joke about a guy who went to his doctor for a fitness checkup. His doctor looked him over, and, knowing the guy played tennis, the doctor asked, 'How old are you?' 'Forty,' the guy replied. And so the doctor told him, 'I don't think you should play singles in your forties.' So the poor guy had to wait ten years before he could play singles again."

"The main thing is to not stop," Vic emphasized. "The problem with many team and college sports is that continued active participation is not easy and often not done because of the need to get nine guys together to play baseball or 11 to play football. Tennis, which requires only one other person, is one of the great activities for keeping yourself fit in later years, and we are seeing more older players now playing as seniors. The secret of fitness in a nutshell is regular exercise. I may skip a day now and then, but I try to exercise daily."

ATHLETIC HISTORY

Vic played competitive tennis from 1948 through 1958, when he retired from full-time competition to work for Goldman, Sachs, a brokerage firm in Philadelphia. During his career, he starred on the United States Davis Cup team (1951–57), won doubles titles at the major international tournaments, and won the U.S. Open and Wimbledon singles titles. He played in the U.S. Open until 1971, when he was the referee, and in 29 years he lost only once in the first round. From 1942, when he earned his first national ranking, until 1966, when he won two significant matches as a part-time player, he ranked in the top ten in America for a longer time than any other tennis player.

Vic was more than just a tennis player; he was an athlete who played tennis. For example, he played basketball as well as tennis (partial scholarship) for the University of North Carolina, and instead of playing tennis during the winter, he played squash. While competing as a part-time tennis player in the '60s, he also competed in squash and won the national seniors (over-40) singles title three years in a row.

Vic started playing tennis when he was four or five years old. Born and raised in a middle-class Philadelphia community where his father had a plumbing supply business, Vic chased balls for his father at a local tennis club which had four clay courts. By age 13, he was winning 15-and-under tournaments. After junior high school, he went to Penn Charter, a good tennis and prep school in Philadelphia, on a four-year tennis scholarship. Winning the Interscholastic doubles in 1940 and the singles in 1941, he may have been the best young player in the country.

After completing the 1942 tennis season at North Carolina and earning his first national ranking, he enlisted in the Army Air Force. In 1946, after returning to North Carolina from the Pacific Theater, Vic played college tennis and the summer circuit, where by 1948 he earned national ranking again (number seven). When he graduated in 1949 and married a classmate, he considered giving up tennis because he had lost time in the service and was 26 years old. However, he decided to play tennis full time.

Vic got a break in 1950 when the United States Lawn Tennis Association (USLTA and now the USTA) sent him, Doris Hart, Shirley Fry, and Art Larsen on an expense-paid trip to South Africa and on through Europe to Wimbledon, where he lost to Budge Patty, the eventual winner, in the semifinals.

In 1951, Vic was ranked number one and was a member of the Davis Cup team. He became known for his attacking topspin lob and rugged match temperament while winning the prestigious singles titles at Wimbledon and Forest Hills and helping the United States team win the Davis Cup back from the Australians. During his prime, he played 23 Davis Cup matches, more than any American at the time, and he was the oldest player (31) to win the national singles for the first time. He teamed with Doris Hart for three years, losing only one significant match while winning three mixed doubles titles at Wimbledon, three at the U.S. Open, and one at the French Open. During the same years, he teamed with Tony Trabert to win four titles at the U.S., Australian, and French opens.

When asked how he achieved success in doubles competition, Vic responded, "The answer is to get good partners, and I had good ones in Tony Trabert and Doris Hart. Doubles partners should have complementary games, should like each other, and should practice together so they can anticipate each other's moves. I think Doris was the best women's tennis player at the time, and we had a simple system; she hit every ball she could."

FITNESS REGIMEN

Vic said, "I sometimes bicycle when I'm not playing tennis. I think cycling and swimming are the best exercises for somebody with knee problems. I've always loved tennis so it's still my main form of exercise. However, partly due to age and mostly to bad knees, I can't run and cover as much court as I'd like."

Vic said he developed a half-hour exercise program a couple of years ago, and he goes through it each morning after getting up. He begins each day with this routine for two reasons: first, he gets it over with, and, second, it limbers him up and makes him feel better. This alleviates the arthritic stiffness he feels after a night's sleep. His routine includes stretching, situps, pushups, and work with a five-pound weight. He designed the weight work to keep his good leg muscles from getting too atrophied through lack of running. "What I'm really trying to do," he said, "is keep my good parts in good shape. I don't want them to go bad because my knees are not so good. This seems to be working; except for my knees, I'm in excellent shape. I don't have problems with my back, arms, or shoulders so I'm still able to play tennis."

"About the only difference in my tennis game," Vic said, "is that I don't run for as many balls as I used to. I still hit the ball well and I get a good workout. Besides playing a lot of doubles, I have a routine with a couple young pros who could beat me if we played a regular game. When I play singles against them, I give them half the court from the center line out, including the alley, and two serves. I get one serve and I can play into their whole singles court. It works out to be a pretty even match. They get a good workout because they have to cover the whole singles court and I get a chance to hit more balls because I don't have to cover so much court."

Vic said, "The biggest problem for me as well as any athlete who's been competitive is to get out and do something when you know you can't do it as well as you used to. I rationalize it; I know I'm not going to get some balls, but what I'm doing is better than the alternative.

With a positive attitude, you can get the value of exercise. It's unending and it's not going to get better, but you've got to keep it from getting worse."

"I have no special diet," Vic said. "I've never been a snacker or a big eater, and I eat only two meals a day. I eat a good breakfast every morning, and that's probably my best meal. I usually skip lunch, and I eat an early dinner around 6 PM. I feel better by eating light, and I don't go to bed on a full stomach. If I get hungry during the day, I eat fruit. I don't limit my food or avoid anything, but I eat moderately. My cholesterol is about 175 and exercise rather than diet keeps it down. I enjoy a drink now and then, but I never drank much when playing competitive tennis. I smoked in the Army, but not since then. My biggest problem is a sweet tooth, which I watch, because I don't burn up the sweets like I did when I was younger."

"My youthful appearance is due to exercise, moderation, and good luck in never getting hurt," Vic added. "I trained hard when I was playing because my game wasn't that good. I depended on feeling good."

MENTAL ATTITUDE ABOUT HEALTH AND FITNESS

"I can't imagine not exercising," Vic said. "I seldom go more than a day or so without some vigorous exercise although I've been troubled with bad knees for about ten years, which is the result of 50 years of pounding on tennis courts. I'm not able to do some things I would like to do if I were still able to run. I try to compensate for this, but it's a little tougher because running is one of the best forms of exercise."

Vic has kept a positive attitude in regard to his arthritis and has tried to help others by serving as a spokesman for exercise and medicine. In 1988, he did a 36-city media tour for Pfizer Pharmaceutical to promote exercise and the arthritis drug he's taking. He said the tour featured exercise and wasn't obtrusively commercial, and he always had a rheumatologist with him to provide a two-prong approach.

"When my arthritis started about 10 years ago," Vic explained, "I didn't do anything but take aspirin by the handful until my doctor suggested an arthritis drug. Now I take one pill at breakfast and that's it. Although this drug doesn't cure anything, it has given me good results by relieving a lot of the stiffness and inflammation, thus enabling me to remain active."

Vic is a good example of what medication and exercise can do to help an arthritis sufferer remain active. "I have a little arthritis in my left hand and virtually none in my tennis hand, proving to me the value of exercise. My hand doesn't bother me, but my knees can hurt with up-and-down movements. Side-to-side movements don't bother my knees."

Vic believes exercise and medication can alleviate the suffering of other arthritis victims. He said, "The media tour touted the value of exercise for people with severe arthritis. The worst thing you can do is become a couch potato and complain that you can't do this and that. This negative attitude can lead to circulatory problems, heart disease, and other ailments which can kill you whereas the arthritis won't. My purpose in doing the tour was to help people with arthritis get on a good medication and then exercise under supervision."

Vic's positive mental attitude and self-motivation are key factors in his personal battle with arthritis, and he expressed his thoughts in relation to what he believes others should do to resolve their problems. "People have to get motivated and get off their duffs to do something about their health problems, whether they have arthritis, age, weight or anything else working against them. The biggest problem people face as they get older is their lack of motivation to exercise. It's not as difficult for a successful athlete to get motivated because it's taken motivation for the athlete to accomplish something and to be in shape to do something well. But it's difficult to get people motivated to exercise when they have lived a sedentary life."

"Somehow people have to motivate themselves," Vic said. "I don't know the answer except that a lot of it has to do with vanity. People should have pride in wanting to look and feel well. Take the guy, for example, who has a big belly hanging out over his belt line. I call this 'Donlops' disease' — his belly done lopped over. I think it's repulsive and I would starve myself before I would let myself look like that. Besides looking awful, the guy can't feel well."

"I can't imagine going through life without exercising," Vic continued, "and that is probably true of most athletes who have accomplished something. Baseball players were notorious for letting themselves get out of shape, but Robin Roberts, whom I knew, was an exception. He took care of himself and he had a long career. Nolan Ryan is an excellent example of an athlete who keeps himself fit. He exercises every day even when he isn't pitching, and it's paying off for him."

Vic's attitude has changed in regard to weight training. He said, "I never did weight training to stay in shape as I associated it with weight lifting and I didn't want to develop that kind of muscle. But if I were a young tennis player now, I would use all the techniques they have designed specifically for muscles used in my sport. There are lots of methods to stay in better shape now."

Personal Fitness Goals

"My goal is to try to stay the same," Vic stated. "This is not possible, but it's something to work towards. I can't do much to improve my knees; maybe I'm wrong, but at this point [I think] they're not going to get better. The reason for a lot of the exercises I do is to keep in good shape those parts that are working well. If I can keep them from getting worse, I'll be happy. The rest of me is in good shape so I don't have any problems. I'd like to keep that going. It's like an old car; it's a constant maintenance job to keep it working. It's a matter of constant vigilance, discipline, and regularity — doing things on a regular basis."

Recommendation for Improved Fitness of People over 40

"Motivation, perhaps based on pride and vanity, is the most important thing," Vic said. "You must be willing to put time and effort into your program over a long period of time to see the results. It's like dieting. People want to lose ten pounds and they want to lose it tomorrow. They don't do it the right way and so a month later they are right back where they were. It's a matter of being properly motivated to do it the right way.

"Take pride in your physical condition," Vic recommends to mature adults who want to improve their health and fitness, "and have the discipline to maintain good eating habits, to exercise regulary, and to maintain proper weight."

"More than anything else, I recommend daily exercise," Vic said. "The more the better, but use common sense. The worse cases are the weekend jocks who sit behind desks all week and don't exercise until the weekend and then try to kill themselves with eight hours of tennis, golf or whatever. I don't think golf is bad, but overdoing your exercise on a weekend results in little more than sore muscles. The main thing is regularity. Although it's not always possible, strive to do some exercise every day. I try to play tennis at least three or four times a week, and the days I don't play I do something like bike riding. Walking is a good way for older people, especially those with arthritis, to start exercising. For example, walking out to the mailbox and back could be a start, and the next day they could walk a little farther. They have to get motivated to start doing something. Getting started is not easy because inactivity feeds on itself as it makes you feel less like doing something. I have found that inactivity for three or four days makes me not feel like playing tennis. The longer I go without exercising, the less I feel like exercising. It's vital that you force yourself to do something on a regular basis."

Jack Staton

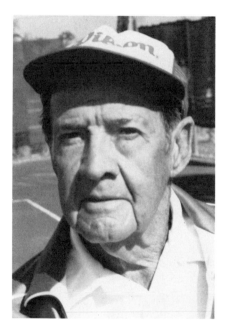

born: November 20, 1909

height: 5' 6'

weight: 150

home: St. Petersburg, Florida

athletic highlights:

• won 55 national senior tennis titles through 1989

• won two grand slams in senior tennis by winning all four national singles titles (clay, grass, indoor, and hard court) in one year

• won all 1989 national singles and doubles titles in M80s (men's age 80-and-over) except the Myrtle Beach clay courts which were canceled because of Hurricane Hugo

• played on the winning 1985 United States Crawford Cup team

• won national clay court M75s singles title while playing at the top of his age group at age 79

• won the European National Championship for his age group in 1985

Jack A. Staton has been a tennis player since 1937. He stays in shape to play tennis and he plays tennis to stay in shape. When asked how he stays in shape, Jack replied, "Just play tennis. With the weather down here we can play all year, thank goodness." Asked to describe his fitness regimen, Jack said he plays tennis. When pushed to describe his warm-up exercises before playing tennis, he admitted, "I do some, but not a lot. Just a few minutes. I don't go through all the rigmarole that some of these guys do." He would not admit to exercising at other times. "No, I don't do any exercises to build up anything more. I think I've already done that. Tennis gives me all the exercise I need. I work around the house, mowing, trimming and other stuff like that, but I don't go to gymnasiums or get involved in that kind of thing." He plays in 18 to 20 tournaments from mid-January through September.

After becoming a winner on the senior tennis circuit in 1954, Jack got a job as a sales representative to promote tennis products for Wilson Sporting Goods. His job, which took him to national tournaments throughout the United States, was to get the best players to use Wilson equipment. In the process, he improved his tennis skills by watching pros teach in the clinics he organized. Because of his job, he watched and played with some of the best, and he has received tips from players such as Jack Kramer, Bobby Riggs, Jimmy Connors, and Guillermo Vilas.

He had one of Wilson's first metal rackets, the T-2000, with him at the 1970 Orange Bowl Junior Tournament in Miami when a young Jimmy Connors asked him where he could get one of those shiny steel rackets. The T-2000 racket that Jack gave to Jimmy became Connors' trademark, and Connors eventually endorsed Wilson products.

Jack has acquired many friends through tennis, and he once said, "Tennis is a sport of a lifetime. One 84-year-old guy said to me after losing a match, 'I'll get them next year in the 85s.' "

ATHLETIC HISTORY

Jack was a halfback on his high school football team in Oak Hill, West Virginia, a forward on the basketball team, and a 440 runner on the track team. In 1933, he moved to Orlando, Florida, with his grandfather, and he played four or five years in a city basketball league.

At age 28, Jack said he decided to try tennis because he wanted to play another sport. Three years later he won his first tournament, the Orlando City Championship, and he earned two more significant wins at the age breaks of 35 and 45. The first of these was the 1944 state championship in the men's 35-and-over division and the other was his first national title in 1954 in the M45s. To this first national seniors title he has added 54 national championships, mostly in singles and in all categories from the M45s through the M80s with one exception, the M50s, which did not exist until he was 55. These national titles include two grand slams, which represent winning all four M65s singles (clay, grass, indoor, and hard court) in 1975 and all four M75s singles in 1984.

Jack has never stopped competing and has continued to win in his 80s while remaining healthy and free of injuries. He has consistently ranked first or close to the top in his age group. For example, as one of the older players in M75s at age 79, he was ranked fourth and he won the senior national clay singles title.

Jack's winning ways at the National Clay Court Championships in Myrtle Beach were interrupted in 1989 by Hurricane Hugo, which washed out (or blew out) the tournament. Having won all national M80s singles and doubles titles, having played this tournament for more than 20 consecutive years, and having won the M75s in 1988, Jack was a favorite to win the M80s and a third grand slam in singles and possibly a fourth in doubles.

After winning his second grand slam, Jack said he was inaugurated into the Florida Tennis Association's Hall of Fame and invited to play against international competition. He was selected for the 1985 United States Crawford Cup team, which won the cup in Brand, Austria, against competition from nine other countries, and he added to this achievement the European National Championship which he won for his age group in Baden-Baden, West Germany.

Despite his success in winning tournaments, Jack insists he never had a tennis lesson. "Actually, I never took a lesson," he said, " but I used to watch the good players, and then I would try to copy their good points. After I took up the game, I made up my mind I was going to learn it."

Jack still makes changes in his game, integrating new shots after practicing them. Noted for his steady play, he believes his strength is his patient ability to hit just one more ball than his opponent.

Another strength, according to Jack, is an edge in stamina over other players his age on the senior tennis circuit. Playing 18 to 20 tournaments each year, he has the endurance to play one singles match and one doubles match each day of the tournament week. (Seniors are not scheduled to play more than that.)

Jack is also not hampered by physical ailments, and his eyes are still good, although he wears glasses for distance. He said, "I don't have any problem physically. No problems with knees, shoulders, and elbows. I've been lucky. But I hit the ball without doing anything crazy with it, and I think that's one reason I haven't had problems. My stroke isn't the greatest, but I'm quick and can get to most balls. My friends tell me, 'You look like Ken Rosewall out there on the court.' It makes me feel proud to be likened to Rosewall."

Jack describes himself as a backcourt player who seldom goes to the net and who hits passing shots when his opponent comes in. He tells a story about a note that he got from Eddie Moreland, who used to be a pro at Forest Hills and a top player who demonstrated techniques at the tennis clinics Jack organized for Wilson. When Eddie picked up a newspaper and saw a picture of Jack going to the net, he wrote a card to Jack and said, "I know you weren't going to the net to hit the ball, so you must have been going to shake hands with your opponent."

FITNESS REGIMEN

Although he is in excellent physical condition, Jack has no special fitness program. "The only thing I do for exercise is play tennis, and I watch what I eat. I'm not a fanatic on exercise because I get enough playing tennis. In regard to diet, I don't do anything different than anybody else except maybe I'm on an oat bran kick. I eat plenty of vegetables, avoid fats and salt, and have a beer or maybe a drink now and then, but not to excess. I eat and drink in moderation, and I just try to have some fun."

Between tournaments, Jack said he plays tennis at least four times a week. "Most of the time I play two-out-of-three sets, and then maybe we'll play some doubles." When preparing for a tournament, he plays a week or two on the type of surface to be used in competition. He belongs to a couple of local clubs, being fortunate to get an honorary membership at the St. Petersburg Tennis Club after winning his first national title.

During a rare moment when he is not playing tennis, Jack might be found fishing for trout near his St. Petersburg home.

MENTAL ATTITUDE ABOUT HEALTH AND FITNESS

Jack's attitude has remained simple over the years. He wants to stay healthy and have fun, and he has fun wherever he goes with his tennis racket. He plays tennis to stay healthy, and as long as he's healthy he will play tennis.

PERSONAL FITNESS GOALS

It's not surprising that Jack's fitness goals relate to tennis. He wants to win tournaments and stay in shape. When he's not playing in tournaments, he stays active enough so that he can quickly get ready to play in the next tournament.

RECOMMENDATIONS FOR IMPROVED FITNESS OF PEOPLE OVER 40

Jack recommends that others should work hard to improve their fitness. "If they just try, anyone can change and improve themselves by really working at it."

"I improve or maintain my fitness," he said, "by staying active and playing all the time, especially with younger fellows. That's what others should do if they want to play tennis or any other sport. They have got to get out there and sweat it out."

3

THE YOUNGER
GENERATION
ROLE MODELS

INTRODUCTION

The "younger generation" role model athletes profiled in this chapter were born between 1928 and 1948. Like the "older generation" athletes featured in the previous chapter, these athletes grew up when competitive opportunities were still limited and few people pursued exercise beyond age 40. These "younger" athletes were in their 20s and 30s when they began to benefit from extensive research into diet, exercise, athletic equipment, and physical techniques.

As adults during the '50s and '60s, the "younger generation" athletes passed through a transitional period leading to significant changes in public awareness and pursuit of physical fitness. They experienced the advent of televised sports, an increasing number of media messages suggesting ways to improve health and fitness, and growing opportunities to participate in athletics due to greater economic freedom.

Under any circumstances, some individuals rise to the top, like cream in a bottle of milk. Bob Mathias, Pat McCormick, and Bob Seagren represent the cream of their generation, achieving Olympic fame at early ages. Although they had good coaching, they did not benefit from the special diets and training which are standard among athletes today. For example, Mathias had a good high school coach who taught him the basic form for each decathlon event, but it was his raw natural talent that led him to become world decathlon champion at age 17.

Bruce Crampton, Phil Mulkey, and Nancy Reed were also champions as young adults. Crampton and Reed were highly ranked for many years in golf and tennis, respectively, and Mulkey held the world decathlon record for five years. Unlike the Olympic champions who ended their competitve careers at early ages, Crampton, Mulkey, and Reed have continued to pursue their athletic careers through their mid-50s.

Sharon Crawford, Judy Dickinson, Damon Douglas, Marion Mehrtash, and George Hirsch are the remaining "younger generation" athletes profiled in this chapter. They represent the large group of people who have established their working careers and then pursued amateur athletics in their spare time. These are the "weekend warriors," as Sharon Crawford calls herself. They seldom let a day go by without training, and their persistence to excel has earned them recognition, awards, and titles during the middle years of their lives.

The athletic accomplishments of the "weekend warriors" were insignificant for the first 30 or so years of their lives. In the late 1960s and early 1970s, about the time when the fitness craze rippled through the United States, all members of this group except Mehrtash strove to get themselves into better shape. As their physical conditioning improved, they entered races and won more than their fair share.

During the 1980s, Marion Mehrtash got involved with sports to satisfy a mental rather than physical need. She wanted to add new friendships for personal pleasure and happiness as she passed through her 40s, which is a difficult period of change for many people. Mehrtash acquired physical fitness as well as mental fitness, and she has won triathlons in her age group.

These "younger generation" role models, like the older athletes, share common traits such as enthusiasm, motivation, and a positive outlook. Similarly, they have worked hard and persevered to achieve goals. Their fitness programs reflect individual objectives and styles based on daily training methods which they enjoy.

Bruce Crampton

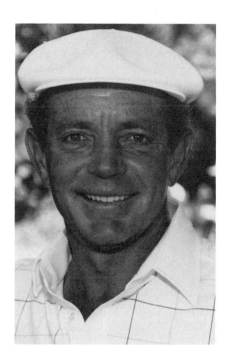

born: September 28, 1935

height: 5' 9.5"

weight: 178

home: Dallas, Texas

athletic highlights:

- won 15 individual titles and $1.3 million on the PGA Tour
- won 15 individual and two Legends titles through 1989 on the Senior PGA Tour
- won the Vardon Trophy for lowest stroke average in 1973 and 1975
- won seven tournaments in 1986 and was named Senior Golfer of the Year
- won $415,582 on the Senior Tour in 1989, pushing his official career earnings above $3 million

"The Senior PGA Tour is great for the game of golf," Bruce Crampton remarked. "Many people have told me that they had stopped watching or participating in golf because they had lost interest in the game. However, the Senior Tour renewed their interest and got them turned on to golf again. They are now playing golf, buying equipment, and watching golf on TV. This benefits charities, and it's great for the sponsoring corporations. Corporate representatives like the Senior Tour because they are often in the seniors' age bracket, and their customers like playing golf with us and being around the sport."

Bruce continued describing the growing interest in the sport he loves so much. "The game of golf is more important than any individual corporation and it's benefiting from increased exposure overseas. The way the Asian, Australian, and European tours have expanded is a direct result of what has taken place in the United States. Live telecasts overseas have been a factor, and I think the American people should feel proud of what their golfers have done to promote the game in the rest of the world. There are now golf courses in communist countries, including a course in China and one in Moscow that has been built or is nearing completion."

The Senior PGA Tour has grown from two $125,000 tournaments in its first year (1980) to 43 tournaments in 1990 with almost $18 million in prize money. With Jack Nicklaus and Lee Trevino joining Arnie Palmer, Gary Player, Bruce Crampton, and many other golfers with recognizable names, the Senior Tour has a bright future to build upon a brilliant first decade. Jim Ferree, one of the tour's leaders in the '80s, was quoted in a *Sports Illustrated* article as saying, "Think about this, golf has had its Hall of Fame playing out here every week. You don't have to go to Cooperstown, or wait for an old-timers game."

ATHLETIC HISTORY

"I played a lot of sports as a youngster in Sydney, Australia, where I was born and raised," Bruce said. "I was a good swimmer, and I played rugby, soccer, cricket, and a little baseball. But once I started playing golf, that was it. It's something I will never master even though I haven't done much else since I was 14. I've enjoyed a little skiing in later years, and I wish I had started skiing when I was younger."

"I started playing golf when I was 12 and the next May, in 1949, I won the district school boy championship," Bruce said. "From that point on I had a bright career as a youngster. I won the boy's district championship three straight years, and in 1951 I won the state school boy championship. Then, at age 16, I was the youngest, I believe, to win the state junior championship, which was for youths under 21. In 1953, I won the junior championship again, beating Bruce Devlin in a long match. Tied after 36 holes, we had a Sunday morning playoff and we tied again as Bruce Devlin holed a 4-wood for a two on the 10th hole. When we played again in the afternoon, I won the title."

In 1953, when Crampton was still 17, he represented Australia in golf matches against New Zealand. However, that same year he missed playing in matches at St. Andrews because Australian team officials decided he was too young to participate. "Because of my young age," he said, "they chose to leave me off the team because they didn't want me around the drinking and I couldn't participate in the social events. I decided then to ask my parents for 12 months to try to improve my golf game before deciding to go on to a university or to set out on a career."

"I turned pro as soon as they (Australian golf officials) decided to leave me off the Eisenhower Cup team," Bruce said, "and I began practicing with Norman von Nina, who was Australia's best player at that time. Norman promised he would take me overseas after I served a two-year apprenticeship. The sporting goods company I worked for gave me a good contract and three afternoons off for practicing each week. Norman took me under his wing and showed me the finer points of golf, including shots around the green and shots from bunkers."

"I played some exhibition matches with Norman throughout Australia," Bruce said. "This was great experience, and we earned enough money to cover the majority of our expenses. In 1956, we began our overseas tour by playing an exhibition in Singapore, the Egyptian Open in Cairo, and the Egyptian Match Play Championship in Alexandria. We went on to Europe to play in the British Open as well as matches in France and Belgium, and then I came back to win the Australian Open Championship."

The news media wondered if Bruce would have won the Australian Open if Peter Thompson, the great Australian golfer, had been in the field. Thompson had just won his third straight British Open title. A few weeks later, in September, Thompson and Crampton played in the same tournament, a five-round match on Peter's home course, Victoria Golf Club in Melbourne. Bruce explained what happened. "We were tied after three rounds, and we had 36 holes to play on Saturday. In the morning, Peter shot 3 under and I shot par 73, so all the clubhouse talk was about how Peter was going to win the tournament. But, in the afternoon, it was one of those days when everything went right; I made 9 birdies, shot a 65 for a new course record, and won the tournament by four shots. This win, tacked onto my Australian Open win and my bright career as a youngster, proved I could compete favorably against Australian players."

"My next goal was to compete against the best players in the world," Bruce continued, "and my Australian Open Championship earned me an invitation to play in the 1957 Masters Tournament in Augusta. I chose to begin play on the PGA Tour in Houston, and I played several tournaments leading up to Augusta. After the Masters, I played in Great Britain and did not play on the PGA Tour again until the next year when I returned to Augusta. I continued to play on the PGA Tour, but it wasn't until 1961 that I won a tournament in the United States. By winning the Milwaukee Open, I was exempted for the winter tour and from that point on I played all the time over here."

During his early years on the PGA Tour, Bruce was nicknamed the

"Iron Man" when he played 37 tournaments straight two years in a row. "The press did that," Bruce explained. "Other players have played as many tournaments as I did. At that time, I wasn't married and didn't have a home over here. I found that if I took time off to spend a week with friends, they would arrange golf games every day and I wouldn't get a break from golf. I decided I was better off playing in tournaments. But, when I went back to Australia, I put my clubs into the trunk of the car when I arrived at the airport, and I sometimes did not touch them for six to eight weeks as I would be burned out. This 'Iron Man' reputation was a matter of being away from home. I didn't set out to earn that title or set any records with consecutive tournament appearances; it worked out that way because I was far from home."

Bruce was known as a golfer who seldom spoke on the course and smiled less often. "It's the way I was trained," Bruce commented. "As a youngster, I was taught to think, think, think — to keep my mind on what I'm doing for the few hours that I'm on the course. My instructor was a great admirer of Ben Hogan, and he told me to take every opportunity to watch Ben, which I did. I saw how intense he was and how he concentrated on his game; I read a lot about his concentration; and, I became another of his admirers. So, I tried to emulate his attributes and apply them to what I'd been taught as a youngster. I was told recently by a friend that Ben respected me during my early career because I was a hard worker. He said Ben had commented that 'when Bruce comes to the golf course, he comes to work.' "

Bruce's hard work, concentration, and persistence began to pay off after he won the Milwaukee Open. During his first five years on the U.S. tour, his annual earnings did not top $8,500. Then he became a substantial money winner, ranking in the top 60 for the next 14 years and winning over $100,000 each year from 1965 through 1975. Bruce said, "I had $100,000 years going, which was really something at that time."

In 1972, Bruce was second in the Masters, second in the U.S. Open, and second in the PGA. The next year he became the fifth man to win $1 million on tour as he added $274,266 to his career total while winning the Vardon Trophy for the lowest stroke average. In 1975, he won the Vardon Trophy again.

Bruce was on the August 1973, cover of *Golf Digest* magazine, and a featured article, "How to Putt Confidently," described him as one of the best putters and an emerging superstar. "I still feel I'm a good putter," Bruce said. "I think that came from playing with the small ball, which is harder to putt with, and I think those of us who played with the small balls have been good putters."

Bruce's earnings dropped to $50,000 in 1976 and only $800 the following year as he lost his concentration due to family problems. "My wife was unhappy with the traveling, and it just wasn't working out," he explained. "She had actually filed for divorce and that bothered me; I couldn't handle it. I became insecure, was playing poorly, and I decided I had to choose between my family and golf. I chose my family and got away from golf. So I got into the oil and gas business for eight years."

"Then, as I approached 50, my wife, my friends, and my fans encouraged me to play the Senior Tour. My youngest son, who was a baby when I quit the PGA Tour, had never seen me play in a tournament, and he and my older boy said they would love to see me play. About that time, the U.S. Congress started talking about changing the tax laws, and the oil and gas business would become more difficult for a small independent operator. The timing was right for me to get ready to play the Senior Tour, and I'm glad I got back to something I knew more about. I still have an interest in the wells that are producing, but I don't operate at all. I enjoyed the oil and gas business; it was a lot like golf except that I had to wait ten days before I knew if I made the cut."

In 1986, his first full year on the Senior Tour, Bruce won seven tournaments and was named Senior Golfer of the Year. After four years on the Senior Tour, he matched his 15 individual titles and surpassed his $1,374,294 in U.S. money winnings on the other tour. In 1989, he won the MONY Arizona Classic in Phoenix and the Ameritech Open in Cleveland, and the $415,582 in winnings pushed his career total over $3 million. Including two Legends titles with his 30 individual titles, Bruce has won 32 U.S. PGA and Senior PGA tournaments.

FITNESS REGIMEN

Bruce is noted for being a non-drinker and non-smoker, and people have kidded him at times about not drinking. "It must be hell to wake up in the morning and know you're not going to feel any better all day," they said.

"I get up every morning and do about 45 minutes of stretching and flexibility exercises," Bruce said as he began describing his current fitness program. "I've been hitting a lot of balls and using the exercise room at the club where I've been practicing. After golf practice, I usually come home and ride the exercise bike for about 40 minutes five days a week. This routine ties in with my workouts on the tour where we have a fitness trailer and the same style bike that I have at home. I usually exercise five days a week when I'm on the tour. I have added light weights to my workout; I use five-pound ankle weights, dumbbells, and a little more than that on the pull-down machines. I use weights every other day mainly to strengthen rotator cuffs and small muscles as a prevention from injury."

"The core of my fitness program was developed for me by one of the physical therapists on the regular tour. When I was getting ready for the Senior Tour, I asked him to devise a fitness program to help me with shot placements and distance. He handwrote a program I have followed religiously. I have added anything worthwhile I've seen on TV or picked up from books like Dr. Cooper's (*Aerobics*). A doctor at PGA West suggested I cross my legs in front of me to take the weight off my back when I do exercises, and this helped a lot. As I learn better ways of doing things, I modify my fitness program."

Bruce explained that the regular and Senior PGA Tours each have a fitness trailer for the players' convenience. Each trailer is well equipped and is manned by two physical therapists. "The trailer is a semitrailer that expands into a nice workout room for us," he said. "It has stationary bikes, two stair-type machines, a cross country skiing machine, weights, and electronic equipment for injuries."

"In early 1989, about 20–25 guys on the regular tour and a similar number on the Senior Tour agreed to be tested for physical fitness," Bruce said. "I felt good when told I rated second to Chip Beck in fitness flexibility based on a test that had us sit with our feet braced against something and stretch our fingertips as far as possible beyond our toes. I also tested about average in every category with the younger players on the regular tour. My body fat is 14% and my HDL/LDL ratio is 2.9. Seeing results spelled out in numbers like this motivates me and makes me eager to keep exercising."

"I try to be careful," Bruce stated in regard to his diet. "When on tour, I have to eat out and attend banquets, and my food selections are limited. I drink juices, eat oatmeal and whole wheat bread, and get lots of fresh fruit and nuts. I try to be sensible without being a nut about my diet, and I don't deprive myself as I sometimes eat ice cream and yogurt. I watch my weight and I cut back on my eating if I find my weight increasing. Last year I went down from a size 36 pants waist to a 34. The people in our fitness trailer suggested I should maintain my weight at 178 instead of 182, so that's what I do."

Mental Attitude about Health and Fitness

"I have been taking health and fitness seriously since I started getting ready for the senior tour," Bruce stated. "Until that time, I was following what I'd been taught as a youngster. My instructor used to tell me that nothing agreed with golf except hitting golf balls. You didn't want to ride a bike or swim or lift a heavy suitcase because it messed up your timing. 'Just hit golf balls,' he'd say, and that's what I did. But modern research has changed that way of thinking, and, when I became aware of that, I looked into what I should do for improved fitness as I got older."

"I've really enjoyed my fitness program, and it's helped me," Bruce emphasized. "Apart from feeling good, it's helped me rest and reduce my stress. It feels good to start exercising, to ride the bike, and to do some things to burn up some stress and frustration. I'm aware now that our bodies or minds emit emulsions during aerobic exercise, and these emulsions make us feel good. I wish I had done this all my life."

"Physical fitness wasn't taught this way to my generation," Bruce commented, "but each generation improves upon the preceding. My exercise program is not going to make me play better, but it will give me the opportunity to play my best. It's also nice to feel good every morning and to not have any injuries. On the Tour, it's evident in the fitness trailer that the players who are most conscientious about regular exercise are the ones with the fewest aches and pains. You seldom see them on the table getting ultrasound, heat, ice, or a therapeutic massage. I think Bob Charles, Al Geiberger, Bobby Nichols, Butch Baird, and myself are the most conscientious about exercising, and we have played well. Among the younger guys who have come from the regular tour to join the Senior Tour, Mike Hill exercises regularly, and I'm sure we'll see more players like Mike who have included exercise as part of their routine. You don't see many older guys working out, perhaps because they were taught the way I was that nothing agreed with golf except hitting golf balls."

Personal Fitness Goals

"I'm aware you can keep chasing that high and you want to do more and more until you tend to get burned out," Bruce said in explanation of his fitness goals. "I pace myself carefully based on what they tell me in the fitness trailer. I learned last year that I was working out too hard and that I should not get my pulse rate above 141 when riding the bike.

As a result of being in better aerobic shape, I don't have to work as hard because my body is getting enough oxygen. To become more efficient, my heart has grown larger and is moving more blood per stroke. Therefore, I don't have to work as hard. I'd been riding at a 150–155 pulse rate, and my body didn't need that. Now that I'm aware of this, I watch myself. If I don't feel like exercising, I don't. I listen to my body, but I'm still regimented."

"I played over 30 tournaments in 1989, but I skipped the last two because I'm working to improve my game. For the first time in 30 years, I'm taking lessons. Hank Haney has a great teaching facility at Steinrich Country Club (Dallas), and I've been going there daily to hit balls. I'm enjoying myself and feeling like a kid again. I'm taking a couple weeks off the tour because I thought my game wasn't ready for public display, and there are more things in life than chasing dollars, titles, and whatnot. I felt that I ought to do something I wanted to do, and I wanted to stay home and work on my game every day and that's what I've done. I may not score any better, but I'm having a ball learning a lot of things I didn't know."

"My goal is to play as well as I can as long as I can on the Senior Tour. I'm motivated and I've got new thoughts as well as a new way of swinging a golf club. My new swing is contrary to anything I was told as a youngster, and I'm excited about it. I want to see how good a player I can be at 60. Although I'm a perfectionist and I know I can never master the game, there's always the thought of going out and never hitting a poor shot. I love the game because it's a constant challenge, and I was born to hit golf balls. But first I must give myself the opportunity to play by staying fit and healthy. Not long ago somebody asked me what was the most important thing in my life, and I said my good health because without that I can't do anything well."

RECOMMENDATIONS FOR IMPROVED FITNESS OF PEOPLE OVER 40

"I think adults wanting to improve their fitness should get advice about a program and should consult with a physician to find out what shape they're in," Bruce recommended. "They should get the parameters for their workouts and should never overdo them. I encourage people to devise a fitness regimen and to make it part of their daily routine; they will never regret it. Many people avoid exercise due to laziness, and they wonder how others find time to pursue their activities. It's a factor of time and priorities. Two hours spent daily on exercising has to come from some area. Whatever they decide to give up, the benefits of feeling good and accomplishing more outweigh the negatives of things given up. I think exercise helps mentally, too, because the brain needs to be stimulated like other body parts. By exercising in the morning and making your brain work to send signals to your muscles, your mind will grow and keep healthy."

Bruce said he made a videotape explaining how he came out of retirement and played so well on the Senior Tour in 1986. "The first quarter of the video showed my exercise program, which was the first time, I believe, that a golfer demonstrated exercises on a videotape. I thought this would benefit golfers or anybody interested in fitness, and I've had nice feedback from it. It was important to me to share this story with anyone who was interested in my comeback, and a good part of that story was my exercise program."

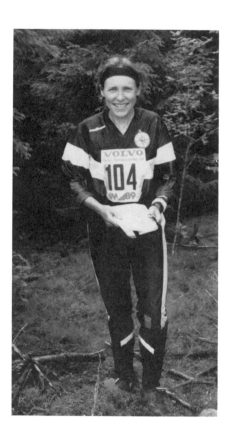

Sharon Crawford

born: September 24, 1944

height: 5' 6.75"

weight: 135

home: Concord,
         Massachusetts

athletic highlights:

- won the U.S. Women's Orienteering Championship eleven times through 1989 and the North American Women's Championship twice (1982–83)

- has been on the U.S. Orienteering Team since 1976 and the Ski-Orienteering Team since 1982

- completed the 1989 Hawaiian Ironman Triathlon

- became a Coureur de Bois Gold medalist for the seventh straight year after completing the elite category of the 100-mile Canadian Ski Marathon

After growing up in Montana, Sharon L. Crawford got a bachelor's degree in liberal arts from Stanford and a master's in mathematics from Montana State University. She then moved to the East Coast to get a job as a computer programmer in the Massachusetts high-tech industry. Except for a two-year break working as a programmer in Alaska during construction of the oil pipeline, Sharon has remained in the Boston area.

"I don't care how many years I've lived in the East," Sharon said, "I still consider myself a Westerner. One of these days I'll move back permanently."

Sharon's yearning for her past may be part of the reason for her relentless pursuit of rugged outdoor activities. For nearly twenty years, she has filled her weekends and vacations with sports such as orienteering, triathlons, ski races, marathons, and mountain climbing. She loves these sports and trains hard to excel, especially in orienteering.

Beginning in 1977, Sharon won the U.S. Women's Orienteering Championship 11 times in 13 years. Factors contributing to her success are athletic ability, physical endurance, competitive spirit, determination to improve, and persistence in training. In addition, her analytical ability is significant because it has helped her navigate well while running cross-country.

"In orienteering," Sharon said, "it's important to think quickly and to make immediate decisions on the run. The fastest runner in the world will take forever to complete an orienteering course if unable to locate the control points. In this respect, orienteering and programming are similar. Both involve analytical thinking that breaks tasks into small steps, measures progress 'on the run,' analyzes information quickly, makes fast decisions, and lives with the results. Immediate feedback on these decisions promotes clear thinking and develops confidence in getting out of tight situations such as those which might be encountered in a remote wilderness."

Sharon competes in the 21–35 age category because she has little competition at higher age levels. "We can compete later in life," Sharon said, "because our minds get sharper as our bodies slow down."

ATHLETIC HISTORY

"I grew up in Montana and lived in Billings from third grade through high school," Sharon said. "At that time there were no opportunities for girls to participate in organized sports. I learned to swim in grade school, played summer recreational softball, hiked, and camped."

"I was nearly 30 before I became an athlete," Sharon continued. "When I started jogging in 1972, I was 20 pounds heavier than I am now and I was out of shape because I had done nothing for fitness while working in Boston. I tried jogging one-and-a-half miles around Walden Pond and made it about one-quarter of the way before stopping to walk. Then I decided to jog around the pond each day, usually before work. I alternated walking with jogging and gradually reduced the walking until I jogged the entire distance, which was a major achievement."

"The same year I started jogging," Sharon said, "I climbed Mt.

Logan in Canada. I had climbed in Switzerland with my brother, but this was my first organized expedition. We flew in by plane, landed on a glacier, and ascended the peak from there."

Sharon has climbed the two highest mountains in North America and the highest in South America. In addition to Mt. Logan, which is 19,850 feet high, she climbed Alaska's 20,320-foot Mt. McKinley in 1974 and Argentina's 22,834-foot Mt. Aconcaqua in 1978. She hasn't done any organized climbing since her South American expedition because she has concentrated her efforts on orienteering and triathlons.

"I got into the sport of orienteering in December, 1973," Sharon recalled. "I saw a PBS television spot for the local New England Orienteering Club's last meet of the year. I thought this outdoor activity involving maps, compasses and hiking sounded like fun. Since I had nothing else to do, I went to the meet, which was held in the Blue Hills south of Boston, and fell in love with the sport."

Sharon began participating in orienteering, cross-country skiing, and marathoning within a year. "In February, 1974," she began, "I ran a local marathon with no training and only one day warning. My brother wanted to know how to register for the Boston Marathon, so I called and learned that participants had to qualify by completing another marathon and that the last qualifying event was to be held the next day. Somehow I got involved in it. I had been running a couple miles almost every day for a year, but I had never run a distance longer than that. Running and walking, I finished last with a time of about five hours. This marathon run led to my joining a running club to improve my training."

In May, 1974, Sharon began her first orienteering season by trying the advanced red course. After three-and-one-half hours, she was forced to quit when time ran out. "About halfway through," she said, "I was overtaken by meet organizers who were collecting the controls."

Sharon's orienteering career was interrupted by a two-year move to Alaska to work as a programmer on construction of the oil pipeline. However, while vacationing in Boston in 1976, she went to Canada to compete in a five-day orienteering event which included trials for the new U.S. Women's Orienteering Team. She made the team and went to Scotland to compete in the world championships. "We had to pay our own way, and it was a great experience even though our team was dead last," she said.

"When I came back from Alaska in 1977," Sharon explained, "I began working hard to learn more about orienteering. Since then, I've been orienteering in Europe almost every summer and in New England every spring and fall, which are the sport's prime seasons in the Northeast. I also participate in some local meets during the summer when I'm not in Europe."

Sharon has competed in every biannual World Orienteering Championship from 1976, when the United States fielded its first women's team, through the 1989 meet in Sweden. "I've gone eight times," Sharon said, "and I am competing well against younger women because of my experience. The women coming up through the ranks of orienteering are faster runners. In a 10K road race, they would leave me in their dust. Although more girls are coming along and getting experience, I have won the U.S. Women's championship 11 times. My six-year winning streak was broken in 1983. Then, after winning four more years, a younger woman who has shown improvement won the championship in 1988. After losing to her, I told myself, 'Okay, I've had my reign; now it's her turn.' But I went to the 1989 championships in California and won again. Of course, it's just a matter of time until I lose my title for good because other women are developing their skills."

"Running speed in the woods is a factor in winning," Sharon said, "and orienteers adjust their running technique to the terrain. I run at about the same speed in woods and on trails. Many orienteers are fast trail runners, but they hardly move in the woods because they are cautious. They don't know how to move their feet or they're unwilling to throw themselves through trees and bushes. In comparison to a good track runner with a smooth style, a good woods runner has a choppy style due to putting feet down in different positions each time."

"In big European meets, I compete in my age category because the competition is fierce," Sharon explained. "In the annual five-day O-Ringen meet in Sweden, my best finish was fourth. In 1989, over 18,000 people competed on more that 100 courses at the O-Ringen meet, and I finished 13th in my age group. My best finish in the world championships was 29th out of 70 at the 1985 meet in Australia, but Sweden had only four participants because that was each team's limit. Sweden and other European countries big in orienteering each have 20 or 30 people who could beat me, but I was first among non-European women."

"With my summer orienteering limited to a European vacation and an occasional local meet," Sharon said, "I have some weekends available for other activities. In 1984, I spent two weekends participating in triathlons. The first one was for women only. Of 102 entrants, I was

101st coming out of the water. Then I passed people on the biking and running events to finish 67th. Afterwards, I thought, 'this would be a good sport if I could swim properly.' "

"I have been competing in two to four triathlons each year," Sharon said. "In 1989, I completed the Hawaiian Ironman after qualifying by winning my age category in the Cape Cod Triathlon. Before the start of the Cape Cod event, I copied upside down on my bib the numbers of all women competing in my age group. Every time I saw a woman who appeared to be my age, I looked down at my bib to see if I was competing against her. I did not want these women to finish ahead of me, and they didn't."

"The Ironman was brutal but a great experience. The hype during the preceding week makes you feel like you're on top of the world, and I can see why people want to do it again. My finishing time was 13 hours and 46 minutes, about an hour slower than my Cape Cod time, and I was eighth out of 25 in the women's 45-and-over age group. There's a lot to learn and a lot of technique involved in triathlons. If I do the Ironman again, I will try to improve my biking time, partly by replacing my four-year-old bike with a better model. I was tired after biking, so I walked up some hills during the run. All I wanted to do was finish as it was getting dark."

"The winter ski season complements the foot-orienteering season," Sharon said, "but I wish it were six months long because I love to ski. I compete in ski-orienteering and long-distance ski races. The latter includes cross-country, which is a good sport for keeping the total body in shape because every muscle is involved. Poling and upper body strength have gained importance as cross-country skiing technique has evolved."

Sharon's favorite ski event is the annual Canadian Ski Marathon, which draws nearly 2000 contestants to its site in Quebec. Sharon said, "It took me four tries before I could do the Coureur De Bois, which is the highest endurance level, in the allotted two days. Participants ski 100 miles cross-country with a five-kilogram pack and camp out the first night. Except for firewood and water, our backpacks include everything needed for camping. In February, 1990, a Canadian and I became the first women to complete the Coureur De Bois for seven consecutive years. I'm the first U.S. citizen to do this. I received a Gold Bar award for each of these seven finishes and the HOECHST Trophy Award for completing this event five times. This latter award consists of a plaque and a permanent bib number. Each year I now wear bib number 36. Of all my awards and trophies, the Gold Bars and

HOECHST Trophy mean more to me because they represent 14 days of skiing, seven nights camping out, and 700 miles."

FITNESS REGIMEN

"The ski season starts after the Christmas holidays," Sharon said, "and I participate in a race or event almost every weekend. The 1990 U.S. Ski-Orienteering Team Trials were in January at Telemark, Wisconsin, and I will go to Sweden and compete in the World Ski-Orienteering Championships. There is no funding for the 6-man, 4-woman U.S. team, so this remains a pay-your-own-way sport. The Canadian Ski Marathon was the first weekend in February; that consumed four days — one day to drive 350 miles to Quebec, two days for the marathon, and one day for the drive back. Meanwhile, I tried to squeeze in a full workweek between weekends. The life of the Weekend Warrior!"

"I work full time during the week," Sharon explained, "but I try to work out at least one hour per day and longer on weekends when I'm not competing. I don't have a regular routine because my workouts depend on weather conditions and the training I need for my seasonal sports."

"When I can, I bike ten miles to work," Sharon said. "This takes about 40 minutes. Since 1988, I have biked straight home after work. When the weather was nice, I used to stop at Walden Pond, which is a mile-and-a-half out of the way, to swim across and back, and then run around it. Including the biking, this triathlon workout took about two hours. I haven't done this workout since I got a membership at a hotel fitness center near my office. Twice a week I take an hour-and-a-half lunch break to swim 1000 meters and use Nautilus equipment at the hotel."

"When I'm not working out at the hotel," Sharon continued, "I often run at lunch time. In warm weather, I run in the woods or on the roads two to four times per week. In the winter, I try to run every Tuesday at a field house, which is available through my membership in a women's track club. A coach is there to help, and I run various distances from a quarter-mile up to a couple miles. Sometimes I run by myself, but I often run with others because it's easier to do it as a group."

"I find training more enjoyable when I have seasonal changes. Thus, if I can ski during the week, I don't run, and this is a welcome mental break. When we have snow, I ski during the week on a local golf course."

"A typical week in November includes Nautilus or swimming on Monday, running on Tuesday, Nautilus and swimming on Wednesday, a noon run on Thursday, Nautilus and swimming on Friday, and a two-day orienteering meet on the weekend. If my weekend event is exhausting, I'll rest on Monday."

"During the last few years," Sharon said, "I've evolved into a vegetarian. For breakfast, I eat whole grain bread, a hot cereal like oatmeal, and maybe some cut fruit to go with it. A typical lunch that I take to work will have plain yogurt spread on bread with a covering of something like lettuce, cabbage, and fruit. For my evening meal, I typically cook a big pot of vegetables with whatever I have grown in my garden. I may add dry herbs to the vegetable stew, and sometimes I will use only potatoes and onions."

"I don't eat ice cream because it has so much fat and sugar that it's not worth it. I eat non-fat yogurt made from skim milk, and I spread yogurt instead of butter on bread. I don't always deprive myself of sweets, and my weakness is cookies. I sometimes buy a high quality chocolate chip cookie from a candy machine at work."

"With the way I like to eat," Sharon said, "I know that my weight would balloon right up if I stopped training. I don't care how much exercise I get, I'm always battling my waistline."

MENTAL ATTITUDE ABOUT HEALTH AND FITNESS

"My thoughts on conditioning are a lot different now than they were when I began jogging in 1972," Sharon said. "Health and fitness have a high priority in my life. Year-round I train for and participate in orienteering, running, bicycling, cross-country skiing, ski-orienteering, and swimming. Often I keep going through sheer stubbornness, determination, and a desire to prove myself, for example, that I can do the Ironman."

"I get popular magazines like *Runners World, Ski,* and *Triathlon.* I enjoy reading the articles to get professional viewpoints on health and fitness. By the time I read about the same subject in each of four magazines, I tend to think there's truth in it. I keep up with technology and research as best I can, and I apply what I can to my program."

"Orienteering is my main sport," Sharon said, "and my mental attitude is important because the sport involves map-reading and navigation while running at high speed. The ability to concentrate is critical while pushing myself up hills, through marshes, and over rough terrain. The ability to push yourself when you're not in a head-to-head race is important because orienteers start at different time intervals and often don't see their competitors on the course. People who haven't raced much don't know what it's like to push that last ounce of energy out of yourself at the end to win a race."

"My medals and trophies represent the effort I put into events," Sharon said. "Because I focus on effort, a results list is more important to me than awards. I want to see my time and the times of my peers. I usually know after a race if I put forth my maximum effort, but a results list shows how my effort fared against others. I think every finisher should get a medal and a results list."

PERSONAL FITNESS GOALS

Sharon plans to continue her fitness program and sporting activities as long as she can. When she slows down and can't compete effectively against young women, she may resume mountain climbing. Her next expedition may be Mt. Everest, the highest peak in the Himalayas.

RECOMMENDATIONS FOR IMPROVED FITNESS OF PEOPLE OVER 40

Sharon recommended the following points for mature adults to improve their fitness:

1. Set realistic short-term and long-term goals
2. Monitor your progress with written records
3. Commit to a regular exercise or training schedule
4. Organize your daily life so that your priority for exercise is high enough to ensure it gets done regularly, like eating, sleeping, bathing, and brushing teeth
5. Have some fun, too

"Maintain a written record of what you do," Sharon recommended. "One of your goals should be to write something in a notebook every day. Your notebook will become your conscience waiting for each day's entry, and each entry will become a result. Your notebook will show the results of your efforts, and you will have something to look at to see how you've progressed."

"When I awake each morning, I think about what I will do for my daily training. I know I will train, but I'm not always sure what I will do. Figuring out how and when to get an hour of exercise each day can become a sort of game."

"It isn't necessary to do a certain number of miles or reps each day," Sharon added, "but it's important to do something. For someone who hasn't been exercising, walking is an excellent way to start a fitness program."

Judy Dickinson

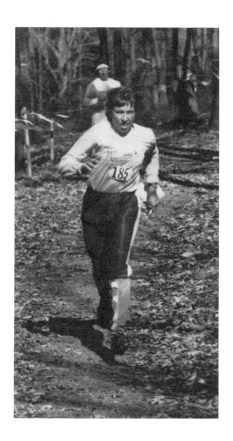

born: March 1, 1941

height: 5' 5"

weight: 135

home: Wayne, New Jersey

athletic highlights:

* completed the 1982 New Jersey Shore Marathon and the 1983 New York City Marathon
* won the 1986 U.S. Orienteering Championship for women 45 and over
* finished third among all women in the 1987 U.S. Orienteering Championship
* was selected for the 1988 U.S. Ski-Orienteering team and competed in Helsinki
* finished 12th in the 1988 World Cup for women 45 and over
* was selected for the 1988-89 U.S. Orienteering "B" team and the 1989 U.S. Orienteering "A" team which participated in the world championships in Sweden

Judith Dickinson is a blue collar athlete. Her father, an avid outdoorsman, taught his four sons and two daughters to hunt and fish. Judy grew up as a tomboy, hunting and fishing with her father and playing sports with her brothers. "We played games like baseball, tag ball, and basketball," Judy said. "Everything we did was rough."

Because of her upbringing, Judy has pursued rugged sports and adventures outdoors. She says she doesn't have a great athletic body, but with intensive training and perseverance she has managed to achieve athletic successes. According to Judy, she compensates for her lack of speed by not slowing down in the woods like her younger, faster orienteering competitors and she uses adverse conditions to her advantage. For example, when fair-weather orienteers complain about rain, heat, or cold, Judy knows she has the advantage because she toughs it out under all conditions.

Judy, who usually competes against women in the 21–34 age group, was the oldest competitor in the 1989 world orienteering championships. "I'm older, and my map-reading vision during orienteering is poor because I'm losing my close vision," she said. "I'm near-sighted, I have stigmatism, and I can't wear glasses when I orienteer because of sweat. The only thing that seems to work is to wear a contact in one eye. The contact gives me distance vision in one eye, and I use my other eye to read the map."

ATHLETIC HISTORY

Besides playing sports and sledding down hills with her brothers, Judy hunted and fished throughout her childhood. "We hunted everything there was to hunt and fished for everything there was to fish," she said. "I would have liked to have been on teams, but there weren't many sports for girls in those days; it was all for boys."

In 1959, after graduating from high school, Judy began learning the martial arts — judo and karate — at a school in town. In 1965, she became an active competitor and part-time instructor in Okinawa Karate when a friend she met in 1959 opened a school.

"I was one of the first women to compete in karate," Judy stated. "When I first got into the sport, the participants were all men who didn't like having me compete against them in the forms and sparring. In order to compete, I had no alternative until a few other women became active and ready for competition. We started having women's competition, and, as more women joined, our women's sport became almost as popular as the men's. Karate is more organized than it was at that time when clubs scheduled their own competitions, which were usually in New York City. I never participated outside the United States, but we had international involvement as Europeans came to compete with our club members. During ten years of participating, I achieved proficiency at the level of third degree."

"After giving up the martial arts in 1975 and before I got into orienteering in 1981," Judy said, "I was into road running and backpacking. I'm not a fast runner, but I ran distance races like the 5K and 10K. Before I quit road running to concentrate on orienteering, I completed the 1982 New Jersey Shore Marathon and the 1983 New York City Marathons."

In addition to running, Judy's main sporting interest for several years was backpacking. She hiked alone for three weeks in the Swiss Alps, and she took several trips with Outward Bound. On one Outward Bound trip, she went to Nepal and circumnavigated the Annapurna Massive in the Himalayas, a three-week trip of about 150 horizontal miles and an unknown number of vertical miles, including an 18,000-foot pass. Judy said this beautiful experience was almost marred by a boulder which smashed to pieces when it fell in front of her on the trail.

"I also went to Peru on an Outward Bound expedition to pick up trash left by previous groups," Judy said. "We went to a city called Cuzco, which was an ancient Inca village, and we carried our food and sleeping gear while hiking for five days along part of the 2000-mile Inca trail. We saw old ruins as we walked along the trail picking up trash for our porters to carry out. Up and down or vertical distance was more significant than distance traveled, so one backpacker was assigned the task of figuring out the change in elevation each day."

Judy described a frightening situation while climbing the Mountain of the Holy Cross, which is between Aspen and Leadville in Colorado. "The mountain is shaped like a rough cross," she explained, "and the north slope has snow fields year-round. People go there for religious experiences. We used ropes and ice picks to climb the snow fields to reach the mountain top which is small like the roof of a house. There was room for about two dozen people, and we planned to have a picnic there. But when we reached the top, a thunderstorm was there. The thundercloud wasn't big, but I told our leader this is dangerous and we started down the other side. I soon heard this metallic noise that reminded me of static electricity, and I saw my ice ax, which had a rubber coating on the handle, vibrating in my hand. The hair on my arms was standing straight up, and, fearing a bolt of lightning, I threw my ax down on the rocks. The storm was generating a field of electricity, but it never made a bolt of lightning because it wasn't big enough.

Judy continued to hunt and fish until the 1980s, when she drifted away from both sports for a variety of reasons. Her involvement in orienteering is one reason she stopped fishing; both sports have the same prime seasons, spring and fall, in the Eastern Coastal region. "In the summertime, there are too many bugs in the woods," Judy said. "Down South they only orienteer in the wintertime because the woods are thick with rattlesnakes. The people who are really into orienteering go to Europe in the summer to participate in several major competitions."

"I spent about half my time running and the other half orienteering for a couple years," Judy said. "After going to a national orienteering meet, I found how exciting the sport is, and I stopped roadrunning to concentrate on orienteering."

"I was on the United States Orienteering Team for the world championships in Sweden," Judy said. "I worked my way up through the system, running in my age group at first. After winning the national championship for my age group in 1986, I competed against younger women and in national team competition. In 1987, I almost made the national team in the trials, and I placed third in the United States National Championship. For the next two years, I was a consistent top-five finisher at national championships. In 1989, my training went well, and I made the national team."

"I had been doing cross-country ski-orienteering for about three years when I was selected to participate on the United States Team in the 1988 championships held in Helsinki, Finland. I did alright," Judy said, "but our team was near the bottom."

"Our orienteering teams finish near the bottom in international competition," Judy said. "One reason is that our federation has only about 500 orienteers active in national competition. We are way behind Sweden and Russia in numbers of orienteers. Our team is getting better, but so are others. Competitive orienteering is about 20 years old, beginning with club championships in the 1960s and world championships in the 1970s. The sport is growing. Eastern European countries have gotten involved and are now comparable to the Scandinavian countries. Russia has one million orienteers, the largest number in the world."

"Because I'm self-employed and my business dies off in July and August, I have no problem getting away to compete at that time. I fund most travels myself. The federation covered our entry fees, uniforms, and travel expenses with money donated from people like myself. We got only a few hundred dollars per athlete. During the recent international competition, most of us went to Europe to train and compete for six weeks. I took a tent, sleeping bag, and camp stove, and I bought food at grocery stores. One-third of our expenses were for groceries because food is more than double our cost here."

FITNESS REGIMEN

"My diet is basically like any athlete's nowadays," Judy said. "I try to maintain a balance of 60 percent carbohydrate, 30 percent fat, and 10 percent protein. Low fat is important. For breakfast I eat foods such as lowfat yogurt with bananas, cooked wheatina cereal, skim milk, and half a grapefuit; for lunch I'll have a bagel with lowfat cheese and romaine lettuce; for a second sandwich I'll have whole wheat bread with lowfat cheese and lettuce; and for snacks I eat carrot sticks, celery sticks, apples, peaches, pears, nuts, and raisins. I eat chicken, fish, and a little pork. About the only time I eat red meat is in something like lasagna. We grow vegetables in our garden, so I eat a lot of fresh vegetables."

"Four or five mornings a week before work, I train at a health club," Judy said. "After swimming 15–30 minutes, I work out on the Nautilus equipment or I ride an exercycle. For orienteering fitness training I am supposed to run intervals in the woods where I get my heart rate up to its maximum. I do 50-second intervals at a fast speed. Doing similar intervals on an exercycle and using a heart monitor, I have reduced my resting heart rate from 49–51 down to about 46."

Judy continued, "I joined the health club after injuring my foot during the U.S. Orienteering Championship in October, 1989. During the meet, I did well the first day and was in second place. The next day, while running across rocky grass-covered ground, I tore a tendon in my foot and had a stress fracture one quarter of the way through. I limped the rest of the way and finished 8th. Before injuring my foot and joining the health club, my morning routine included yoga, situps, and push-ups for one hour to improve flexibility and strength. I did that for quite a few years."

"As a wholesale florist, I trim and collect forest products for use in the floral industry. I carry heavy bales on my back as I walk through the woods all day. After work, I train by running through woods because it doesn't do much good to train on roads. I run up and down hills, jump fences, and cross stones. About 80–90 percent of an orienteer's training should be done in the woods or on rough trails."

MENTAL ATTITUDE ABOUT HEALTH AND FITNESS

"I injured my neck when I was young," Judy said, "and I've had a problem with my spine. As a result, I've realized that I've had to keep myself strong. I also had to be strong to compete in the martial arts. I've always loved to train, and sports are like gravy on the top. Training has become part of my lifestyle, and, because I was fit, I've been able to do things that other people couldn't do."

"The mental aspect is 90 percent of any sport," Judy said. "My experience in orienteering is an example. During team trials, I competed against tall, lean women in their 20s who ran track in high school and college. They were fast with ideal runners' bodies, which I don't have. On a track or road, I wouldn't stand a chance running against them because I'm not fast. It's a different story in the woods. In orienteering, it doesn't matter how fast you run, you will never win if you don't have the mental abilities to handle navigation."

"Orienteers run through brush, jump over logs, run up and down mountains, and run over stony ground," Judy explained. "The fast runners lose their speed when they get into the woods, but it doesn't make any difference to me because I run through the woods at the same speed as in open terrain. I know where to put my feet, partly because I run through the woods after work and feel right at home. I'm not intimidated by brush, cold, rain, or heat, and I use adverse weather and course conditions to my advantage, especially when they bother my competitors. I tell myself, 'Boy, these things don't bother me. This is my day.' "

"People often get depressed during the long, dark winters in Scandinavia," Judy explained. "To combat this problem, researchers found that recreational exercise helps relieve depression. People who engage in sports like skiing and orienteering have high self-esteem and are not prone to alcoholism and depression. Scandinavian countries are big on sports, particularly winter sports and sports you can do for a lifetime. Each town has a big indoor swimming pool for everyone's use, not just for children and athletes. Cross-country skiing is popular. Ski trails are everywhere and people of all ages use them."

PERSONAL FITNESS GOALS

"I want to keep going as long as I can," Judy stated. "I think it's important to read about people who have been successful later in life. A good friend in town took up running when he was 70, and now he's 80. He runs a local 5K race in about 35 minutes, and by the time he finishes they are getting ready to start a 10K race. He goes right on to run the 10K in about 70 minutes. Enjoying sports at any age is like putting money in the bank. It's fun doing them when you are young, but 20 or 30 years down the road it will pay off with better health."

Recommendations for Improved Fitness of People over 40

"It's never too late to start improving your physical fitness," Judy advises. "I live with my mother who is 82 and a good example. About ten years ago she was told to go on a low cholesterol, low salt diet because she has high blood pressure. Besides following this diet, she has been walking since then, and she recently joined a health club to take up swimming. She swims about 45 minutes to an hour four to five days a week. As a result, she changed her appearance and she looks great, proving that it's never too late."

Damon Douglas

born: January 11, 1934
height: 5′ 9″
weight: 160
home: Greenwich, Connecticut

athletic highlights:

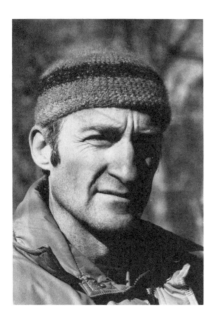

- completed Hawaiian Ironman in 1984
- tops in H55 (men's 55–59) orienteering
- won the U.S. Orienteering Championship for men over 50
- set record for the quickest traverse of the 34-peak Catskill Range, completing the peak-to-peak run in four days, ten hours, and some minutes
- won the Liberty-to-Liberty (Statue of Liberty to Liberty Bell) triathlon for his age group both times he entered
- finished second in the Karrimor International Mountain Marathon (about 50 miles) in Scotland
- won his age group every time in the Katterskil Spring Rush, completing nearly 80 miles in about seven hours via ski, run, bike, portage, and canoe

Damon Douglas is an athlete with many endurance achievements such as 100-mile mountain runs and "ironman" triathlons. He developed the stamina and fitness for these endeavors over a period of 12 years, beginning at a time when he was overweight and unfit. His perseverance in gradually improving his physical condition led to his ultimate success as an athlete.

Damon is modest about his accomplishments. "I have trouble thinking of myself as either a role model or a champion athlete," he said. "At age 34, I weighed 209 pounds (I'm 5′ 9″). I had gone through school and early adulthood avoiding all forms of exercise. Somehow I got hold of myself and lost five pounds each year for the next twelve years. I've done the Hawaiian Ironman and some hundred-mile mountain runs, but I only win when the competition doesn't show up."

COACH OF U.S. ORIENTEERING TEAM

Damon's athletic accomplishments in orienteering led to his appointment in 1987 as coach of the United States Orienteering Team. "It's mostly a mail order business because the team members live all over the United States," he explained. "I encourage the members to train; I produce light papers on bicycling, diet, using the track, and heart monitors; and, I monitor individual correspondence. The team is divided into levels; the top team has 5–10 men and 5–10 women, and a larger lower level brings the total number of members up to about 50."

"My main duties are to field teams in international competition. In 1989, we competed in Sweden. The men's relay team finished 16th out of 25, and the women's finished 19th out of 20. International orienteering has been discouraging to Americans because we're not good at it."

"Our problem is manyfold," Damon continued, "beginning with too few orienteers. The sport of orienteering does not fit our culture. For example, our land laws are different; we don't use land the way they do in Europe. Orienteering is also not the type of sport that Americans go for because members are not rewarded instantly and there's no spectator aspect. It's a funny kind of sport because nobody is allowed on the start line except the competitor. You see your competitor leaving for the start line, and the next time you see him he is popping out of the woods after punching the last control. Another factor is transportation. Our sites tend to be remote with only a few accessible by public transportation while a city like Stockholm has about 70 sites reachable by bus or tram. It's hard to generate the numbers of enthusiastic contestants that Europe has. We have fewer than 7,000 members in the United States Orienteering Federation (USOF), and we have about 9,000 people who orienteer in registered meets during the year. Sweden has about 140,000 orienteers in its eight million population."

"Most European countries support orienteering with training programs," Damon added. "Scandinavian and most Eastern European teams get an average of one week in training camp each month. The countries provide funds for transportation, room, and board. We fund ourselves when we try to have a training camp, and we have not been able to assemble everyone on our team. We do the best we can, but we don't have the people and money needed to put together a good training program. We see some team members at national meets, but, for example, I didn't have the time and money to go to the 1989 U.S. Championships in California. We encourage people to train in Europe, and I try to arrange training for our team members with Europeans at their clubs."

ATHLETIC HISTORY

"As a six-year-old child, I was quite a swimmer because our neighbors, who were good friends with my parents, allowed me to use their pool," Damon said. "Although I was swimming at a year-and-a-half, I never trained and was barely able to compete when I was 10 or 11. When I couldn't make the junior high school swimming team, I developed a tremendous distaste for athletics. I went through college avoiding anything related to athletics, taking the easiest physical training or the minimum possible."

"In 1968, at age 34," Damon said, "I was fed up with myself. My diet was horrible; I ate mostly cheese, hamburgers, and ice cream sodas. I started a conditioning program, and I kept a little diary in which I had written six reasons why I wanted to improve my health. These reasons included shortness of breath when I got up to give a speech (I was in sales at the time), drowsiness after lunch, being winded when I got to the top of one flight of stairs, and a bad physique, with my stomach hanging out over my clothes. When I would tire or allow my program to lag, I would read my diary and I'd get going again."

"I tried the Royal Canadian Air Force exercises for a couple months and banged up my back. They were horrible. Then, when I was in a store looking for something better, I saw Dr. Kenneth Cooper's first book, *Aerobics,* which had just come out. I bought a copy and started to exercise without a plan."

"I took the Cooper's self-administered physical fitness test," Damon continued, "and I was in the lowest category. Following his program, I tried running around a city block, and I could not get to the end of the block without stopping. I eventually ran around the block, then two blocks, and kept going, progressing at a slow rate."

Damon said he lost 60 pounds and never went on a diet. "I lost almost exactly five pounds a year for 12 years. It was steady and not planned. I cut cream out of my coffee as a first step, and I don't remember what I cut next — maybe sugar out of my coffee. I did a lot of little things like that, going a couple weeks and then cutting something else. I got down to 140 at one point, but my trim weight was around 148–150. For awhile, about 1984, I was almost one-hundred percent vegetarian while maintaining a low-fat diet. Throughout these years the transitions were gradual. I never made a sudden change."

"I continued to increase my running," Damon said, "and I entered my first race, a three-mile time-estimation race, in 1973. Two years later I ran my first marathon — the Niagara Marathon. Since then I've run many marathons, including the Boston Marathon a couple times. I moved on to ultras, longer distances like the JFK 50-miler and the 100-mile Wasatch mountain endurance run in the Wasatch Range in Utah."

"Along the way I picked up biking, which is by far my best sport. For example," Damon explained, "when I did the Hawaiian Ironman in 1985, I was 800th out of 1100 in the swim, 300th in the bike, and 600th in the run. I did poorly in my age group, which is tough because of the retirees. There are two classes of participants: those who work and those who are retired. The retirees cream those of us who have to work because it takes a lot of training for the Ironman."

"I've done longer, multi-day races," Damon said. "In 1980, my colleague, Marshall Childs, and I set a record for the quickest traverse of the Catskill 3500 in New York. Called peak-bagging, this event required us to cross under our own power all 34 Catskill Mountains with elevations over 3500 feet. We completed our peak-to-peak run in four days, ten hours, and 24 minutes, covering 135 horizontal miles and over 7 vertical miles during 70 of these 106 hours. Four of the peaks were untrailed so we had a lot of bushwhacking."

"I got into orienteering in 1974 when I responded to a notice in a newspaper. I founded a club in North Carolina and another in Western Connecticut when I moved back in 1982. I then got more involved as the sport is as big in western Connecticut as anywhere in the United States. I've done well; I won the U.S. championship in my over-50 age group, and there are four or five of us in my age group who can beat each other any day."

"I've done odd multi-event races like the Liberty-to-Liberty," Damon said. "You start at the tip of Manhatten Island near the Statue of Liberty, swim two-and-a-half miles across the Hudson River, bike

110 miles to Philadelphia, and then run a marathon in the city, finishing with a run up the 'Rocky steps' at the art museum and Liberty Bell. I entered the race twice in the 1980s and won my age group both times."

"Another interesting race," Damon reminisced, "was the New Zealand coast-to-coast. Starting at the Tasman Sea, we biked to the foothills of the Alps, ran up and over the Alps, kayaked down to the flats, and bicycled to the Pacific Ocean. About 220 kilometers long, the winners had times around 14 hours, and I was about 6 hours slower."

"An incident I observed at the beginning of the New Zealand race is an example of our competitive spirit. The race starts on the west coast where, it rains all the time as the winds pick up moisture crossing the Tasman Sea from Australia. As the wind hits the Alps and rises, it creates heavy rainfall, and few people live in the region. Because the race started before dawn with a short bicycle ride, we had to camp out. A few of us had rented small vans, but most people slept in tents. That night it poured; it was horrible, and the van shook back and forth. I slept, but I was conscious of the strong wind and heavy rain hitting the van. When I got up and went out in the morning, the camp appeared to have been devastated by an earthquake. Tents were knocked over, and I waded through water. Then I noticed movement in a collapsed tent. I saw the zipper open and a guy climb out wearing nothing but a t-shirt and shorts. With the rain pouring down on him, he saw me and smiled and said, 'Great day for a race!' "

Damon had done various long-distance races with partners, who are required for safety when staying out all night. In 1987, he and his son did the 65-mile 24-hour endurance race near Calgary, Canada. "That was a tough event," Damon said. "The Karrimor International Mountain Marathon in the fells of Scotland was another interesting orienteering race. My partner and I had to run with packs, which were required, while covering about 50 miles in two days. This race required a combination of navigational skills, mountaineering, and stamina. The finish was funny. My partner and I were the first veterans to finish, and my partner fell flat on his face in a mud puddle after crossing the finish line. Although we finished first, we placed second because some older guys won on their handicaps."

"Another interesting race I have always enjoyed and won in my age group is the Katterskil Spring Rush," Damon said. "The race starts with a short uphill run to your skis and is followed by 4 miles of downhill skiing, 15 miles of running, 50 miles of biking, a two-mile canoe portage, and 7 miles of canoeing white water to the finish. In 2 years of competition before going solo in 1984, my partner and I finished second and third in the open division. In my first solo race at age 50, I beat everyone over 30, outperformed 137 two-man teams, and finished fifth overall with a time of seven hours and two minutes."

"I have done many different kinds of events," Damon concluded. "I've raced with canoes, snowshoes, and skis, both cross-country and downhill, and I've competed in small local races that combine canoe, bike, swim, and run events. I claim to have raced in every self-powered sport but speed skating."

FITNESS REGIMEN

"I have backed off on exercising quite a bit since I started coaching," Damon said. "Coaching, which I find enjoyable, takes some time, and about all I do for fitness is run. I go to bed around 10:00, and I get up at 5:25 weekday mornings to run before work. I like to run at the track twice a week, once for what I call my turbo run and once for sprints. My turbo run consists of 20 minutes at my 5K or 10K race pace, which is an eight-minute mile. I would like to run at seven, and I used to run at six. I'm slowing down fast. My sprint session consists of quarter or half miles at a seven-mile-a-minute or better pace. Weekdays when I don't go to the track I run four miles at an easy eight-and-a-half-minute pace."

"I worked behind a desk at IBM for 23 years and couldn't take it any more," Damon said as he explained his current employment as a surveyor. "Working as a surveyor complements orienteering because it has made me more agile and comfortable in the woods and it has improved my map sense. As a result, I can beat faster runners in my age group."

Damon said orienteering meets are seldom canceled, and he looks forward to 10K orienteering events almost every weekend. His wife, who is athletic but not competitive, participates as well. "Orienteering is good in that respect as we both go," he said, "and it's an individual sport when we get there."

"In a recent two-day orienteering meet, I ran all the way on Saturday, which is really good," Damon said. "I ran up steep hills and, because of my experience, pushed it down over rocks. Many people can't run across rocks and don't have the stamina to push it up hills. On Sunday, I followed my perfect Saturday run with a perfect start, finding the first three controls, which were difficult. The fourth control was a cinch and I blew it, so I stood around trying to figure out where

I was. It's hard to navigate at high speed, but I can read the map while running. I may have to slow down, but I read on trails where the terrain is good or while going up hill in a crouched position."

"As for diet," Damon explained, "I watch the fat, particularly if I'm training for an event. After my morning run, I drink carrot juice, take vitamins C and E, and eat boiled whole oat grain with yeast. I think the value of oxidants is important. Carrot juice has made a big difference in my ability to recover from stress. I eat some sweets, but not much except for an occasional binge when I eat half a cake. I have to watch my cholesterol because my family has a history of heart problems and high cholesterol. I have high cholesterol even with my exercise and my low fat diet, but my HDL stays very good."

MENTAL ATTITUDE ABOUT HEALTH AND FITNESS

"Of the Several Tongues of Mountain Feet," an article describing the record-setting peak-to-peak Catskill 3500 run of Childs and Douglas, was printed in the *Woodstock Times* on August 28, 1980. In response to the writer's comment about "seeing more of nature by walking," Damon wrote to explain why he runs in the mountains. Excerpts from his letter, which appeared in the November 26, 1980, issue of *Woodstock Times,* provide insight to Damon's thoughts of fitness, nature, and pleasure.

> [I wonder] why I run through the mountains when others walk to "relax and contemplate the natural beauty."
>
> Running gives me a choice; I can rest, walk or run. Even under the most competitive conditions, there's always time to pause. At one point in our Catskill Mountain record-setting run, rather than break a shimmering spider web, glistening with dew backlit by the morning sun, Marshall checked his speed so abruptly that I ran up on his heels. We concluded that such a work of art should be allowed to live on and cautiously detoured around through the woods. There's always time to pause and admire, and even while running, musing comes easy.
>
> Would we have seen that spider's web, or the bear, if we hadn't been running — covering two to three times the distance of the fast walker? Volume doesn't count much with me in and of itself, but volume means greater chance of exploring the fringes of the mountain universe. I don't think I will ever see my fill of fungi; each one is an individual. At our speed, how many more of these heavenly creations do we have the good fortune to admire.

The crux of mountain running for me seems to boil down to enhanced awareness — awareness of myself and my environment. Awareness of self is on many levels from the very physical concern for an embryonic blister on the right big toe to perceptions of where I fit in the scheme of things. If you run all day in the mountains you must pay attention to your body — feel your heart beat, listen to the calves and thigh, watch the color and smell your urine. The body responds — the swish of blood coursing through the arteries, the laughter of legs powering up the Devil's Trail from the Tombstone. The body demands good food, and I see that it gets it. The care of the physical body seems to blend continuously into care of the mind. Mountain running seems to clear my head of self-deception and bring acceptance of the real person I am.

Awareness of self leads to awareness of environment. The exertion of mountain running tunes up all my receivers. How to describe the sound of the silence of the woods, the sight of the trillium patch on the way up to Doubletop from Graham, the taste of the wayward insect, the feel of light drizzling rain. But if I had to pick one reason why I run it would probably be because of my nose. It must be that the high oxygen demand turns the nose on to full power. At my desk I ache for the smell of moldering leaves, of lichened rocks, of mountain water. Imagine running along the trail from Overlook to Devil's Kitchen. The charge up from Mead's has filled your blood with ketones so your head is already floating a dozen feet above your body. Just enough rocks on the trail to keep your concentration sharp, but the running is easy and all the pieces are in place. You turn a corner and blam, your eyes are blinded by a blaze of rhododendron and your nose explodes. You veer to let overhanging branches whip your face and shoulders with magic dew. How far is nirvana?

What's it like when a day of running ends and I come down out of the mountains? Though my thighs are not always able to lift the foot high enough to avoid stubbing that right big toe, I am strong. With my limbs caked with mud and my clothes soaked with sweat, I am clean. Though fatigue pulses through every nerve, I am whole. And as to living longer? My birth certificate shows that I've been around for 46 years, but the mountains and I are eternal. We will visit together as often as I can manage. And one peaceful day, I will return home forever.

PERSONAL FITNESS GOALS

"I'm bothered by the fact that I never seem to have goals," Damon lamented. "I really don't have any. When I retire in about ten years, I want to do the Hawaiian Ironman again, and I'd like to do a trail race in Tennessee. I don't operate by setting goals, and that bothers me because I think it's a mistake. I keep going, so the mistake isn't bad. In a way, I have vague goals to keep improving and keep going."

RECOMMENDATIONS FOR IMPROVED FITNESS OF PEOPLE OVER 40

Damon said his advice is really thought out and important for people to understand.

GO SLOWER AND FARTHER THAN YOU THINK YOU CAN

"Go much slower than you think you can," Damon recommends. "I think it's disastrous for people to start an exercise program and go at it too hard. They are apt to come back in a couple months with a sprained this or a dislocated that and be out of it."

"Likewise," Damon advises, "go much farther than you think you can. It's a long run, and people stop before they should. Just about anybody can do the Hawaiian Triathlon if they want to, and they could do it with steady progress."

"I offer the following conflicting advice to all who will listen:

1. Do much less than you think you can. Take it easy. Give all your body parts — muscles, tendons, cardiovascular system — a chance to develop in harmony with each other. Raise your work load very slowly. Think in long terms, like years and decades.

2. Do much more than you ever thought you could. Keep on making the small incremental gains. It sounds like compounding interest. Repeated small percentage gains over time add up to huge differences in the long term."

"My last recommendation," Damon advises. "is to perform with some group. It's people help. I belonged to a bicycle club, but the only groups I have now are the orienteering groups, which is why I do that most. If a running club was handy, I would probably do that more. I thought of retiring and forming a retirees athletic club, a local club for older people. The bicycle club has a 'great years division' for older people who want to race but can't keep up with younger people."

"Orienteering is fun," Damon said. "I wish more people could enjoy it. Those of us who are 'gung ho' should do more to encourage others. We should encourage people who want to improve their navigational skills and to have a nice day in the woods. I teach a clinic for beginners at orienteering meets, which are held on weekends. It's great to see the older people come out, and I try to orient the clinic so they can enjoy the sport without feeling they have to bang through the woods."

"There's a masters world orienteering championship every other year," Damon added, "and it has five-year age groups which allow for all competitors. You ought to see these 85-year-olds when they cross the line. Boy, they look good!"

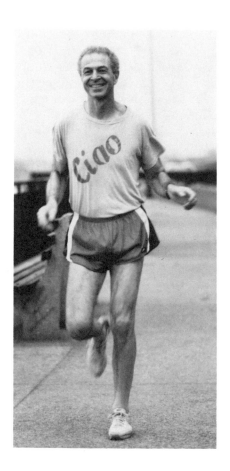

George Hirsch

born: June 21, 1934
height: 6′ 1″
weight: 155
home: New York City, New York

athletic highlights:

- competes in mid- to long-distance events, finishes strong, and wins some age group races
- ran a 2:38 Boston Marathon at age 44
- won the over-50 age group with a 2:59.52 time in the 1989 San Francisco marathon

Although he describes himself as a "middle-of-the-road runner," George A. Hirsch does not challenge traffic in both directions. Proud of his accomplishments, which include strong finishes and occasional wins in his age group distance races, he is realistic in comparing himself with others."

I was never real good," George said in describing his running. This modesty may stem from realism gained in his position as publisher of *Runners' World,* an enviable combination of profession and favorite pastime resulting in familiarity with world-class runners. Besides featuring outstanding runners in his magazine, George has run in races with the world's best marathoners and mid-distance runners, and he includes many of them in his circle of friends.

George, according to acquaintances who descibed him, was a tough "screw-the-weather" fanatic who used to run regardless of the weather. They said he is a "horrible trainer runner, but put a number on his back and he becomes an animal."

George said he was not a great athlete when growing up in New Rochelle, New York, and he was unspectacular in team sports. After graduating from Princeton, where he was a quarter-miler, and Harvard Business School, he served with the United States Navy in Italy. After a brief naval career, he worked for Time-Life International, traveled a great deal, and started magazines in Japan and Argentina.

George returned to New York and settled into the publishing business in 1967, starting and publishing the *New York Magazine,* the nation's first city weekly. His second venture, *New Times,* gave underground writers a mainstream forum from 1973 through 1979. A year before *New Times* folded, George turned his fervor for running into a third successful publication, *The Runner,* which lasted until it was absorbed in 1987 by its competitor, *Runners' World,* with George as publisher.

Those who know George have used a variety of words that provide an interesting portrayal. He's said to be optimistic and enthusiastic, never bored, and psyched every day of his life. Always delighted and never complaining, he lives in the present, likes to focus on objectives, and doesn't give up easily. Intense, organized, thoughtful, professional, stable, sensible, sane, tough, and caring complete the portrait except for one thing — he likes to cross the finish line.

ATHLETIC HISTORY

George Hirsch is a sports enthusiast who as a youth tried to find an athletic activity for which he was well suited. He could run well but he was never good enough to fulfill his needs. "I never played sports," he said, "but I tried everything. I was never a gifted athlete."

George found it difficult to do well in sports like basketball and tennis. "I shot baskets until long after dark hoping that lightning would strike," he explained, "but I was cut from the basketball team the first day I tried out as a freshman."

"I haven't had a whole lot of achievements," George said, "but athletics has provided good fun and good health. I jump into lots of races in New York or Central Park or wherever I happen to be traveling. I'm relatively strong, winning or finishing high in local age group races, but I'm not a real champion in my age group nor a factor in a big masters-type event. My 1989 performance was good, highlighted by winning the over-50 age group in the San Francisco marathon. My time was 2:59.52. I ran about 20–25 races, which is more than in recent years, and they included three marathons and middle distance runs such as 5K, 10K, and 10 mile. I ran a few 10Ks in the 38s, but I've run faster."

George said he ran the 440-yard dash and the 880 in high school. "I ran the quarter (440-yard dash) in about 52 seconds and I never broke 2 minutes in the half-mile. I ran in college, at Princeton, with similar unimpressive results."

As a naval officer stationed for three years in Italy, George did nothing to stay fit, he said. After leaving the navy, he ran a little while attending Harvard Business School.

By the time he was working days, nights, and weekends founding *New York Magazine,* George was out of shape and his weight was up to 175 or 180, 25 pounds more than it is now. Needing exercise, he resumed running in 1967 and soon found recreational and competitive enjoyment.

At first, George said he had difficulty running any distance. Nevertheless, he set the Boston Marathon as a goal, and he began by running around the block for about five minutes. His objective was to complete the race, which he did in 1969 with a time of 3:26. "That made me a long-distance runner," he stated.

George's next goal was to run the Boston Marathon in less than three hours. "I was much better prepared in 1970 and ran it in 2:54. I trained hard, mostly running with no real speed work or track workouts. The training formula that works best for me is a mix of easy running and moderately hard steady running. I'm in favor of track work for others, but not for me, partly because there aren't many tracks in New York City. I often run in Central Park, which is my country club." Nearby is his East Side triplex home which has a workout room with a sauna and shower on the lower level.

At age 44, George enjoyed his best year as a marathoner, running several races and achieving a personal best of 2:38 in the Boston Marathon. During that race, he remembers running 16 to 17 miles with Joanie Benoit, until she gradually pulled ahead and won the women's race.

Fitness Regimen

In describing his diet, George said, "I'm more conscious of nutrition now than five years ago, and my cholesterol is down over 100 points through diet and exercise. I can now enjoy excesses, but not every day. I used to eat ice cream every night, and I now restrict bagels and cream cheese to weekends. I eat meat less frequently, buy skim or 1% milk, and drink a few beers, but not a lot. I have had a bunch of shifts in my diet, nudging a handfull of things in the right direction and not being hard on myself."

"I try to run five or six days a week, mostly in Central Park, and I compete a fair amount. My work requires a lot of travel, and I am always jumping into races which I look for and find wherever I happen to be. I run in some races for fun and I train for others. I like the feeling that I worked hard, and I also like the lower end of an age group. For example, at 54 in the 50s age group, you have to monkey around with the frisky 50-year-olds."

George said he experienced a back problem in late 1989, and he began treating it with rest and exercise. He took time off from competition and started doing daily exercises such as bent leg situps that are designed to help alleviate back problems.

Mental Attitude about Health and Fitness

George's attitude has changed since he began running more than 20 years ago. Thinking about significant changes, he said, "I've become very conscious of fitness and health, especially my diet. But I'm not flawless; I have too many milkshakes and that sort of thing. I'm quite knowledgeable about nutrition, which I take seriously. If I overindulge, I don't overdo it day after day after day."

With his increasing age and experience, George has become more casual about his running because he knows he's a runner for life. "If I want to swim or bike or go to a movie today, that's fine; the long haul is what counts," according to George.

George continued to expound on his beliefs. "I don't care if you're Bill Rodgers or an accountant living in Pittsburgh, you can't keep improving (as you age) and you begin to put it in perspective. You wonder if it's worth training hard for 16 weeks and putting all other things in a secondary position in order to run a marathon two minutes faster."

Conversely, George points out, "You can stay fit if you run three or four times a week, three or four miles at a pop. We were all running beyond fitness, and it wasn't necessary."

PERSONAL FITNESS GOALS

George said his fitness goal is "to slow down as gradually as possible, year after year."

His plans for 1990 include less running, partly because he began the year with a lower back problem that lessened the amount of running he could do. He was also a year older, and younger guys coming along in his age group would make it more difficult to be competitive. "You have to do it early in your age group if you're going to do well," George said. "I will certainly look for some fun races."

RECOMMENDATIONS FOR IMPROVED FITNESS OF PEOPLE OVER 40

"To quote NIKE, 'Just Do It,' day after day," George recommends.

He advises developing a simple, uncomplicated fitness program with realistic goals. The program should include exercise 5 to 6 days a week, even when traveling and during periods of heavy schedules and stressful situations, and the goals should be readjusted often to keep them doable. He suggests setting time goals or goals within an age group.

Bob Mathias

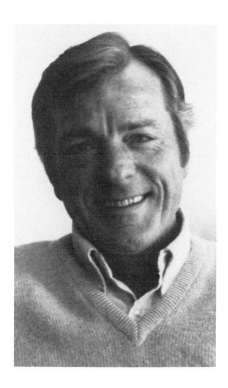

born: November 17, 1930
height: 6′ 4″
weight: 220
home: Fresno, California
athletic highlights:
- won the decathlon in the 1948 Olympics in London and in the 1952 Olympics in Helsinki
- played halfback on Stanford's league championship and Rose Bowl football team
- received AAU's Sullivan Award as the Outstanding Amateur Athlete of the Year
- elected to the National Track and Field Hall of Fame in 1974
- elected to the San Francisco Bay Area Hall of Fame in 1980
- became a charter member of the U.S. Olympic Committee's Hall of Fame in 1983

In 1948, Robert Bruce Mathias, a 17-year-old fresh out of high school in Tulare, California, won the decathlon in London to become a national hero and the youngest person to win an Olympic track-and-field event. Four years later in Helsinki, Bob repeated his decathlon victory as he won the event by the largest margin in Olympic history.

Bob was interested in trying out for the 1956 Olympics, but he was declared a professional and therefore ineligible because he made a 1953 motion picture called "The Bob Mathias Story." His 10th and final decathlon competition was in the 1955 All-Service Meet. At the time, Bob was a captain in the Marine Corps, and he was talked into competing. He trained to win and he did, concluding a fabulous undefeated decathlon career.

Bob's success and fame led to his becoming the first athlete to make goodwill trips for the State Department. As a goodwill ambassador, he visited towns and villages in more than 48 countries to talk to school kids and give clinics and demonstrations. He became a friend of presidents and an acquaintance of world leaders, a four-term U.S. Congressman from California, the first director of the U.S. Olympic Training Center in Colorado Springs, and the executive director of the National Fitness Foundation.

When asked how difficult it was for him to handle the transition from a 17-year-old high school student to a star, Bob replied, "Well, I don't think it was difficult. My coach would tell me to take one event at a time. I was surprised at the outcome of the 1948 games. I certainly didn't expect to win the Olympic decathlon. When I returned home with my first gold medal, there were parades in my honor, and I had to give talks and speeches — things I didn't like to do because I'm a shy guy. I've been giving a lot of talks and speeches ever since. If you put it into perspective, every day is a new day and a challenge. I always thought that was fun to do and I did it, but what am I going to do tomorrow?"

Bob handled his fame well because as a youth he had learned from his family the need to understand and be compassionate with all people. The family backyard, which had a hurdle, shot and discus pit, parallel bars, and high jump rig, was a neighborhood playground and a learning center for Bob, his two brothers, and his younger sister.

ATHLETIC HISTORY

"In high school, I was a three-sport athlete," Bob said. "I played football, basketball, and track for four years, which kept me in shape because I was always doing something. Then, two months out of high school, I won my first decathlon. It was a tremendous experience for a 17-year-old, and it happened at a fast and furious pace over a three-month period."

Bob's track coach, Virgil Jackson, heard that the decathlon, which consists of ten events held over a two-day period, would be included in a Los Angeles track-and-field meet the week after Tulare's high school graduation. Coach Jackson wasn't sure what the ten events were, but he thought the competition would give Bob something to do after graduation.

Bob began his track career as a freshman at Tulare High School. He threw the shot and discus because his older brother, Gene, had competed in those events. In his sophomore year, he began running the hurdles because he thought it was fun. By the time he was a senior, he was also high jumping and running the relays, and he had long-jumped once.

Natural athletic ability and some experience were positive factors for Bob. On the negative side, Bob had no experience in half the events, the school did not have a javelin, and rules were different at the national and international level. For example, the shot weighed 16 pounds instead of 12, and the hurdles were 42 inches high instead of 39. To help resolve these differences, Bob's dad bought a javelin for him, and three-inch hurdle extensions were made in the school's craft shop.

A rule violation in the 1948 Olympics caused Bob to lose a 45-foot put when he was disqualified for leaving the shot put circle from the front. "Coach Jackson and I didn't know about the international rule," Bob said. "and my Olympic coach didn't tell me about it. I guess he assumed I would know something like that. I had good basic training, but there were a lot of things I didn't know."

"During those couple months prior to the 1948 Olympics," Bob explained, "it was track season, and Coach Jackson taught me the basics of the ten decathlon events. I had done the long jump, high jump, high hurdles, discus, and shot, so we had to work on the running events, javelin, and pole vault. Coach and I would stay an hour-and-a-half or two after the regular afternoon track session to work on the events I hadn't done before. In those days, nobody knew anything about weight training, special diets, and other fitness-related things. Weight-lifting was off limits because coaches believed it hindered athletes by making them muscle-bound, and decathlon training excluded the 1500 meters so that it would not hinder development of the other events. We were supposed to perform well in the first nine events and gut it out in the 1500 meters. There wasn't the kind of coaching and training then that there is now, but we worked hard and I was fortunate to have a good coach who knew the basics in all the track-and field-events. In fact, my teammate, Sim Iness, won the discus in Helsinki in 1952, and he learned his basics from Coach Jackson, who was a heck of a good coach."

The week after graduation from high school, Bob won the decathlon at the Pasadena Games. A few days later, Coach Jackson told him about the national track-and-field meet, which also served as the Olympic trials, and they decided to go when the Amateur Athletic Union agreed to pay their expenses. Three weeks after his first decathlon win, Bob went to Bloomfield, New Jersey, where he won the national event and a berth on the Olympic Team. Three weeks later he won the Olympic gold.

"I wasn't used to major competition," Bob said, "and I didn't know who my competition was. If I had known, I probably would have been scared to death. There wasn't any television then, and I didn't know a thing about foreign athletes. Most athletes had only one decathlon to compete in each year, and it was hard to get news about that one."

"I was too young to be intimidated," Bob said, "but support from spectators helped in the high jump when I missed the bar twice at a low height. If I had missed a third time, I wouldn't have had any points, and that would have put me out of contention. Part of the crowd, evidently some Californians on a tour, started hollering, 'C'mon Bob, c'mon Tulare' when I was getting ready for my third try. When I stopped and waved at them, I forgot how nervous I was. I made the jump and went on to get more points by making higher jumps."

"A similar thing happened to me in the 1952 Olympics," Bob added. "My first two javelin throws were lousy. Before my last throw, Jack Weiershauser, my track coach at Stanford, and some American fans started to chant, 'Oh Bob, hey you, don't forget to follow through.' This support helped, and I had a good throw. I think the knowledge that someone was rooting for me helped me relax. Being down on the field all day, I would tend to forget things and get tense. By taking my time and waving at people in the stands, I would relax and perform better by doing what they told me to do — follow through. My brother Gene also helped me relax by coming down from the stands and sneaking onto the track to talk with me during waits of two or three hours between the jumps and pole vault."

"After the 1948 Olympics," Bob said, "I went to prep school and then Stanford. My track coach at Stanford was a low hurdler who knew nothing about the weights and the jumps, so I had to get outside coaching to help with those events. I ran the hurdles, pole vaulted, and threw the shot and discus for Stanford. Sometimes I high jumped and ran relays. When the school term ended in June each year, I trained for and won the AAU National decathlon."

"Decathlon competitions were few and far between," Bob said. "The AAU, which was the governing body for just about everything, had one national decathlon a year. In 1949, I competed in our national meet, and then I competed in a meet in Switzerland. I had two decathlon competitions that year, and the next year I had only one. Overall, I competed in ten decathlons and won them all."

Bob wanted to play football in college because that was his best high school sport, but as a freshman in 1949, he was too busy traveling and making personal appearances. He played running back the next two years and helped his team win the league title and a place in the Rose Bowl. Despite his success in football, he did not play as a senior because he chose to train for the 1952 Olympics, where he improved his marks in all ten events.

FITNESS REGIMEN

"My main exercise is tennis," Bob said. "I tried golf, but it wasn't enough exercise for me. I started playing tennis when I was working in the motion picture industry in Los Angeles. I needed exercise because it makes me feel better, and I chose tennis, which I think is the best way to stay fit. I love tennis, and I play singles and doubles, whatever match I can get, at least once a week."

"I love doing manual labor for exercise," Bob stated. "I have property in the mountains about an hour from Fresno, and I have done a lot of physical work up there during the last couple years. Today, I worked about nine hours clearing brush, driving a tractor, and hiking."

"As for other exercise," Bob continued, "I've always walked a lot, especially in cities during my travels. I have never liked jogging because it was part of my training and it seems like work to me. In addition to walking and tennis, I played racquetball for the seven years when I was director of the Olympic Training Center."

"I have no special diet," Bob said, "and I've never been overweight as I try to keep my weight down. I eat less these days although I have a wife who's a helluva good cook. We eat low cholesterol food, and my recent cholesterol count was 207."

MENTAL ATTITUDE ABOUT HEALTH AND FITNESS

"I need lots of exercise, and I don't need much food," Bob said. "I have to exercise regularly, be selective in my foods, and eat in moderation."

"I believe people should do whatever they want to do that's fun for them," Bob stated. "I think the activity I enjoyed most was running the boys and girls camp in the mountains near the property I now own. Beginning with a boys camp in 1962, I had the camp about sixteen years until I sold it. It was a private summer camp with sports and camping events for kids 8 to 15 years old. If they were there four, six, or eight weeks, you could see their progress. I really enjoyed them."

Bob sold the summer camp after he was appointed director of the Olympic Training Center. While serving seven years as director, he enjoyed seeing young adults develop their athletic skills.

"I gained a lot of good experience seeing the athletes progress even though I wasn't a coach or actively involved in the coaching," Bob said. "Each team brought in its own coach. I got to know the girls on the 1980 womens' volleyball team during their two-and-a-half year stay at the Training Center, and I saw their disappointment when they didn't go to Moscow because of the 1980 boycott."

"The Olympic Training Center is a great idea," Bob continued. "It's not a place for Olympic athletes but a place for potential Olympic athletes. Olympic athletes are older and out of college; they have their own coaches, and they don't go to Colorado Springs to train. The Training Center is for the high school champions and other such athletes whose skills are almost at the national level. It's a great idea because the athletes get together and develop the Olympic spirit while meeting people from other sports. I think this charges them up and makes them work harder. They don't stay at the Training Center year round; they might go for one, two, or three weeks. While there, the best coach in the United States will coach them, and that superb coaching will rub off onto others when they return home. It's a great learning experience. People are continuously coming and going. When I left after seven years, 10,000 athletes had trained at the Olympic Training Center, and that's a lot of people. I don't know the number of Training Center athletes who went on to become Olympians, but I'm sure a lot of them did."

"I've been to every Olympics since 1948 except Moscow," Bob stated. "I love them. That's my hobby, and I want to go to Barcelona in 1992. I do a lot of public relations work to promote the Olympics, I get involved with the United States Olympic Committee in all kinds of fund raising activities, I'm on one of the Committee's advisory boards, and I get involved in any decathlon activity. I'm also on a local committee in Fresno, which will host the national junior track-and-field championships in 1990."

Personal Fitness Goals

"My fitness goals are to maintain my weight, keep my muscle tone, and eat well in moderation so that I feel good," Bob said. "Other than that, I don't have specific fitness goals or a regular regimen, but I know when I feel good."

Recommendations for Improved Fitness of People over 40

"My recommendation for anyone over 40 is to find an exercise that is fun to do and then do it consistently," Bob said. "My wife tried aerobics classes and quit. She got the Jane Fonda tape and exercised at home until that got boring. Now she plays lots of tennis, which she enjoys, and she is in great shape. People should have fun exercising, whether it's walking around the block, playing tennis or racquetball, or doing whatever is convenient. In the long run, people have to enjoy what they are doing because it's hard to do something like aerobics every week if it's not enjoyable. The average person should enjoy whatever exercise he or she does. Joggers and runners enjoy their sports, and I think that's great."

Pat McCormick

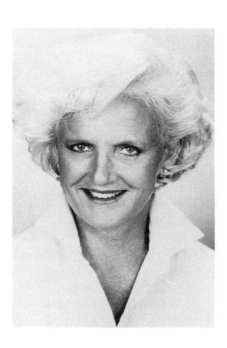

born: May 12, 1930
height: 5′ 4″
weight: 130
home: Seal Beach, California
athletic highlights:

- won four Olympic gold medals in 3-meter springboard and 10-meter platform diving — two in the 1952 Helsinki, Finland games and two in the 1956 Melbourne, Australia games
- won 27 national diving championships
- member of the United States Olympic Hall of Fame
- awarded the James E. Sullivan Memorial Trophy in 1956
- won the Babe Zaharias Trophy and the Thurman Munson Award

"Do something for your community," Patricia McCormick stated while talking about things adults should do to improve their health and fitness. "I think that's what life is all about. We should all try to make life a little better by helping another person or an animal or our environment. Helping everyone and everything is too much for our government to do, and individuals have to pitch in to do what they can."

Like other former Olympians, Pat has worked to support the Olympic spirit and athletes in the United States. As a volunteer member of the 1984 Los Angeles Olympic Organizing Committee, she used her life story as a motivational speech. After the Olympics, she developed her story into an inspirational program which she presents to business groups and students of all ages.

"I'm often on the road speaking to kindergartens, colleges, and businesses," Pat said, "and I love what I'm doing. I have a good program for kids. I go through the process of what it takes to be a winner. I identify with their self-esteem and self-confidence, which is important to fight drugs. I show films, the Olympic flag, Olympic torch, Olympic gold medal, and I tell stories. When I'm working with the little kids, I get them involved in my program by playing Olympic games. My program for corporations carries the same message, but I tailor my speech to meet their needs."

ATHLETIC HISTORY

"I have always been athletic," Pat said. "I love to ride horses, I body surfed as a little girl, I played football with my brothers, and I participated in kicking and throwing contests. I have done quite a bit of swimming, and the swim team occasionally drafted me. I swam well in AAU events of 50 yards."

"I started diving seriously at age 14," Pat explained. "Someone happened to see me diving at Alamitos Bay, near Long Beach, and asked me to go up to the Los Angeles Athletic Club to try out for the diving team. I made the team and got to watch Sammy Lee and Vicki Draves, two great divers who trained at the Club. That's when my dream started."

Pat said there was no diving facility at her school, Wilson High School in Long Beach, and she didn't go to college after graduating from high school. Her goal was to make the 1948 Olympic team.

"As with any beginner," she explained, "I started training about twice a week. As I progressed from next-to-last finishes to next-to-next-to-last, I built my training up to about six days a week and about four hours a day. During a heavy schedule, I'd be in the water 8 to 12 hours a day. It's no secret that anything worth doing takes a lot of effort."

"After training hard for the 1948 Olympic team, I missed making it by one-hundredth of a point," she exclaimed. "That failure motivated me to do something no one had done before. Standing there crying, I decided I wanted to go to the next two Olympics and win four gold medals. The next day I started working toward my goal, and I worked for it every day until I accomplished it. Greg Louganis recently tied my record with four gold medals, but I'm the first person and the only woman to do this, which is fine."

Pat married diving coach Glenn McCormick before the 1952 Olympics and gave birth to their first child eight months before the 1956 games in Melbourne. She trained throughout her pregnancy, swimming a half-mile a day up until two days before her son was born.

After winning two gold medals in 3-meter springboard diving and two gold medals in 10-meter platform diving, Pat retired from competitive diving and went to college. "I wanted to finish my family, and there was no reason to continue diving. At that time, there wasn't the money in sports there is now, there wasn't much competition for women, and there weren't many scholarships available. I wanted to get back to school, so I went to City College and then to Long Beach State, where I graduated."

During a seven-year period from age 19 to 26, Pat said she lost only once while winning 27 national diving championships (Amateur Athletic Union) and 3 Pan American titles.

After retiring from diving, Pat gave birth to her daughter, Kelly, who won a silver medal in the 1984 Olympics and has continued to compete. "I don't go to many meets to watch Kelly," her mother said. "I bowed out of that when Kelly decided to go into diving because I realized people would make comparisons between us. Kelly and I became the only mother-daughter in Olympic history, and it was brutal for a little while until we learned to handle it. The only time I go to a meet is when Kelly calls and says, 'Mom, I want you there.' She usually invites me to national meets and the Olympic games and trials, and I sit way up at the top of the stands and cry like all the mothers do. I have always emphasized to Kelly that the medals are only measures, and how you get there is what counts. She's comfortable with that."

FITNESS REGIMEN

"Being fit is probably one of the most important parts of my life as an athlete," Pat stated. "I swim most every day, lift weights, do stretching and isolated exercises, and do walk-jog. Actually, I have two forms of workout to keep me in shape. When I'm real busy and on the road, I try to do one of them. The first one is swimming. The second, which I can always do, includes walk-jog, isolated exercises, and stretching. For fun, I love to ski, body surf, and scuba, and I have a wonderful quarter horse that I ride three or four times a week. I also play golf; I was on the amateur circuit for a while, and I got to be quite a good golfer. With these sports I'm competing against myself. Sports like tennis require a good partner, otherwise it's frustrating to play."

In describing a typical day, Pat said, "Two of every three mornings I am in my pool at 6:45 where I swim until 7:30. Then, I work with weights until 8:45. After that I do stretching and isolated exercises, walk-jog my dog around the pier, and get dressed for work at 10:30. I ride my horse in the evening."

MENTAL ATTITUDE ABOUT HEALTH AND FITNESS

"I feel very, very grateful that I have the health to do the quality things that I want to do in life," Pat stressed as she explained her mental attitude about fitness.

"Quality years are important," Pat added. "Isn't it amazing how times have changed? Long ago when a person got to be my age, that was about it, health-wise, due to deterioration from disease and ailments."

"I think adults who avoid exercise get in the habit of not doing anything," Pat commented. "When I was in Spain for six weeks, I walked every day and swam when I could. But, I thought, 'Gosh, you could get out of the habit of exercising,' and when I came home I had to say, 'This week I'm going to start with my weights.' I thought, 'What if the average person doesn't know you have to get sore and it's a pain in the kazoo to get up early for about four days? But, after four days, you start feeling better, you're proud when you do, and then exercising gets easier.' "

Pat said, "These adults need role models to tell them that if you do this, you've got the whole world by the tail. This helps them perform better."

"Recently," Pat recalled, "there was a good segment on TV about older people, and it showed that really old people can get in good shape. It got into scientific things like oxygen in the bloodstream. It showed people in convalescent homes who were on exercise programs, and it showed how much better they felt and how they were building their muscles. That's what fitness is all about. Isn't it neat what can be done and what is being done?"

PERSONAL FITNESS GOALS

"Good health is one of my motivations," Pat said. "In addition to feeling good, I would like to squeeze another 30 years out of my life, and I can do it only by keeping fit."

In her motivational program, Pat tries to change attitudes. She believes the greatest dream in the world is the highest goal, and she teaches people the following five-step process to reach it:

1. Have a dream
2. Work
3. Don't be afraid to fail
4. Surround yourself with greatness, a loved one, a coach, or a hero
5. Continue stepping up from the victory stand

RECOMMENDATION FOR IMPROVED FITNESS OF ADULTS OVER 40

Pat's fitness advice for adults over 40:

1. Work out 1 to 2 hours a day
2. Stay involved in some sort of work
3. Do something for your community; give something back
4. Work with kids in some capacity

"The key word is consistency," Pat stated. "Older people who want to improve their fitness don't have to be fancy. They don't have to lift weights. They don't have to swim. They don't have to walk. But, they have to do one or two of these exercises. Whatever they decide that fits into their ability and their frame of mind, they've got to set up a routine to do it almost every day. If they choose walking or swimming, they should add a fun sport, too, whether its shuffleball or shuffleboard or tennis. There are no restrictions. Enjoyment and consistency are the keys."

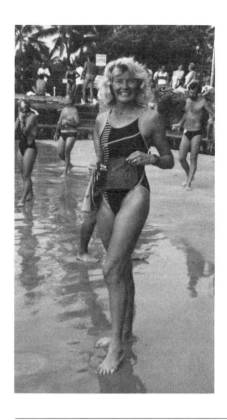

Marion Mehrtash

born: May 14, 1941
height: 5′ 7.5″
weight: 133–136
home: Gardena, California
athletic highlights:

- completed the Hawaiian Iron-man Triathlon in 1986, '87, and '89
- won medals in marathon and triathlon competition, mostly seconds and thirds in age group
- finished first in age group in all three Los Angeles Triathlon events

Marion Mehrtash took up sport in her early 40s, not to become fit but to make friends. At 44, she became a serious competitor as she began training for marathons and triathlons. Although she trains hard and competes to win or be among the top three finishers in her age group, she enjoys the social aspects of sport and the beauty of nature. Her sport provides pleasure and happiness during the transitional middle years of her life.

"The sport of triathlon makes me feel free, like the ocean is mine and the next 26 miles are mine," Marion said with emotion emphasizing every word. "The Hawaiian Ironman is perfect for me. I awaken in the morning and do nothing but sport until nighttime. There's a lot of socializing going on and it's fun. I meet many great people and international people. When I see people walking during the 26-mile run, I encourage them to keep going. 'Hey, come on!' I call to them. 'You've run 21 miles already, you can do five more. What's the big deal about it? C'mon, move it!' I get to know these people by talking to them. Maybe I lose five minutes and maybe I lose a medal, but maybe my encouragement got another person to the end of the road. I think the greatest feeling in doing any sport comes from making somebody achieve more than they thought they could. I see many newcomers who are where I once was, worrying about finishing the race, but I did and they will."

"You have to take the good with the bad," Marion philosophized. "Swimming has always been the hardest part of the triathlon for me. After learning to swim through the big waves, I went through a period when I was getting seasick. In a two-mile swim from pier-to-pier, I was one mile into the swim when I started to throw up. By the time I approached the second pier, I was at the two-hour mark and we were only allowed two hours and ten minutes to complete the race. I had a few friends there and the crowd on the pier began calling my name. 'Marion! Marion! Go, go!' they yelled. With their encouragement, I completed the race, but I must have looked horrible because they said I looked five hours dead. If it had not been for my friends' encouragement, I would not have finished my first pier-to-pier swim and I would not have gone to Hawaii because I had never swum 2.4 miles."

Marion explained that friends helped improve her running and biking, and she attributes development of close relationships to distance sports. "In distance sports, people get close to each other and really see each other's soul. I have run marathons to pace friends. One friend thought he couldn't run a marathon around our peninsula, but I helped him run his best marathon ever by chit-chatting with him every couple miles. This is the real fun of sport, and you reminisce about the days when you helped pull somebody through and when somebody pulled you through. Winning medals along the way is like a pat on the shoulder."

ATHLETIC HISTORY

Marion grew up in Bremerhaven, West Germany, and came to the United States in 1958. She was always active, riding bikes with the children, mowing the lawn, and swimming. Then, after turning 40, she became involved in athletics.

Marion explained how she came to realize she had no friends to call her own. "My friendships included business acquaintances and friends shared with my husband," she said. "I thought how sad it is that I don't have anybody for myself, and so I started playing tennis to collect people. I was literally out there collecting people to form my own group of friends, and I found that sports are a wonderful way to meet people of all ages."

"I played tennis about four years," Marion said, "and I was good enough to be welcomed on the court. I played on a team with four gentlemen, and I met another player I run with on occasion. My young tennis partner tried to train me for competition, but I never played that well, which is a reason I quit the sport. I am more relaxed with running, biking, and swimming."

"I started running in 1985," Marion said. "In December, when I could run five or six miles, I joined a local running club. I was naive about competitive running and training, and when I heard club members talk about marathon training, I decided to train for a marathon too, although I hadn't the foggiest idea of what was involved. Two months later, in February 1986, I ran the Long Beach Marathon in 4 hours and 20 minutes, and I was excited about having run a marathon."

Marion said her next major event in 1986 was the New York City Marathon, which she got into via the lottery. She then tried a small triathlon and finished third. Finding triathlons to be fun, she drifted from the marathon to the triathlon.

"I was playing tennis when I decided to go for the Ironman," Marion said, "and I told my tennis friends I wouldn't be playing tennis anymore because I was going to train for the Hawaiian Ironman. They looked at me and said, 'We're going to Wimbledon next year.' I thought, 'You'll see!' I showed them as I qualified for the Ironman by lottery and also by placing in the Monterey Triathlon. Because I wanted to qualify, I competed in Monterey, which I thought would be the hardest place for most women because the water was only 51 degrees. I qualified, which made me proud, and I finished the Ironman in 14 hours, 55 minutes, and 59 seconds. I had a wonderful time."

"In 1987," Marion said, "I went crazy doing a triathlon, 10K run, or marathon almost every weekend. I wanted to do well in the 1987 Ironman, and by that time I had the nerve to enter the Bakersfield Triathlon, which was a difficult place to qualify because it had many tough contestants. I had enough guts to try to qualify there and I succeeded. I went to Hawaii two weeks before the Ironman and had an absolutely lousy time. I missed my friends and was lonely, and I barely bettered my 1986 time."

Marion skipped the 1988 Ironman, choosing to try the Alcatraz Triathlon instead. "By that time, I was deep into triathlons. However," she admitted, "although I can swim long distances, I'm a lousy, slow, terrible swimmer. During the Alcatraz swim, the current was the highest and heaviest in seven years. Anybody who could complete the swim in an hour or so made it across, and everyone else was fished out of the water because the current got too strong. In the blink of an eye we were fished out of the water, put in a dinghy, and ferried across the current. Then, because the current was so viscous, we were allowed to jump back into the water to continue and be legitimate finishers. I jumped into the water a second time, which was tougher to do than the first time, and I finished the Alcatraz Triathlon, winning a gold medal in my age group."

Marion said she has run the Boston Marathon once (1987) and the Los Angeles Marathon twice. In 1989, she returned to Hawaii for the Ironman and had a wonderful time, although she was hobbled by an injured ankle. "I had a running accident four weeks earlier when I was blinded by a car's lights and I jumped aside over a stone divider. I thought I needed to avoid the car coming toward me. I ripped both sides of my ankle, causing swelling and problems that will take about nine months to heal. My doctor wanted the cast left on six weeks, and I said, 'Forget it, because I'm going to do the Ironman.' I explained why the cast had to come off, and he thought I was nuts. We got the cast off two weeks before the Ironman, and I babied my foot as I combined walking with running to finish the race."

"I have won a lot of medals, mostly seconds and thirds in triathlons," Marion said. "In 1989, I finished first in my age group in the Los Angeles Triathlon. First, second, or third place doesn't make that much difference to me. I finished sixth in my age group in my second Ironman, and I was 17th out of 25 in 1989 while competing with an injured foot. The top five finishers almost always have trainers and put more hours into training than I do because winning and being number one means everything to some women. I want a more balanced life, and my purpose is to have a wonderful time, to socialize, and to be healthy. If I should also get a medal, that would be great."

FITNESS REGIMEN

"I train from 5:00 in the morning to 8:00 or 8:30," Marion said, "and I'm usually in the office by 9:45 at the latest; I work until 5:00 or 6:00. During the winter, I swim three mornings a week in the ocean, and the mornings between swims I lift weights at the health spa. This is my time off from competition, and I try to put my body back together because it gets messed up and a little skinny from all that running. I try to put a little weight on, get a little muscle back, and work on my leg strength. In January, I get more serious about training, do more biking and speed work, and begin thinking about the next race. By the end of January, I begin my evening training while maintaining my morning swim. I build up my running in preparation for the first marathon of the year. After the marathon, I maintain my running and build up my swim until mid-April. For the next couple months, I swim, run, and bike intensely, working on long distances. Before triathlon competition, I switch my focus from long to short distances."

"My diet changes with my training," Marion said. "It's not so much because I want to eat healthier, it's that I give my body what my body wants. I eat a lot of fish, vegetables, and fruit, and I drink a lot of juices and fluids. During my winter training, I eat heavier food because my body wants more fat to protect itself from the cold water. My weight varies from 133 to 136 pounds, depending on activities. I carry less weight when training during the summer or preparing for a marathon."

"In the spring when I'm training hard, I eat lighter foods that are heavy with carbohydrates. I eat grapefruit, spaghetti with little on it, bread, potatoes and other such plain food every couple hours, and I'm constantly nibbling. I use a little cholesterol-free margarine. My cravings change during heavy training and my eating habits are like those of a squirrel."

"Men outnumber women in the sport of triathlon," Marion stated. "Although more women are getting involved in the triathlon, it is still tough for women to find the many hours needed for training no matter how wonderful or modern their husbands are. People ask me, 'When do you clean the house?' I don't have anyone to help me clean, cook, shop, or entertain, so every moment of my life is filled. The only time I do nothing is when I sleep. It's hard for me to keep the house going, cook, shop, and train at the same time. It's easier for a man to train better because he doesn't have to worry about the house and cooking when he comes home from work. Although my husband is used to me jumping out of bed at five o'clock, he has told me, 'You don't have to go every day.' But I have to go every day because I will never get back into the ocean if I don't. Training is not always fun."

Marion said, "I don't train much alone; if I have to, I do. My husband lifts weights almost every night and he runs about six miles a day, but we don't train together because I run faster and longer. I have six or seven wonderful male friends, all married and varying in age from 25 to 66, and I enjoy training with them and being with them. That's how I socialize. I don't train much with women because I don't want to listen to their nagging; I hear enough of that in the office. When I want to train with my best triathlon training partner, who is 66, I call and if his wife answers, I ask her, 'Well, I was wondering if I can have your husband tomorrow night to kill him a little bit with some running.' If he's available, fine; if not, that's too bad and I go by myself."

"I have some males friends I run with, some I bike with, and some I swim with. The hardest training partner to find is one who is willing to get up at five o'clock in the morning to swim in cold water. It's easier to find a running or biking partner. Of my three swimming friends, one of them shows up for sure so I have a babysitter in the ocean."

Marion has had accidents while training. Besides injuring her ankle a month before the 1989 Hawaiian Ironman, she described two biking mishaps involving run-ins with stationary objects. "I rode into a parked Volkswagen and I got a neck injury," she said. "Another time I fell asleep on my bicycle and ran into a sign. I was training for my first Ironman and was intent on getting my mileage. While riding up a steep hill, I fell asleep after seeing a 'man working' sign, and that's the last thing I saw until I awakened with my nose against it. At that point, I couldn't do anything but gently fall over. It's idiotic to push hard when tired, and I've learned to respect the sport more."

"The triathlon is a great sport because it consists of three events and you can meet many different people," Marion said. "You stay healthy all the time. If my legs hurt from running too much, I bike more; if my knees hurt from biking, I swim more. Thus, the same muscles do not get pounded over and over during training. The triathlon is a healthy sport, but training is tiring because so much effort is required for all three activities. My training never stops; it just intensifies or goes in different directions. It's a way of life."

MENTAL ATTITUDE ABOUT HEALTH AND FITNESS

"I'm married to a gynecologist, and I do all the computer work for our three medical clinics," Marion said. "I work hard and am not a housewife who can train and have the opportunity to do nothing. In our medical practice, we find women who do not take the proper hormones to replace those their body no longer produces. It is essential for women to have a proper hormone balance before engaging in any activity, and they must establish their own personality. They must learn that life is not wrong when they think of themselves, and their husbands must learn to give them free time. The women must not feel guilty when they protect their free time. Most women cannot get themselves to say, 'I'm going to the club and pump weight,' and then leave their poor neglected husbands to make their own breakfast or to eat later in the evening. From a husband's viewpoint, it's a small price to pay for a happy, healthy wife who likes herself."

"In my husband's practice, I have seen women who are cranky during their menopausal years, and I knew I needed a personal activity to make sure I never got cranky. Most women are cranky because they have nothing of importance to do. They get this empty nest syndrome when life's pressures increase and their lives are busy but not fulfilled. Their husbands have careers, and they feel sorry for themselves because their careers ended when their children no longer needed care. They don't realize that a new life has begun and they can make themselves happy by finding something other than needlepoint work, something where they can have their own friends. I think that's important."

"You need somebody to help you get up and train in the morning," Marion stated. "It's not easy to awaken at five o'clock, push your bike outside, and say 'here I am.' The weather may be cold, rainy, and miserable, but you have to go if your training partner is waiting for you. Training partners also provide encouragement. 'Hey!' one partner will say, 'let's go. We are going through this together, and we're going to make it fast.' For example, five minutes after I began a 100-mile bike ride, it started raining. After biking 25 miles, we talked about going on with the ride, and we decided there's no sense turning back because we were already wet. I changed into dry clothes 25 miles later, and we completed our ride while 90% of the people did not. Despite the bad start, the bike ride was one of my greatest because the scenery and sights were spectacular. I saw clouds going over the hills, lightning in the sky, and cows and horses grazing in the fields. Beauty is part of the sport."

Explaining her competitive attitude, Marion said, "I see and enjoy nature while competing because I don't wrap myself up in thoughts about my competitors being five seconds faster than me. I try to go as fast as I can, to be as strong as I can, and to do my best. If someone along the way tells me a competitor is a couple turns ahead and I can catch her, I go for her no matter how tired I am. If I catch her and find another lady closing in on me, I will go faster. The two of us will try to shake each other, and that's when the real race begins."

"There is much beauty in nature, and you have to be aware of your surroundings while competing and training. While swimming in the cold ocean this morning, we saw an incredible view of the rising sun dressing the Santa Monica Mountains in gold and red colors. The ocean was clear enough to see the bottom, and we felt like we could touch the sand. We seemed to be dolphins swimming back to paradise while the waves pushed us, but this was training. Afterwards, I was so cold that I asked my partner to stay until I got my car door open. My hands and feet were like ice, and I could barely move the the key. Since nobody was at the beach or in the water, you need a partner to be safe."

"I love to bike along the ocean and watch the breakers," Marion said. "Riding between the ocean and hills north to Malibu, I forget about my house and all the work to be done while enjoying the fragrant smells and colorful sights. There's always time for work, and there's no excuse for a woman saying she cannot go out and do some sport. The best diet program won't help a woman if she sits at home because she will still feel miserable. Most women, especially when they are around 50, have hormone changes and need something to do. I have advised many women to walk or run, to enjoy nature while talking with people they see working and exercising. People are always outside working, and many take the same walks every day. I see a lady walking her dog every day. She's been doing it for years, and maybe she doesn't have anyone to talk to except her dog. By saying, 'Hello, it's a nice day,' my partner and I may be her only human contact. It seems as though she looks for us every other day as we run down the strand."

"Many women in their 50s think life is over for them when their kids are gone," Marion explained. "Some women sit and watch TV while others go back to work or become volunteers. They can also take up sport, get their bodies in shape, make themselves pretty, and get a doctor to organize their hormones. The women will then be wonderful wives and in tip-top shape for their husbands. They will feel relaxed with their anxieties gone, and their lives and everyone else's will be happier."

Marion remarked, "Fitness is fifty percent mental; it's from your head to your toe. You like yourself if you have a feeling of well being. If you don't like yourself, you may have a gorgeous figure and still feel depressed. The sport of triathlon has made me feel better about myself; I feel like I have accomplished something. It makes me feel that I can swim through big thick waves and back to land where I can deal with any cranky lady who comes into the practice and tries to make my day miserable. 'Hey,' I tell myself, 'I can take care of her. No problem. I've had my fun and I feel great. What can I do for this woman to make her feel great, too?' My attitude is positive because I am fit, and others feel good about me because I feel good about myself."

"I admire athletes who are over 70," Marion said, "and someday I hope to be the oldest woman in one of these events. Life is not over after 60, it's just another phase. I have several male friends who have done all sorts of things like ride bikes across the country to show the world that someone over 60 can do a lot more than be a couch potato thinking about aches and pains. I sometimes have so many aches and pains that I wonder if its from old age or overexercise. When I train hard, my shoulders may hurt from weightlifting, my legs may hurt from biking, and my knees may hurt from running. My whole body may hurt, but that's a way of life. I could complain about it, but the aches and pains often fade with each day's exercise. It's important to learn the difference between injury pain and exercise pain because they need to be treated differently. Either way, pain can be healthy because it makes you feel you're still alive."

Personal Fitness Goals

"My personal goals are to be happy and to make friends," Marion said. "I don't exercise for fitness, and I honestly don't think about fitness. I think more of staying healthy, and fitness comes automatically as a wonderful by-product. Being fit makes you feel healthy, vibrant, and alive."

Marion planned to begin her 1990 season with the Los Angeles Marathon in March and continue it as usual with distance events through to the Ironman in October. Since she did not finish number one in her age group in 1989, she would have to qualify for the Ironman, and she planned to do this at the Bakersfield Triathlon or some triathlon in Southern California. She was also pointing for the German Ironman scheduled for July 14, 1990 in Roth, Bavaria. "That's why I'm training in cold water," she said. "I'm a weak swimmer, and I understand the river water is cold."

"I hope my interest in distance sport will always be there even if I give up competition," Marion said. "It's great to go on a long bike ride with friends. My basic emphasis is to get people out of the house to enjoy the fresh air, to greet the morning sunshine, to see the clouds in the sky, to listen to birds, to feel wind go through their hair, to meet with friends, and to be healthy and happy with what the world has to offer."

RECOMMENDATIONS FOR IMPROVED FITNESS OF PEOPLE OVER **40**

For people over 40 to improve their fitness, Marion recommends: "Eat a proper diet, including meat, vegetables, grains, and fruits. Get a good night's sleep and wake up with the first rays of sunshine. Enjoy the morning by taking a walk, slow at first, and say, 'Good morning' to friends and strangers you meet. Continue walking each morning and walk longer each day."

Marion suggests a gradual progression for people interested in pursuing sports and making friends. Using her experience as an example, she recommends, "Find a neighborhood running group, start running a little, and make some friends. Join a health club, pump a little weight, learn to swim, start biking with others, and make more friends. Do a short triathlon and see how many people you get to know in your age group. Then improve your performance at another triathlon and see some of the same people again. Be sure you visit your doctor to ensure your health is fine for your sport, lose some weight if you have to, and, above all, have a great time. Realize you are not old at 40 plus; buy a triathlon magazine and read how well the 'old folks' are doing at 70 years and over. You will learn there is no such thing as an old man or old woman; they only get wiser and so will you if you take care of your health."

"A lot of people make themselves old," Marion stated. "When I was in Germany last year, I found people who literally practiced being old. When people over 40, thinking of themselves as old, say, 'I can't get out of bed so fast anymore, I can't do this, I can't do that,' I say, 'For God's sake, run a little, move a little, walk a little, and you'll feel vibrant.' I met a German friend I had not seen in 30 years. He's three years older and fit. We walked in the hills of Austria, and it was beautiful. Many times he said he used to run, and I said, 'What do you mean, you used to run? What makes you think you can't run now? Let's run.' We ran up and down the hill, and then the man felt great about himself. By the time we ran down, he had forgotten his age, and he said, 'I have never had such a wonderful time in the mountains with anybody as I had with you.' His wife couldn't believe what a happy husband I brought back, and she remarked about how young and happy he appeared. Meanwhile, I was thinking, 'If you would move your body a little more he would be young and happy with you.' We had dragged her halfway up the mountain until she panted that she couldn't walk any farther even though we had stopped to make sure she got fresh air and could see how pretty the hills were."

"If 80-year-old people can run the marathon, why can't you?" Marion had asked her German friend. "All you need do is lose five pounds and start walking, lose two or three more pounds and start running, and soon you can do it. Well, I got a letter from his wife yesterday, and she said her husband is going to run in the 1990 New York City Marathon. This is the success of sport; it's not the medals you bring home."

"Go out and do it," Marion encourages. "You can be out there having fun with the crowd. It doesn't matter if it takes you four hours or five hours to run a marathon if you have set this goal for yourself and you make it. Your goals should not be limited to making money or climbing the corporate ladder. There are many healthy opportunities in life, and people with healthy attitudes live longer because they are relaxed and they have a wonderful time enjoying life."

Phil Mulkey

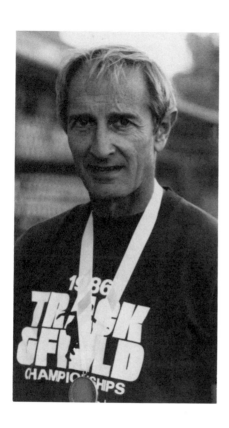

born: January 7, 1933
height: 5′ 11″
weight: 165
home: Atlanta, Georgia
athletic highlights:

- selected to participate in the decathlon on the 1959 Pan Am and 1960 U.S. Olympic teams
- broke Rafer Johnson's world decathlon record in 1961 and held it until Bill Toomey bettered it five years later
- won a Missouri State Golden Gloves Boxing title
- was named to the pre-season Regional All-American Basketball Team at the University of Wyoming
- won a Tennessee State Diving title
- won four gold medals in track and field at the U.S. National Senior Olympics in 1989

Each year Phil Mulkey adds about 100 medals to his collection, which he estimated to be about 3000 through 1989. He puts the medals in shoe boxes labeled by year, and he stores them in a closet. "What else can I do with them," he says. "There are too many to display in my house, and how would you choose a selective few to display?" He also stores a large number of trophies in his basement. "It's shameful the way I have them stored," laments Phil.

"I may have more medals than anyone else because I have competed in so doggone many events and meets," Phil said. "I compete like the dickens to win a medal, especially if I think someone may beat me, but the game is over the instant I get the medal. Although the medal is meaningful, winning it doesn't matter when the battle is over. I have paid a heavy price for my world championship medals and trophies because the training I put into winning them was phenomenal."

"Nobody cares about how many medals you've got," Phil stated as he continued explaining his philosophy about competitive athletics for fitness. "If you're a former Olympian, your competitors want to beat your butt. They want to beat me, and I don't want to be beaten. It works out well and is as exciting as heck. We bet beers and soft drinks on a single jump, and we'll give astronomical odds if we're feeling good. It's a wonderful way to spend a good part of your life staying fit."

ATHLETIC HISTORY

Born and raised on his family's farm in the foothills of the Ozarks, Phil did not participate in sports until his sophomore year at a small rural high school in Missouri. "I didn't even know what sports were," Mulkey claims. Then the school's track coach said he needed someone to run the mile in the county meet the next day. Mulkey volunteered and then ran about three miles to prepare for his first track event. Although he had only one day to prepare, Mulkey finished second and won a silver medal.

As a 15-year-old 100-pounder, Phil read about 17-year-old Bob Mathias winning the decathlon in the 1948 Olympics, and he began reading books on fitness and diet relative to athletics. He continues to read about the subject, he said, because research is ongoing.

In his junior year, Phil said he began competing in the sprints, jumps, and throws. Although weighing only 120 pounds, he did well in the throws, particularly the shot put. As a junior and senior, he qualified for the state meet in the shot put, winning the event his senior year, when he weighed exactly 133 pounds. He made the finals in the sprint relay, the 400 meters, the long jump, and the discus. He wasn't able to medal in any event except the shot, but he was beginning to show some all-around aptitude as a decathlete.

After high school, Phil said, "I joined the Army where I did moderately well competing in track and field. I finished third in the high hurdles in the All-Army Championships and second in the intermediate hurdles in the All Armed Forces Championships."

Phil completed his military commitment and earned honors as a regional All-American while attending the University of Wyoming on a basketball scholarship. However, disenchanted with the athletic program, he quit basketball and left Wyoming for Memphis State University, where he graduated with honors in education. While at Memphis State, Phil worked to support his wife and four children, and he decided to concentrate on track and field as an individual rather than be part of the University's program.

Phil said he qualified for the 1952 and 1956 Olympic Trials in the decathlon, but he did not make the team either time. "The 1952 decathlon trials were held in Tulare, California, Bob Mathias' home town," Phil remembered. "I know Bob quite well. I used to hang around him at the trials. He was only two years older than I was, but we were a world apart."

In 1960, Phil competed in the Olympic decathlon trials for the third time and finally qualified for the United States team as the runner-up to Rafer Johnson, the eventual winner in Rome. Unfortunately for Phil, a pulled groin muscle in the pole vault took him out of the running for a bronze medal.

"The year following the Olympics," Phil said, "I broke Johnson's world record with 8049 points, which is still a moderately good score by any of today's standards. My score lasted until Bill Toomey broke it about five years later, and I believe it still ranks about 15th best among American athletes."

Phil continued to compete on a national level, winning the national decathlon championships in 1964 and 1965. However, his scores weren't that good, and he retired from serious track-and-field competition. "But I could not walk away from track and field," he said, "and I played around by going to open meets where I could enjoy competing without having ambitions for much success."

During his first seven years of track and field after age 40, Phil said he won 32 gold medals in masters national championships in the pentathlon, 400-meter hurdles, high hurdles, long jump, triple jump, pole vault, shot put, discus, javelin, and 60-yard dash.

FITNESS REGIMEN

"My weight varies about 10 pounds, increasing some during the off-season, which is September, October, and November." Phil explained, "I splurge a little bit and let all my muscles and bones get back together. Then I start a mild indoor exercise program in December and continue at that level until about March when I go outside and begin to bear down a bit."

Phil described his diet as moderate. "I am neither strongly opposed nor strongly for any sort of regimentation. I maintain a good, well-balanced, basic diet, watching what and how much I eat. I listen to my body and follow some of the things I read about nutrition. For example, I minimize my fat intake and try to make a nice blend of carbohydrates, proteins, and other nutritional requirements. I don't think anyone should go off the deep end on any kind of diet because there are no secrets out there on how to lose weight."

"My training includes a little work with weights because I think resistance is needed. I do some stretching and running. Mostly I work on my technique because that will make the difference in the end."

Phil has found time for competition and training throughout his adult life, and his current speaking schedule is flexible and well-suited for training. In regard to the time required for training and for his work as a motivational speaker, he said, "I'm not working hard now, but I still have responsibilities. As far as training goes, I try to train every day I feel like it. If I train hard three days back-to-back, I will skip a day because I know it's getting too much for me. On the other hand, I try to train when I can because there are times I won't get a chance to go out. Hit-and-miss training works for me because three or four hard days a week is about all I can handle at my age, and training harder is retrogressive. I train at least two or three hours a day because I have many events to cover."

"I've had injuries almost every year," Phil said. "I don't think anyone can participate in many events and meets without being injured. I haven't suffered anything worse than pulls and strains, and they haven't kept me out of action. Although my performance when I'm injured may not be what I want, it's still kinda' fun trying to get through."

MENTAL ATTITUDE ABOUT HEALTH AND FITNESS

According to Phil, "anything is possible and success is a surety."

"Health and fitness are what life is all about," Phil said. "That's all that matters when you get right down to it. Power, prestige, and money won't buy good health, and the agony of living with poor health isn't worth it. My athletic program is a marvelous excuse for staying fit. As disciplined as I am, I know I would not stay as fit without it. I'd probably stay reasonably fit, maybe 90%, but I'd rather be 95%, and that extra 5% is hard to make yourself acquire unless you have some reason for doing it."

"Winning is not that important to me now," Phil states, "but it is important to feel healthy and to feel that I have performed as well as I possibly can. Anything less than that is disappointing."

Phil's positive attitude toward health and fitness carried over into his career. As a motivational speaker, he has presented a wide variety of winning-philosophy topics in keynote addresses and sales seminars. He also conducts group workshops on image development.

PERSONAL FITNESS GOALS

"My goals are to stay fit and to do as well as I can each year," Phil said, "especially in the national and world championships. That's broad and ambiguous because I know they're only the means to the end, which is great fitness. The means to getting there involves camaraderie, spirit of competition, enthusiasm, training, and any honors won. I want to keep going as long as I can, and there's no reason not to. You never graduate from this program; you just go on to another level."

"I'm looking forward to the 1991 Masters World Championships in Turko, Finland," Phil said. "The 1989 World Championships in Eugene, Oregon had 5000 athletes over 40, and I call them athletes because these people do not fool around. When they go to the games, they go to compete. This was the biggest track meet in the world; it was bigger than the United States National Senior Olympics, which had 3500 athletes."

Phil's track-and-field schedule for 1990 included four major meets, beginning with the Masters Indoor Championships at the University of Wisconsin in late March. The other meets planned were the Outdoor Championships in Indianapolis, the Pan-Am Games at Trinidad, Tobago, and the National Decathlon Championships.

"At each track-and-field meet, I will compete in about nine events," Phil explained. "I always try ten events — all the jumps: high jump, long jump, pole vault, and triple jump; the throws: shot, discus, hammer, and javelin; and the hurdles: high and intermediate hurdles."

"I've won the national indoor and outdoor shot the last two years, which is surprising because I weigh only 165 pounds. I'm obviously not that strong, but I have a good technique for throwing the shot, probably because it was the first event I practiced each day when I was training."

Phil explained that the satisfaction of a major goal led to improved habits and excellent health. "Making the 1960 Olympic team satisfied one major goal and meant more to me than breaking the world decathlon record the following year. A by-product of my Olympic adventure was a carry-over of good health habits developed from many years of disciplined training."

Phil derives enjoyment and ultimately fitness by competing in track-and-field events. Although he is a fierce competitor, it is his way to achieve his fitness objectives. "After winning an event," Phil explained, "my feeling of pride dissipates quickly and I start thinking about my next objective. For example, at the nationals a couple years ago in Orlando, Florida, I beat four reigning champions, all from the United States, to win four gold medals in a diversified set of events. That thrilled me because my goal was to beat these guys in the high hurdles, pole vault, long jump, and shot put. I was primed and ready so my success was gratifying. After coming home with the medals, the satisfaction of that goal became history for me and I began to think about next year."

"I feel the same way about world records," Phil said. "The records come and go; I'll set a few records and then someone breaks them. It's fun to go for records, but I don't keep track of them. Records are a little flair that makes competition interesting, but they are not a big part of my goal so I don't put much emphasis on them, at least as far as remembering what they are. I've had my share of world records, and I probably hold some now, especially in the decathlon."

RECOMMENDATIONS FOR IMPROVING FITNESS OF PEOPLE OVER 40

In his fitness message to older people, Phil warns, "Good health is a full-time job that never runs out...you don't retire from this one!"

"You need to be concerned with what you eat," Phil stated, "but you shouldn't go off the deep end about it. There's all kinds of diet and health stuff that's supposed to be magic. However, in lieu of that, I recommend that you ask a dietician to give you a basic diet that contains good combinations of foods."

"Don't eat too much," warns Phil. "During the track-and-field season, I stay away from sugars and sweets because they add the extra pounds. During the off-season, I splurge a little."

"In addition to eating the right amounts of the right foods, you've got to exercise consistently, although not necessarily every day. You've got to do your stretching because those old muscles get stiff and tight, and you've got to put some power in what you are doing. When I resume my training schedule after the off-season, I do a lot of work on the treadmill because it's smooth. As I progress beyond the treadmill, I'll run a fast 200, 300, or 400 meters. Then I'll rest and run again."

"I'd like to see everyone involved in some kind of sport," Phil continued. "Some people over 50 sit back and say they are too old. That's a huge mistake. The sport doesn't have to be track and field; it can be anything. Those who do not pursue some activity may be sorry in the end. Many people avoid exercise like it's a dangerous plague, but it's essential to stay fit because the body, which is in a degenerative state, is losing cells, strength, and reflex action. We can slow the degeneration by demanding that the body stays fit. The body is responsive to the old 'use it or lose it routine.' If it finds it isn't needed, it quits on you."

"When I was younger," Phil said, "and I pulled something like a shoulder muscle, I would spend more time working on my legs. If I pulled a hamstring, I'd work more on my shoulder girdle. Thus, when something bad happens, you can turn it around and make something good out of it."

10 TIPS FOR HEALTHY COMPETITION

As a spokesman for Holiday Inn, one of the major sponsors of the United States National Senior Olympics in June, 1989, Phil was featured in promotional material distributed for the games. One pamphlet included the following tips for the senior athletes:

1. **Beat the heat:** Try to keep out of the sun as much as possible. Keep your fluid level high. Drink all you want and then some.

2. **Stiff muscles:** No matter how inviting, stay out of the hot tub. Cool off after your event in the pool.

3. **Sore joints:** Pack them in ice for 20 minutes, take a breather, and do it again.

4. **Injuries:** Check with your doctor. It may be more serious than you think.

5. **Energy level:** Eat comfortably, but don't overdo it.

6. **Tension:** Accept it — it's all part of the game.

7. **Technique:** You've trained well and are well-prepared for this event. Stay confident and relaxed.

8. **Stress:** The best way to beat it is to get plenty of sleep.

9. **Attitude:** Be happy! Have a good time 'cause this is fun.
10. **Good overall health and well-being:** That's exactly what these games are all about. Take the spirit home with you.

According to Phil, more companies like Holiday Inn are needed to sponsor events for large numbers of seniors to compete at comfortable levels.

Holiday Inn promotional material for the USNSO games contained the following comment: "It's never too late to start," Mulkey emphasizes, "because the moment you begin is the moment you start feeling better. I'll bet there are a lot of people out there who, had they known they were going to live this long, would have taken better care of themselves! And since we're not really sure of the time left for each of us, doesn't it make sense to begin now?"

Nancy Reed

born: April 21, 1933
height: 5′ 6″
weight: 135
home: Winter Park, Florida
athletic highlights:

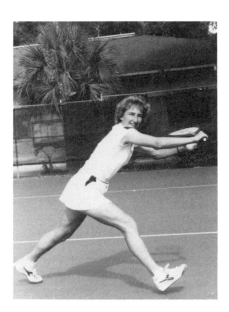

- nationally ranked tennis player during her career at Rollins College in Winter Park, Florida
- invited to play international tennis on the Young Cup (women 40 and over) and Bueno Cup (women 50 and over) teams
- at age 54, won the European singles championship for women over 50
- in 1988, ranked 13th among World Veterans for women over 50
- in 1989, ranked first in U.S. singles and doubles for women over 55 and ranked second in singles for women over 50
- won about 75 national and international tennis titles through 1989

Nancy C. Reed grew up in the Washington, D.C. area and graduated from high school in Bethesda, Maryland. As a youth and young adult, she had the disadvantage of living in an era when schools and governments did little for women's athletics. However, she had the good fortune to attend one of the few high schools that permitted girls' athletic teams to compete with local schools, and she played on these teams. Also, her participation in summer recreational sports led to a tennis career beginning at age 15.

In 1970, at age 36, Nancy played in the U.S. Open for the last time. Her good but undramatic tennis career went into "forced" retirement, meaning that she was too old to compete with young adults and there was little tennis competition available for adults over 35.

However, the late sixties and early seventies marked a new era of national interest in sports and physical fitness. Dr. Kenneth Cooper's book *Aerobics* was published in 1968 and more people learned that they could push their bodies to physical feats of strength and endurance well past age 40. Programs and opportunities for women improved, and the tennis boom of the sixties led to senior tennis and "money tennis" in the seventies.

Nancy, having recovered from a knee operation, turned 40 in 1974 and took advantage of the new opportunities available to her as a senior woman. Unseeded, she played and won her first national senior tournament at the Houston Racquet Club, and she has subsequently been a top-ranked player in her age group.

ATHLETIC HISTORY

Nancy said, "I was fortunate that my high school in Bethesda, Maryland, had girls' teams and competition with local schools. I played basketball, soccer, field hockey, and volleyball through high school, having started with these sports in summer recreational programs which had no organized competition."

"I started playing tennis in summer recreation when I was 15," Nancy said as she began discussing her tennis career. "I won a little playground tournament and thought I was great, so I entered a tournament right away and lost badly, and that made me determined to improve."

"After high school," Nancy continued, "I went to Rollins College in Winter Park, Florida, where I studied biology and played tennis for four years. My friends went to the University of Maryland and my parents wanted me to go to Boston University, where my mother had gone, or to William and Mary. I had heard that these schools were nice, but those were the days before you visited campuses and I wanted to play tennis. Rollins offered year-round tennis and a women's team, and those were my primary reasons for choosing Rollins."

Nancy said, "During my college years, I worked during the summer while playing competitive tennis, and I participated in women's sports other than tennis. I played on the Rollins basketball team, which competed with schools throughout the state, and I played intramural volleyball and some softball."

"After college, I returned to the Washington, D.C. area where I taught biology, played recreation basketball and volleyball, and got married. I worked until I was enough money ahead to pay the cost of traveling to play tennis. Since these were the days before 'money tennis,' I had to pay my travel costs to Wimbledon and other tournaments. The Australian Open was out of the question, being in the winter and before the days of indoor tennis. At age 28, I had saved enough money and I started playing tennis again on the national level."

Although Nancy resumed her tennis career at a late age, she played the summer circuit for nine years and was always ranked in the U.S. women's top 25. She played Wimbledon twice and played in the U.S. Open at Forest Hills from age 21 through 36, except for her five-year break from national tennis after college. During the summer, she played the grass court circuit, which ended the season at Forest Hills. Although she wanted to play in the French and Italian Opens, she said there wasn't time to prepare for surfaces other than grass, thereby keeping her out of these major tournaments.

The second hiatus in Nancy's tennis career came when she retired after the 1969 U.S. Open because of her age, 36. "After a tough match you don't come back as easily the next day," she said. "There was nothing of interest to me in 1971–72 because today's senior tour had not been started. A tournament for women over 40 had gone on for years, but the first real tournament for senior women started in 1971 at the Houston Racquet Club with four age divisions: 35 and over, 45, 50, and 55. Nancy had recovered from knee surgery in 1970 and entered the Houston tournament in 1973.

Senior tennis started to blossom in 1973 and so did Nancy's tennis career. She won her first national title, the women's clay court singles in the 35-and-over division, when she entered the Houston tournament. She won despite being unseeded in the tournament and unranked for 3 to 4 years.

Since resuming tennis at age 40, she said that she has won about 75 national and international titles, including at least one major singles and doubles title in each of the four age divisions through her current 55s group. She has been a dominant player on grass and clay surfaces. For example, in 1988, when she became eligible for the 55s division, she played singles and doubles in the 50s as well as the 55s, winning all four of the grass court titles and the two clay court titles in the 55s bracket. "I skip the national tournaments played on hard surfaces," she explained, "because I believe my body will last longer by staying off hard courts during national competition."

Some grass court wins are memorable to Nancy. She said, "A couple of wins that meant a lot to me were the national women's 45 on grass courts at age 53 and the national women's 50 at age 56. The international cup matches — the Young Cup for women 40 and over and the Bueno Cup for women 50 and over — and the 1988 European Championship in Baden-Baden were also big wins for me. In the European Championships, I won the women's 50 singles and teamed with Mary Ann Plante to win the women's 50 doubles. This was quite an accomplishment because it was a large tournament and, at age 54, it was tough giving away those years to younger players."

In order to satisfy her passion for tennis, Nancy has had to find employment to fit her schedule. After resuming tennis at age 28, she continued to teach because she had all summer off. Although she took a job where she had approval to leave in mid-May before the school term ended, she still found the teaching period to be too long and she couldn't concentrate on her game. When "money tennis" developed in the early seventies, Nancy quit teaching school to give tennis lessons and to manage tennis clubs. She is still giving a few lessons, but she has been self-employed in recent years, managing retail businesses and rental housing with business partners. Being self-employed is important, she said, because she wanted the freedom to play more tennis at any time during the day.

FITNESS REGIMEN

"I play tennis almost every day," Nancy said. "Rain or a tough workweek that leaves me tired may result in my skipping a day. I play matches, but not always tough matches, and I practice. Sometimes I will only give a lesson, but I seem to need or crave exercise every day. If I'm going to play in a major tournament, I will spend the prior two or three weeks playing four tough matches a week with friends or people I know. I can't play too hard before a tournament or I won't have the stamina to get through it. When I practice, I spend about one-and-a-half hours on the usual drills for serving, volleying, hitting down the lines, and so on."

In describing her training, Nancy said, "I've really trained hard. In addition to tennis, I like to take walks and I spend nearly three hours a week on special exercises. Some people do cross-training to prepare themselves, but the only thing I do is ride a stationary bike for 15–20 minutes at low resistance or run a series of 20-yard wind sprints. I ride three times a week and run three times a week, alternating the days for these activities. I don't do distance running because I learned it does not help my game and my joints can't take the pounding. Although I haven't found the need for weight work, I may consider using light weights if I find myself losing too much power as I get older."

"Before I play a match," Nancy said, "I spend at least ten minutes stretching. I have tried stretching after a match and have found that it doesn't help me. The thing I find helpful after tennis is my outdoor whirlpool, which I adjust to any temperature less than 100 degrees."

"I have been following the same diet for about 20 years," Nancy said, "long before the big interest in diets began, but I changed one habit about four years ago. I stopped drinking soft drinks. I will have an occasional soft drink if I need the caffeine to pep me up, but otherwise I have stopped. I usually get caffeine from two cups of coffee a day max. I'm careful with what I eat, and I eat three meals a day. I tend to have cereal, bread, and milk for breakfast as opposed to eggs; for lunch I have vegetables and carbohydrates; and for dinner I have a protein of some kind. I'm not opposed to eating moderate amounts of red meat, and I eat fish, which is plentiful in Florida. I try to have a well-balanced diet that includes red meat. I enjoy drinking beer, so I haven't ruled alcohol out, but I drink it in moderation. I don't add salt to foods, and I have no craving for desserts, but I will eat some."

In summing up her health regimen, Nancy noted she has been relatively free of injuries. She injured a knee playing basketball in college and had it operated on in 1970. She said it took almost a year to recover from that surgery, which is one reason she doesn't run distances like some players.

Nancy, who has not had children, said she has kept her weight about 130–135 throughout her career, although she doesn't weigh herself daily. She said she feels too weak at a lesser weight. Quickness, which is related to strength and weight, is one of her assets, she said, and she must have quickness to win.

Nancy concluded her fitness regimen thoughts with an observation that interests her. "I found that the men I have played tennis with during the last 15 years are losing their strength and are coming back to me; our matches are closer now."

MENTAL ATTITUDE ABOUT HEALTH AND FITNESS

"I don't think I could live with myself if I weren't fit," Nancy said. "If I start to get a little heavy, I immediately take steps to take the weight off, and vice versa, to stay at my best weight."

Nancy said she is seeded number one in many tournaments and other players are therefore out to beat her. In order to maintain her competitive edge, she doesn't play matches every day because it takes too much concentration to win a match. She said, "Playing singles and doubles against men and women two or three weeks before a tournament helps by giving me confidence that I can hit the shots."

PERSONAL FITNESS GOALS

"My goal is to make sure that tennis is a lifetime sport for me," Nancy stated. "I want to keep going."

Nancy wants to keep going like so many older people who are currently active in many ways, including sports. While talking about this, she remarked, "It's so gratifying what people are doing now in their older years."

RECOMMENDATIONS FOR IMPROVED FITNESS OF PEOPLE OVER 40

"There is nothing like a little success to motivate people," Nancy said, who uses this motivational factor when she gives tennis lessons. To get people into the game, she wants to let her older students see how much fun it is. "You can't just tell them to work with weights and to run; they need to be convinced first that tennis can be a lot of fun."

"I've given tennis lessons to a lot of people who have taken up the game in their 40s, 50s, and 60s," Nancy explained. "I find the important thing is to give them as quick and instant gratification as I can by getting them into a game situation. To do this I teach them some basics and don't worry much about their form. It takes about two weeks or four lessons to get them to this point, and then I tell them how to improve their game, how to run after the ball a little better, and how they can stay in the whole set. Then I start talking to them about things such as their diet and weight or perhaps doing some running or a little work on a stationary bike or rowing machine or anything that will appeal to them. I find they are more motivated if they have a goal to aspire to such as winning another game or two when playing their opponents. As they get better, they are more apt to stick with a conditioning program so they can play better."

For people with some tennis experience, Nancy advises them to practice with others 10 to 15 years younger, work on mental aspects of the game, improve their flexibility, and enter age-group competition regularly.

Bob Seagren

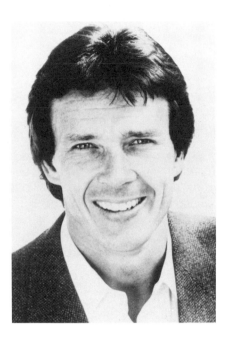

born: October 17, 1946

height: 6′ 0″

weight: 180

home: Los Angeles, California

athletic highlights:

- won a gold medal in the pole vault at the 1968 Olympics in Mexico City
- won a silver medal in the pole vault at the 1972 Olympics in Munich despite being forced to use a borrowed pole
- broke a mental barrier in vaulting, the 17-foot indoor vault, at the 1967 AAU indoor championship in Albuquerque
- won six AAU titles and four NCAA titles while breaking 15 world indoor and outdoor records between 1967 and 1972
- earned fame and $40,000 in winning ABC's first Superstars competition in 1973

In the early morning hours on September 5, 1972, eight Arab guerrillas of the Black September terrorist group invaded the Olympic Village dormitory of the Israeli team. The Arabs killed two Israeli athletes and took nine others hostage; 23 hours later a shootout ended with the deaths of a German policeman, five guerrillas, and all hostages.

Robert Lloyd Seagren, the world's leading pole vaulter but a disappointed silver medalist in Munich, was traveling in Italy with his family while the international drama was unfolding. "I had no idea what was going on," Bob explained, "and I couldn't believe it when I read about the massacre in an English-language newspaper. I played Foosball in the rec center with a few members of the Israeli team the evening before this happened. About 8:30, I went to my dorm and to bed while they walked into all kinds of problems. At dawn, I had not heard about the hostage situation as I drove out of the Village's underground area to get my family from a local hotel. We began a three-week trip driving around Europe, and about two days later, I found out what happened. It was sad to have such a fine Olympics spoiled by this tragedy."

ATHLETIC HISTORY

"My first competitive pole vault was in seventh grade," Bob said, "and I continued to jump through junior high, senior high, and college. I played baseball until my junior year in high school, when I stopped to focus my efforts on pole vaulting, which I enjoyed as an individual challenge with well-defined goals for success. My prospects for a baseball career faded, and a trip to Canada during my senior year whetted my appetite for bigger and better opportunities in pole vaulting."

"Pole vaulting is like golf or any other sport," Bob said, "where you gradually improve your performance as you perfect your technique. Speed and agility are key factors in vaulting, and body movement must be coordinated with the bending fiberglass pole. If you have a natural feel for pole vaulting, you can work to improve your technique. If you don't have a natural feel for it, you'll probably never learn the event."

"I began vaulting at 2 feet and jumped 15 feet my senior year in high school," Bob said. "As a senior, I competed against Paul Wilson, a vaulter in the Los Angeles area who was one year younger and jumping about 16.5 feet. After a bad loss to Wilson, I began to train seriously."

After high school, Bob went to Mount San Antonio Junior College and then the University of Southern California. "My JC coach was Don Ruh, a super guy and a motivator," Bob said. "He got me in shape, and that helped me set my first world pole vault record.

"The 17-foot indoor vault was a mental barrier in vaulting," Bob said, "and, after many close misses, I broke it at the 1967 AAU indoor championship at Albuquerque. As soon as I broke this psychological barrier, it became an easy jump. Five years later I went 18-feet outdoors, but I wasn't the first to do it."

In 1968, Bob won a gold medal at the Olympics in Mexico City with a vault of 17' 8.5". However, a few days before the Olympic qualifying trials in Lake Tahoe, Bob was in the hospital paralyzed from the waist down. His Olympic goal and athletic career were in jeopardy.

When he drove to Lake Tahoe for the trials, Bob thought he had an automatic qualification for the Olympic team because he had won a major competition in Los Angeles. On Saturday, a week before the Olympic trials pole vault competition, he learned that the Los Angeles winner no longer received automatic qualification. While warming up, Bob bent to touch his toes and heard his back pop. "I shot up in the air and fell face down in the grass," he said. "The pain was excruciating and I was numb from the waist down. I had a cracked vertebra."

Bob was taken to the hospital and put in traction. "I thought it was all over," he said. "Not being able to move my legs for a couple days was scary. There seemed to be no way for me to make the Olympic trials. I was still in pain and couldn't move on Monday, but I could move my legs on Tuesday. I was amazed at how fast it went away after that. On Wednesday, I sneaked out of the hospital and went to training head-quarters, and the next day I began jogging. On Friday, I tried pole vaulting with an easy jump of 16 feet. The next day I set a world record in qualifying for the Olympic team."

Bob learned that hyperextension causes the cracked vertebra to move and pinch a nerve, causing everything below that point to shut down. "Doctors showed me various pelvic exercises to strengthen the surrounding muscle tissue, and I did them. I haven't had a severe problem since the 1968 Olympic trials, but once in a while it will hurt when I do something insignificant like sneeze."

Bob won a silver medal at the 1972 Olympics with a vault of 17' 8.5" amid controversey that resulted in most vaulters having their poles declared illegal. Four weeks later the poles were approved. Meanwhile, Wolfgang Nordwig of East Germany won the pole vault when he was allowed to use his pole, which was not affected by the ban. Wolfgang had not adapted well to the type of pole that was banned, so he continued to use his old pole, while East Germany lodged a complaint about the pole preferred by most vaulters. Adriaan Paulen of the Netherlands was the head pole vault official who made the decision, although he had no experience as a pole vaulter.

"Looking back on this is sad," Bob said. "I wasn't the only one affected. Seventeen of the 25 competitors were handicapped. I fared better than the others. The decision to ban these poles irritates me because the old poles and the new poles or the black poles and the green poles, whatever you want to call them, were the same except for slight differences that would not affect the outcome of the event. What did affect the outcome was the purposeful decision to not make available poles of certain sizes. I did not have a pole to use that I needed for my body weight and speed. I had to use a pole that was made for a vaulter who was lighter than my weight and who ran at a slower speed on the runway. I had to make a drastic change in my technique to avoid breaking the pole. Thus, I competed in the 1972 Olympics at three-quarters speed while the guy who won was probably at 100 percent. That's where the disadvantage was. Some of the affected athletes couldn't adjust while I was able to adjust to some degree."

Bob won six AAU titles and four NCAA titles between 1967 and 1972, while breaking 15 indoor and outdoor world records. After the 1972 Olympics, he competed on the pro circuit. "The last world record I set was 18′ 5.75″ in the 1972 Olympic trials. I jumped 18′ 9″ as a pro, but the pro results were never sanctioned as world records. The pro track tour, which was underfinanced, lasted only four years."

Bob retired from the pro circuit in 1976, and that was the end of his pole vaulting career except for a commercial or two a year later. "I haven't jumped since," Bob said, "because pole vaulting is not something you go out and do for fun on a weekend. It's not like tennis or golf. It requires specific training and is too involved to be a weekend sporting activity. I have no desire to jump in a senior-type event. I enjoy doing other things such as tennis, golf, running, and cycling. Vaulting was fun when I was at my best and in top physical condition, but I don't think I would get the same enjoyment doing it on a casual basis."

Following the 1968 Olympics, when he wore his roommate's Puma shoes while winning the gold medal, Bob promoted Puma products for 18 years. In addition to representing a variety of products, he has hosted television specials, appeared on many top-rated television series, and co-starred with Deborah Raffin in "Willa," a 1979 CBS-TV movie. In recent years, he has been host of "The Home Restoration and Remodeling Show," and he acts as a consultant for a firm that specializes in lifestyle and segmented marketing.

In 1973, Bob won ABC-TV's first "Superstars" competition. In addition to $40,000 in prize money, he earned more fame than he did as a pole vaulter. This win led to similar celebrity events in subsequent years. In 1974 and 1975, he finished second in "Superstars," and he won the first "World Superstars" in 1977. He was second the following year. For the 10th anniversary of "Superstars," Bob competed in and won the veterans division. Then he was entered in the finals with the younger athletes. "I would have done well in that if I hadn't been knocked down in the bicycle race by Mark Gastineau. I was leading going into the bicycle event and my strong events were coming up. Despite losing ten points in the bicycle race, I went on to finish the competition in the top five. I've let ABC executives know I'm always ready to participate even if it's against all young guys."

"A similar type of competition is Jim Hershberger's MVP," Bob said. "I've participated every year he's had it, beginning in 1984. Ten events in one day is greuling with a lot of wear and tear on the body. My only complaint is that Jim has changed the events each year to his competitive advantage, but it's his money and his game so I guess he can do whatever he wants. The MVP is not a big spectator event, drawing only a couple thousand people because it moves around quite a bit. There has been some local television and maybe some cable service. I will be there with bells on my toes if Jim has this again and invites me."

Bob's voice rose and he talked faster while recalling exciting competition like Hershberger's MVP. "I had fun," he said. "I thrive on that kind of stuff because I love competition. The prize money was not my motivation. I like to do different kinds of things like that. It's great to get out and test yourself against other people with all things being equal. Hershberger's MVP and "Superstars" were like candy; they are fun, challenging, and a great way to get mental and physical enjoyment."

FITNESS REGIMEN

Running has been an important part of Bob's athletic career and fitness program, but that may be changing. "I've always run a lot," Bob said, "and the faster I was on the runway the better I would vault. I run today, but I don't sprint, and jogging is my mental therapy. However, as I got older, I found that jogging four to six miles a day causes wear and tear on my Achilles tendons and knees, so I'm alternating jogging with cycling. I try to jog three or four times a week and cycle the other days. A 20–25 mile bike ride seems to accomplish the same purpose."

"I'm not fanatical about exercise, and I miss an occasional day because of my work and travel schedule," Bob said, "but I enjoy exercise of any kind. It's good therapy for mental tiredness, especially after a day at work. Coming home and doing some physical activity revitalizes me and gives me a positive mental attitude. After a while it becomes a way of life."

"I've enjoyed playing tennis for many years," Bob said. "I play a lot of the celebrity weekend tournaments in different places. In reference to club level play, I'm probably a strong 'B' player. Doubles is a good social game which I've been enjoying more in recent years, and it's a good form of exercise. I also play golf, but the sport doesn't give me any physical exercise unless I walk the course."

"I've never been a big weightlifter," Bob said, "but I try to maintain my upper body muscle tone. I have some gym equipment in my home, but it collects more dust than sweat. Weightlifting has always been my downfall because I have never enjoyed it, and it has thus been the hardest thing for me to do."

Bob doesn't have a regular routine, although he exercises on a regular basis. "I don't like to run in the same place every day," he explained, "so I run in different locations like the beach and the hills. If I'm ready to exercise and the tide is out, I'll run on the hard-packed sand near the water. At other times I run through the hills where I have some favorite trails and fireroads."

"I don't have a special diet, but I'm not a big eater," Bob said. "Sometimes I'll eat only one meal a day, and I never eat three, which probably makes me the reverse of what good health is all about. I'm never hungry in the morning, so it's easy for me to skip breakfast. If I eat anything, I will have fruit, coffee, or juice. I don't get hungry until after the lunch hour unless I exercise, which stimulates my appetite. I'll eat lunch occasionally, which may be my first meal. I'm content to eat light during the day, exercise in the early evening, and have a nice dinner afterwards. My main course is usually fish or chicken as I've cut down on my red meat consumption during the last 10 to 15 years. I watch what I eat, and I try to have decent meals."

"I weighed between 175 and 180 during my athletic years," Bob said, "and my weight stays the same without a conscious effort. I'm lucky that I'm not a heavy eater and have never had a sweet tooth. I'm not big on candy, but ice cream can be a weakness."

MENTAL ATTITUDE ABOUT HEALTH AND FITNESS

"I'm a firm believer in being fit for life," Bob stated. "God willing, I will always exercise because I enjoy it; I believe it's a way of life. The key to being physically fit is having a well-developed cardiovascular system; that's what fitness is all about."

Personal Fitness Goals

"As long as my health stays good and I have no illnesses to preclude it," Bob said, "I am going to be doing something physical. I'll cycle and swim more, making them a part of my daily exercise, because they produce less wear and tear on the body than running."

"I'm developing a little device with a good friend, Doug Burke, who was a silver medalist in water polo in the 1984 Olympics," Bob said. "This device, which we call 'Swm-Gym,' allows you to do distance swimming in a small backyard pool. By attaching Velcro surgical tubing to your ankles and something like a diving board post, you can swim without making frequent turns and without having your movements restricted. When you swim hard, the surgical tubing stretches and you move forward a little. As you slack off, it drags you back. Because you are stationary in the water instead of moving forward, your swim stroke has more natural resistance and you do more to develop muscles and cardiovascular endurance. We are testing 'Swm-Gym' with the United States Swim Federation in Colorado Springs to compare caloric burn in a short time with regular lap swimming and to determine if conditioning and strength can be developed at a faster rate. Testing 'Swm-Gym' myself, I find that swimming with this device for 20–30 minutes is like spending an hour or more doing regular lap swimming."

"We're planning to market 'Swm-Gym' through pool manufacturers," Bob said. "This device can help people make better use of their pools and encourage them to exercise. Swimming is the best form of exercise because water forms a natural girdle, there's less wear and tear on joints, and there's no pounding. It's good for people of all ages."

Recommendations for Improved Fitness of People over 40

"Be active," Bob advises his parents and other adults over 40. "I encourage my parents to exercise because physical activities, including a walk around the block, provide benefits through increased heart rates. The heart can't sit idle; it's a muscle that has to be exercised. You can have a well-developed cardiovascular system if you have a regular non-strenuous program to cycle your heart through a series of ups and downs, getting your heart rate up a little bit and bringing it back down. That's all you have to do."

4

Jay Lehr & Friends

Introduction

According to Marion Mehrtash, who is one of the "younger genera-tion" role models you can read about in this book, sports friends and training partners provide mental therapy for each other, including the motivation to exercise. "Make friends," she recommends to people over 40 who want to improve their fitness.

Jay Lehr has made friends through his life-long involvement with athletics. Two of his friends, Jim Bennan and Bill Malarkey, are profiled with him in this chapter for two reasons. First, their physical fitness achievements and regimen are worthy examples with interest-ing perspectives. Second, they enhance the idea of friendship as a positive factor in achieving a healthy attitude and body.

Jim and Jay, who swam on high school and college teams, met at a swimming pool while they were in the military service. After a 20-year separation, they met again, having followed separate paths to the Hawaiian Ironman. They have gone on to accumulate impressive numbers of completed events.

Bill and Jay became acquainted nearly 20 years ago through bike rides and Nautilus training. Sharing parallel problems, they had to give up some sports after developing arthritic knees. After turning to cycling and training as replacement sports, Bill and Jay found signifi-cant improvement in their arthritis due to cycling.

Bill, Jay, and Jim are "fit, firm, and 50" because they love to train, they exercise daily, and they use time efficiently. Despite other commitments and busy schedules, they find time for daily exercise because their fitness priorities are high. As an example of making time, Bill and Jay log hundreds of indoor bicycle miles each year while reading job-related material or watching television, and Jim cycles to and from work.

In considering Jay, Bill, and Jim as role models, they should be recognized as trainers rather than triathletes or cyclists. They are not national champions in any sport, and they put physical fitness training in the primary position on their priority lists. Although Jay claims to be non-competitive, he competes in many ways while striving for and achieving his fitness objectives. The point he wants to make is that winning and good scores are of lesser importance than physical fitness.

Jay and his friends, who look great despite their "over 50" ages, work hard to develop their appearance along with endurance and strength. The appearance factor should not be overlooked because vanity is a prime motivator for beginning and staying with a fitness program. People who want to look good and who do something about it enhance their chances for healthier, longer, and more productive lives.

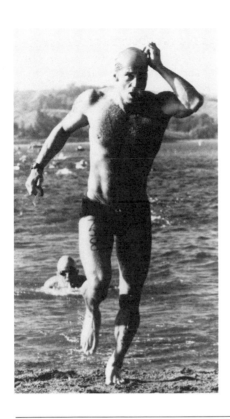

Jim Bennan

born: April 3, 1939

height: 6′ 0″

weight: 163

home: London, England

athletic highlights:

• set Illinois state high school swimming record in the 200-yard butterfly

• completed nine Hawaiian Ironman Triathlons

• completed a number of marathons, cycling and swimming races, and short triathlons

"My name is James Bennan, and I'm a friend of Jay Lehr. I hope you won't hold that against me. I have known Jay since 1957 or 1958. We met at a swimming pool when we were both in the military."

"I agree with Jay's methodology on fitness," Jim said. "Anyone can do it. The idea that a mature person seeking improved fitness should become a 'Jack Lalanne' can cause more harm than good. When these mature people look at superfit adults, I think they often say, 'That person's a physical fitness nut and that's all he does. There's no other facet to his life or personality and that just doesn't interest me. I think I'll just sit here or I'll continue to play golf and get my exercise that way.'"

"It seems that the 'over-40' group consider themselves to be on the road to fitness if they participate in the sedentary sports such as golf and bowling," Jim said. "However, these sports, and even a quick game of tennis, do not promote cardiovascular fitness. One of the best books I have read on the subject of fitness is *Fit or Fat* by Covert Bailey. This book, which can be easily understood by the layman, explains the road to fitness and some dietary rules and regulations."

"I believe people need role models," Jim said, "and the role models should be from everyday life. Their objectives and pursuits have to blend with the population at large."

ATHLETIC HISTORY

James M. Bennan, whose basic sport is swimming, described his athletic evolvement into a triathlete and a fit male over 50. "My athletic history goes back to 1952 when I began swimming on my high school team, which was a dominant power in Chicago and the state. At that time, I weighed about 130 and was of average fitness. The team was coached by Dan O'Brien, who was a great influence and stabilizing factor in my life, especially after my father died when I was a sophomore."

"Dan attacked swimming with a verve, and he created excitement," Jim explained. "I don't think I ever had a practice that wasn't exciting. Dan treated swimming almost like a business rather than an extracurricular activity. One thing I enjoyed was our break halfway through practice. Dan would stop our activity and talk to us. We would be on one side of the pool, and he would be on the other. Dan, who had a reputation throughout the world as one of the innovators and masters of swimming, would give us some pearls of wisdom and talk about stroke technique or the business of swimming. At that time his high school program was feeding swimmers into the systems at Big Ten universities and Eastern schools."

"I was a butterfly swimmer and I swam 200-yard events at the high school level," Jim said. "In the summer, Dan and the team would stay together. We would enter American Athletic Union [AAU] meets and swim all distances up through the college events, which were 200, 400, and 1500 meters. In my senior year, I set an Illinois state record in the 200-yard butterfly."

"I never made All-American, but I came close," Jim said. "I think I would have made it if I had used some training methods that are being accepted today. One thing that interested me in the late fifties was the idea that weightlifting was verboten for swimmers. However, Al Wiggins, a big man who was a sensational swimmer at Ohio State, brought himself up on weights, so the application of weight training was not foreign to the swimming body. I also used weights through high school. I liked the way weights made me feel, and I think working with weights was a terrific accomplishment."

"After high school," Jim continued, "I went into the Marine Corps for three years. I stayed fit and did a few swimming events until I was discharged. Then I went to the University of Notre Dame and started playing football. I loved it, but I never reached the pinnacle I should have because my progress was slowed by not having played high school football and not having learned the technicalities. I continued to swim, moving up from the 100-yard butterfly to the 200, which was a killer for me. The 200-fly is a difficult event, and I did not train at the high level necessary for the event. Although my swimming suffered and my football never took off, I wouldn't have done it any other way. I was active with football in the fall, swimming in the winter, football practice in the spring, and swimming all summer. My weightlifting was prominent in both sports."

Jim said he moved to California after college and gained some weight, probably up to the high 170s, by not doing any athletics for two or three years. Then he became active again. "I started with long-distance ocean swimming," he said. "I swam everything from one-half mile swims around piers up to seven or eight miles. The events were sponsored by the AAU, which began interjecting running parts into the races and introduced me to running in the mid-1970s. There might have been a swim-run-swim, a run-swim-run, or something like that which paralleled lifeguard events. In 1978, I entered my first triathlon in California as a relay partner, and I did a swim and a run portion."

"My weight dropped back into the 160s," Jim said, "and the physical activity helped my mental state through the process of a divorce. I was living in San Diego and knew Tom Warren, one of the fellows who did the original Ironman. I had followed Tom's career as a runner, swimmer, and cyclist, and I read the *Sports Illustrated* article after Tom won the race in 1979. I had not run a marathon at that time, but I had done some cycling and decided the Ironman would be a goal."

"The first time I entered the Ironman was in 1981. There were about 300 competitors in those pioneering days, and nobody knew anything about long-distance conditioning. During the race, we had to be weighed at five different points because the race directors were worried about loss of body fluid. If we lost five percent of our body weight, we would be withdrawn from the race. Times have changed from 'Gee, I think I can do it' to 'Let's race it.'"

In summarizing his athletic history, Jim said, "I have completed nine Hawaiian Ironman contests, a number of single marathons, some cycling races, and short triathlons. I have competed in pool and ocean swimming races, both short and long courses."

FITNESS REGIMEN

"My weight has fluctuated between 161 and 165 for years," Jim said. "I can track back through ten years of my training logs and see that my weight has averaged 163. An important measurement is the male waistline because that seems to be the critical area for accumulation of fat. While body weight can remain the same, body mass can fluctuate. My waist is 31–32 inches, depending on where I measure myself. Recent body fat tests done via calipers and underwater immersion measured my body fat at levels under ten percent."

"My diet is restricted," Jim said. "About the only time I eat red meat is when I have spaghetti, and I don't eat eggs, cheese, or milk. I eat few dairy products, and I try to stay away from fried foods and caffeine. I stopped drinking coffee and tea a couple years ago, but it's difficult finding substitutes in a social situation, and it loses some of its effect while fumbling around for a glass of water. I drink beer and wine except for the six- or seven-month period prior to the Ironman. I don't think giving up alcohol helps me, but it's part of an overall feeling of dedication and conditioning that possibly makes me feel better."

"I try to eat five pieces of fruit a day," Jim continued. "I may have an apple and an orange mid-morning, and I'll have two or three more pieces of fruit mid-afternoon. For lunch I might have a turkey sandwich on a whole-wheat bun with lettuce and tomato. I may add a little mayonnaise but no butter, and I drink something like orange juice. For dinner I always have baked potato, a salad, and something else."

"For exercise," Jim said, "I try to run every day on pavement or streets, and I am consistent in averaging 40–50 miles a week. I don't do a high percentage of grass running. I usually have one injury per year, and the injured member is usually in the back of my leg — a calf or hamstring. I seem to suffer the injury after I start cycling heavily, so I may develop an imbalance between my frontal quadricep muscles and the muscles in the backs of my legs."

"I moved to London three years ago and began cycling to and from work, which, as the crow flies, is about ten miles," Jim said. "However, I usually stretch that into a 20-mile ride each way by cycling in a nearby park. On a typical day, I get up at 5:30 A.M. and am on the road by 5:45 or 6:00. After riding into downtown London, where I'm due by

7:00 or 7:30, I lock up my bike and run. If I don't have a luncheon appointment, I'll run again. I swim two or three times a week after my morning ride and my run."

MENTAL ATTITUDE ABOUT HEALTH AND FITNESS

"I consider myself a closet triathlete," Jim explained. "I don't manifest the accomplishments or spend time talking about them because people dislike the discussion, particularly if they're not in tune with it. Since they find it boring, I try to stay away from the subject. I also avoid wearing my training gear like some kind of badge. Sitting around the house in bike shorts two or three hours after a ride is perceived by others as triathlon time. For example, if someone were to ask your wife, 'What did he do today?' Your wife would say, 'Well, he rode his cycle all day.' My guideline is to not wear gear after training."

"I think my attitude about health and fitness is contagious," Jim said. "Although I try to keep a low profile concerning my physical activities, I get a lot of questions from younger and older men. They want to know how I got into it, how I do it, and what kind of bike I buy. They ask to be taught this or that, and they express interest in swimming, running, or cycling with me. I think people get to know me and then let their guard down enough to ask for help because they are not happy with their fitness. I seem to have more problems with smokers. Smokers look at me and think I'm a nut; I look at them and think the same, and I doubt there will be much communication between us. I think those who are concerned about their fitness will always have questions for me when they find out what I'm doing or see me training. I tell them I am fit because I've trained for years, and then I'll give them my recommendations."

PERSONAL FITNESS GOALS

"My personal goals are to continue the level of fitness I have," Jim said. "Periodically, I look at my training regimen and reevaluate where I will change some things I have been doing. I will continue to run, but I'll try to vary the running and add variety into the swimming or cycling so I won't do the exact patterns every day. Doing the same thing daily can be deadly. Some people are turned off fitness because they get bored or burned out trying to do the same 45-minute workout every day."

"I hope I can continue doing events like the Ironman," Jim added, "and I don't see why not. I have reached this degree of fitness, and my swimming background allows me to concentrate on running and cycling. The run is difficult for me because I'm not a graceful runner and I lack the leg speed to be a strong distance runner."

RECOMMENDATIONS FOR IMPROVED FITNESS OF PEOPLE OVER 40

"Anyone can do it," Jim advises the 'over-40' group on the subject of improving their fitness. Achieving fitness can be fun, and you will feel better when you are fit. You will also gain self-esteem and encouragement by knowing that friends and family realize you are on the road to fitness."

"If you start with a series of small accomplishments and work forward that way, you will be successful," Jim proclaimed. "One of the best things you can do if you're on the road back to fitness is to have front, side, and back view photos taken of you with as little on as possible. Cast a critical eye at those photos and see if you are happy with them. If you don't look good on the outside, you know your inner parts are not working well even though you might consider yourself fit."

"I have found weight measurements and photos to be a real spur to people," Jim added. "In helping people become fit, you have to get them moving and you have to create an interest. You can't bump into someone and tell them to take off their clothes so you can take Polaroids of them. You have to get them to that first point, and that is the most difficult step to take. They need to realize the difficulty of this first step, and you have to encourage them to take it. If you can get them to realize exercise is fun and a better alternative to sitting in front of the television, they will get more out of it. However, it's difficult to get people to take that first step."

"One of the difficulties in getting started is getting over the first hurdle, which is where to go and what to do to get into a fitness program. Do they go to the 'Y' or another similar place? The sedentary person trying to get up from the couch may find gyms and health centers intimidating and will not go to one. What they need to do is make a decision to start a road back to fitness, and the road starts in front of their house. It starts by walking from their house to buy milk if the store is two or three blocks away. The next step is to plan walks because walking is the way back to fitness. You have to walk before you can run. One of the major problems is when people see others running and decide they have to join a 'Y' or fitness program when they are not ready for it. After a short time, they get bogged down and bored. However, by varying the distances and locations of their walks, including brisk 20- to 30-minute walks at lunchtime, people will begin to see progress and the rest of the world will open up for them."

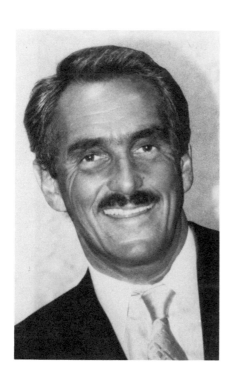

Jay Lehr

born: September 11, 1936
height: 6′ 3″
weight: 185
home: Columbus, Ohio
athletic highlights:

- lacrosse All-American honorable mention goalie at Princeton in 1957
- finished 400th in the 1968 Boston Marathon
- completed nine successive Hawaiian Ironman triathlons through 1989
- completed at least one skydive per month since 1978
- completed 25 high-altitude skydives in one day in 1988

A visitor entering Jay H. Lehr's home sees two unusual sights which personify Jay's athletic interests and his distinct personality. Stepping into a narrow two-story foyer, the visitor sees a stairway to the second floor and a hall leading to the rear of the house. At the end of the hall and fastened at regulation height to the upstairs balcony is a basketball backboard and hoop. Given a basketball, the visitor could shoot a free throw.

To the visitor's right is a living room, and to the left is a dining room without a floor. Instead of a dining room table, the room has a trampoline through which the visitor can see part of the finished basement where Jay has an office and a well-equipped fitness room. The visitor knows this is not the home of an ordinary man.

Jay enjoys the distinction of being different, and he differentiates the small number of fit athletes such as himself from the population by referring to the majority as normal people. According to Jay, a small percentage of people are hard trainers and earnest athletes, and they are dedicated to maintaining their bodies in excellent physical condition. The members of this select group, including the athletes profiled in this book, can be viewed as role models by "normal" people seeking improved physical fitness.

Having developed a demanding and beneficial fitness program for himself, Jay pursues a productive "thrill-a-minute" lifestyle that gets results. With boundless energy derived from a healthy body and a strong drive to get things done, he sleeps only five hours a night and he works whenever he can while doing something else such as traveling, eating, and exercising. "I get 19 highly productive hours out of each day," he claims. Due to his industriousness and proficiency, he has time to train several hours daily while fulfilling his duties as executive director of the National Water Well Association and functioning as an international leader and academic in the ground water industry.

Jay's athletic and fitness accomplishments are an example of what older adults can achieve through proper diet and exercise, and he has influenced people of all ages to improve their physical condition. As a younger man, before an advanced case of arthritis crippled his knees, he provided opportunities for adults to enjoy exercise on a regular basis by establishing amateur athletic programs. After rehabilitating his arthritic knees and gaining wisdom in the process, he emerged in excellent physical condition and decided to share his fitness program with men and women over 40 who have similar dreams of youthful vigor and vitality. Through years of athletics, Jay's mental attitude has been an essential factor in achieving success.

Jay's dramatic improvement in his physical condition proved to him the tremendous benefits of exercise. With knowledge gained from new techniques and experiments with his body, he began writing and lecturing to tout the benefits of exercise and fitness for mature men and women. He gives more than 30 talks a year for service clubs, schools, and fitness centers, and he assists Ross Laboratories, a division of Abbott Laboratories and a major manufacturer of nutritional products, in health maintenance workshops.

ATHLETIC HISTORY

Jay has participated in team sports and endurance activities throughout his life, and he enjoys pushing his body to the limit while training every day of the year. "However," he admits, "I have no special athletic talent except swimming."

"I'm a naturally gifted swimmer," Jay said. "I started swimming when I was 3." As a proficient swimmer, he swam on school teams through his freshman year in college, when he tired of it.

Jay strove to exceed in school sports despite a two-year disadvantage in physical maturity with his classmates. Having skipped two grades, he graduated from high school and college at the ages of 16 and 20, respectively. "Being younger than my classmates, I had to work harder to make teams, and then I found myself sitting on the bench. I played soccer and baseball in high school. As a freshman at Princeton, I swam and played soccer and lacrosse. After my freshman year, I dropped swimming and soccer for ice hockey and football. I did well as a goalie in lacrosse, receiving honorable mention on the All-American team."

After graduating from Princeton, Jay played football and swam on various teams while serving two years in the United States Navy. Leaving the Navy to join the graduate program at the University of Arizona, he found time to play lacrosse and semi-pro baseball, but he declined an offer to try out for the San Diego Chargers' expansion football team.

Jay became the first person in the nation to earn a Ph.D. in hydrogeology, and he soon forged a career as America's leading spokesman for ground water. His successful professional career didn't compensate for the many years he spent keeping the end of the team's bench warm. Having failed to achieve his sports objectives as a young man, he developed an obsession for athletics and in his middle years decided to fine-tune his physical fitness.

"I was driven partly by my intensive personality," Jay said, "and partly by a love of sports. Not having reached my potential as an athlete, I wanted more time to see what I could do."

Since adults had limited opportunities to play competitive team sports in the 1960s, Jay formed teams and leagues so he could play. He started a lacrosse team in Arizona, and *Newsweek* magazine referred to him as the father of Western lacrosse after he developed the program throughout the Western states. His interest in lacrosse led to joint appointments in academics and athletics when he coached the sport at the University of Arizona and The Ohio State University.

As a professor and coach at Ohio State, Jay took over and expanded the Columbus Lacrosse Club, an active men's organization of former college athletes. He played for and coached this club for ten years.

Jay began three community sporting programs in Columbus, Ohio.

These programs gave men in their 20s and 30s opportunities to continue playing sports when their skills would not allow them to continue as professionals.

1. The Central Ohio Men's Hockey Association has six to eight teams and has continued for 25 years. Jay managed it for 10 years, and he continues to play.
2. The "Heart of Ohio Football League" grew to a size of ten teams with over 300 adults playing tackle football. Jay played for 10 years, until arthritic knees ended his football career and temporarily suspended his hockey career.
3. The Columbus Masters Swimming Program has continued to expand since Jay developed it in 1970. Jay swam on teams that broke national records in the medley relay and 200-meter freestyle relay for men in the 35–39 age group.

Jay's sports activities caused severe damage to his knees, beginning with a hockey injury in Arizona and leading to four knee operations and arthritis. From 1974 to 1979, he wore heavy steel braces on his legs and spent 40% of his time on crutches. Like any true athlete, Jay was not a quitter. He continued a rigorous fitness routine, biking and walking when he was able and using Nautilus weight-resistant workouts to build strength.

Jay ran the Boston Marathon in 1968, when the number of runners exceeded 1000 for the first time, but he gave up running in 1976 when his knees could no longer take it. "I went back to playing ice hockey," he said. "Strangely enough I could skate despite my bad knees."

In 1980, Jay read a *Sports Illustrated* article about the annual Hawaiian Ironman Triathlon. Fascinated by the idea of swimming 2.4 miles in the ocean, biking 112 miles along hilly sun-baked roads, and running 26 miles, he decided to participate in a triathlon. Confident about swimming, which is the first leg of the triathlon, Lehr began training for the bike and running events. However, since he couldn't run due to his bad knees, he learned to race walk. Curious about whether or not he could complete a triathlon, he laid out a course in Columbus, Ohio and used newspaper publicity to invite others to join him. Nobody joined, so he competed by himself. "It wasn't all that hard," he relates. "Of course I was incredibly slow." Proving to himself that he could complete the Ironman, he decided to enter the February 1982 event in Hawaii. His goal was to finish, which he did despite walking the marathon wearing leg braces. The following October he completed the Ironman a second time, decreasing his time by 1.5 hours. In 1989, he completed his ninth straight Ironman.

After rehabilitating his knees in the early 1980s, Jay was able to run marathons, including the Ironman, without leg braces. In recent years he completed the New York Marathon and several Columbus marathons. In 1989, he recorded his best time in the Columbus Marathon with a 3:39 run.

Jay continues to enjoy many sports in addition to running, cycling, and swimming. Playing year round, he has maintained a competitive position in ice hockey, where his team has won the Ohio Men's League championship the past two years, and he still plays a limited number of lacrosse games for senior teams. An active skydiver with 700 jumps, he holds two state records. One record is for jumping every month for the past 12 years. The other record is for high-altitude relative work formation dives in one day. On May 3, 1988, he jumped 25 times from over 10,000 feet in 12 hours.

FITNESS REGIMEN

Through diet and exercise, Jay reduced his body fat to eight percent. "I have essentially a no-fat diet with 75 percent carbohydrate and 25 percent protein," he said, "and I take multi-vitamins daily to supplement my potassium and vitamins A, B, and C. The week before an endurance event, I consume little protein and I drink six quarts of EXCEED High Carbohydrate Source."

For the last nine years, Jay has trained daily to prepare himself for competing in the Hawaiian Ironman Triathlon. He tries to work out every morning and evening. For example, on a typical weekday at home, he rises at 5:00 A.M. after five hours of sleep, exercises for three hours, and arrives in his office by 9:00. His basic weekday routine includes weightlifting 2 hours, biking 90 minutes, and running 30 minutes. On weekends, he runs one hour and bikes two hours each day, and on one day he lifts weights for two hours.

Jay supplements his basic exercise routines with anything else that he can fit into his schedule. At least one weekend each month he skydives to continue his 12-year record of consecutive monthly dives. Two days each week he works out on the trampoline in his dining room, and once a week he plays ice hockey. From May through October, he takes a 100-mile weekend bike ride. At the beginning of summer, he swims one mile a day five days a week, and in past summers he has doubled the number of laps to build up for the Ironman.

MENTAL ATTITUDE ABOUT HEALTH AND FITNESS

Jay, who believes lifespans are predicated by genes, explained his thoughts on fitness and longevity. "My father and mother died at 75. I feel fairly confident, if my parachute continues to open, I will last to 75. I don't have one single delusion that anything that I'm doing will extend my life much past that age. If I extend it for a few years, great, but if I don't, it doesn't matter. What really matters is how I feel today, tomorrow, and next year."

The road to fitness is unlikely to be free of pain, and no one is more aware of that than Jay. His active lifestyle has led to many painful experiences, in particular knee injuries suffered from ice hockey, football, and trampolining. Four knee operations took their toll; then arthritis, as part of the aging process, developed in his knee joints, causing them to deteriorate. Calcium deposits built up in the joint and inflammation brought on fluid accumulations. In describing his knee joints, Jay said, "Each movement caused roughness to rub against roughness. I found it difficult at times to get up from my desk because the pain was so severe."

While training for the Ironman during the early 1980s, Jay found changes occurring within his knees. Low-stress exercise had a beneficial effect as it polished the inside of his knee joints, which are now relatively smooth, as proven by x-rays. "In the following two years, through rigorous training, my arthritic condition improved as a result of techniques I developed. For example, I biked at a high RPM and low-load on my knees, and I did unique exercises with Nautilus leg equipment. After a couple years of these workouts, I was able to begin running to a limited extent and eventually resumed running with little or no disability."

Seeing an improvement in his knees, Jay began a serious rehabilitation program and focused his scientific mind on the minute details of physical fitness for his body. He learned the benefits of non-stressful exercise, and the fitness program he developed has made him one of the world's best-conditioned athletes in his age group.

Jay believes his excellent physical condition allows him to function well on five hours of sleep, and, with limitless enthusiasm, he continues to analyze the results of moderate and rigorous exercise on his body. Having conquered severe knee problems to complete nine Hawaiian Ironman Triathlons, he has demonstrated mental toughness and perseverance in overcoming weaknesses to achieve goals.

Personal Fitness Goals

Jay may have competed in the Hawaiian Ironman for the last time because his interests are shifting to bodybuilding. His new goal is to compete in the Mr. Ohio contest in four or five years and not to look out of place on the stage. When looking at himself in the mirror, he doesn't think he looks his age, and he believes it's conceivable that one day he can acquire an excellent body.

Recommendations for Improved Fitness of Adults over 40

Jay has achieved victories and gained wisdom that he wants to share with others who have similar dreams of youthful vigor and vitality. He has no secret formula for achieving fitness, and he does not pretend to be a substitute for a medical professional. His message is simple: it's not too late to achieve your desired level of physical fitness if that is your goal and if you work each day to achieve it. Success depends on your state of mind and not your age.

Jay's basic advice to adults over 40 is simple. "Eat no fats, exercise daily, and lift light weights."

"Eat no fats," Jay recommends. His intent is to avoid all fats because they can inflict the most potential harm on the body. Do everything you can to prevent them from creeping into your diet.

"Exercise daily," Jay stated, "to get an aerobic workout and to develop positive habits. You need aerobic exercise to develop a strong heart muscle and a good circulatory system, and you must develop high-priority habits to negate a myriad of reasons for improper eating and not exercising. Whether you are a beginner or advanced student of physical fitness, you must modify habits because continuation of current habits will not achieve improvement."

"You can develop positive habits through repetition," Jay said. "Get up a half hour earlier each day and do an aerobic exercise. Ride an exercycle, swim, run, or walk for 30 minutes each morning. Don't worry about speed or distance, but spend 30 minutes on your activity. In the evening, before dinner if possible, exercise for another 30 minutes."

"If it hurts, stop," Jay preaches. "Exercise at a level that your body finds comfortable. If your body feels like going fast, let it go; if it does not, don't push it. Your objective is to develop good exercise and nutrition habits which, in turn, will develop good fitness. However, you will be less inclined to develop a habit when you associate pain with the activity. Proceed with your activity on a regular basis and allow your body to set a comfortable pace or rate."

"In order to replace negative habits with positive ones," Jay said, "you must have goals that you want very much to reach and you must avoid boredom, which kills more individual fitness programs than any other factor. Therefore, it is essential to perform a variety of enjoyable exercises on a regular basis without worrying about speed and repetitions. Competitive sports are a wonderful addition to a fitness program because they add enjoyment and prevent boredom."

Jay said the concept of daily exercise without discomfort or pain and without timing or counting reduces the sources of possible negative information. Working out at the same time each day is best because this removes the decision-making aspect and therefore another possible point of negative input. Using this approach, daily exercise can become an enjoyable habit.

"Mental and intellectual obstacles must be eliminated," Jay continued. "A positive attitude must be built, and every aspect of the subject must be internalized such that little memorization of technique is required. You can attain a positive approach through mental programming from daily repetitions of exercise."

"Lift light weights three times a week," Jay advises, "to maintain muscle strength and tone. This applies to women as well as men. Since the purpose is not to build bulk but to make you look better and feel better, get a set of dumbbells and use them regularly."

Jay believes everyone wanting to improve their physical fitness should use a simple methodology to get started, regardless of age and current level of physical fitness. "A simple and enjoyable conditioning program will endure through the aging process. Set a goal, find an enjoyable way to exercise, and develop a simple low-cost program with small milestones that will achieve your long-term goal," he suggests. "After launching a 'no fat, light exercise' program and developing good daily habits, personalize your program to acquire specialized results. For assistance, many good fitness books on nutrition and exercise are available in libraries and book stores."

Jay's recommended approach to achieve physical fitness is a lifetime program which will not ensure longevity, but it should improve health and productivity. A healthy mind and body are the greatest benefits of sports and fitness.

Bill Malarkey

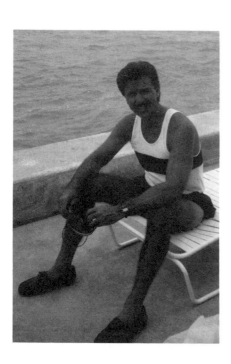

born: April 9, 1939
height: 6′ 1″
weight: 182
home: Dublin, Ohio
athletic highlights:
- played basketball and football at University of Pittsburgh
- in 1988, biked 240 miles in one day to cross Ohio from border-to-border, east to west
- in 1989, biked 230 miles in one day to cross Ohio from Lake Erie to the Ohio River
- in 1989, biked about 3300 miles outdoors and rode a stationary bike about 2700 miles

William Malarkey, M.D., is certified in internal medicine and endocrinology, which is a specialty of internal medicine and deals with thyroid, pituitary, and other such problems. He is Professor of Medicine and Physiological Chemistry and Director of the Clinical Research Center at The Ohio State University. In the late 1970s, Bill became acquainted with Jay Lehr through their mutual interests in athletics, and they have since become good social and biking friends.

"Jay is amazing!" Bill states. "I first met him at a Nautilus fitness center about 1975, and I remember his braces and limping and our discussions concerning his knee surgeries. Although I knew little about him and his knee problems at the time, I thought, 'Geez, in about five years this guy won't be walking.' It's amazing what he's been able to do with those legs. There's a message there, and I'm not sure anybody understands what it is, except we know that inactivity is not helpful to diseased or normal parts of the body."

"Jay told me his last set of x-rays looked pretty good, and that's hard to believe. I know he's got a fairly good pain threshold, but if there's no mechanical movement in his knees, he can have the greatest attitude in the world and nothing's going to happen. Jay said his knee sockets have been worn smooth by high revs with no resistance on his stationary bike, and it must be something like that. Somehow the exercise must inhibit the processes of inflammation, perhaps by creating hormones. I have noticed similar improvement in my knees, which now have less decrepitation and pain. It's amazing, just amazing."

ATHLETIC HISTORY

"I came from an athletic family," Bill said. "My father was on the University of Pittsburgh's 1937 national championship football team. Athletics and football were an important factor in our family and a tradition in our community, a suburb of Pittsburgh. I went to a high school attended by several children of former Pittsburgh teammates, and I spent much of my day playing sports. I played football, baseball, and basketball through high school, and our teams were successful in winning championships."

"In my junior year," Bill continued, "we played in the Western Pennsylvania championship football game in Pitt Stadium, and Mike Ditka, who became my teammate at Pittsburgh, was on the opposing team. My sport was basketball, which is what I really wanted to play at Pittsburgh, but they talked me into playing football also my sophomore year. I played guard in basketball, and I played quarterback and defensive back in football. Those were the days when we went both ways. I only played football one year because I didn't enjoy it as much as basketball. I played basketball until my senior year when I decided to work with an interdenominational youth group after being accepted into medical school."

"I wasn't active in athletics while going through medical school and internship," Bill said, "but I kept in shape by jogging and weightlifting after I went into the Navy. In the 1960s, there were few competitive opportunities for people over 25, and staying in shape wasn't a popular thing to do. You seldom saw people jogging or exercising. There was little data then on exercise, but what we had indicated the importance of a daily structured exercise routine. My informal routine of running and a little bit of weightlifting kept my weight down."

In the early 1970s when Bill was about 32 or 33, he said that new research data substantiating the importance of exercise motivated him into more aggressive workouts. "I played competitive tennis on a local club's team year-round, both indoors and outdoors. I played tennis for about ten years, and then I started having some knee trouble, which is a consequence of many basketball and football injuries. I found that cycling was good exercise for bad knees, and, because I enjoyed the sport, I got into an aggressive program, including bike tours."

In 1988 and again in 1989, Bill biked across Ohio in one day. His riding companions were Jay Lehr and Bob Holmstead, a middle-aged biker whose leukemia went into remission after his spleen was removed and after he resumed strenuous workouts on his bike. According to Bill, these endurance tests, which took about 15–18 hours to complete, and the training in preparation for the rides, "probably put me in the best physical condition of my life. I'm sure I can do a lot more now than I could when I was 20 years old."

"In 1988, we biked across Ohio from east to west," Bill explained. "We rode from Bel Air, Ohio, which is across the river from Wheeling, West Virginia, to the Indiana border at Richmond. We followed Route 40 much of the way, except for the early going in eastern Ohio when we rode about 100 miles in the mountains. Before this ride, I didn't realize how hilly it is there. From the hills and across the flatland we rode against a lot of headwinds, making that a rigorous 240-mile 18-hour ride."

"Last year we biked south from Lake Erie to the Ohio River. Our starting and ending points were the Ohio cities of Vermillion and Portsmouth, and the distance was about 230 miles. The elements were against us that day because we had a lot of rain, making our early morning hours dark and uncomfortable."

"Our bicycle maintenance guru from Columbus' Campus Bike Shop, Dave Heuser, accompanied us on both tours across Ohio. About every hour the driver stopped so we could get food and fluid from the van. When it was dark, the driver followed to give us some headlights because our bike lights didn't provide enough light in rough terrain. The van also protected us from the rear when we were in heavy traffic."

"We were impressed with our strong finishes on both trips," Bill stated. "We calculated a usage of 8000 to 9000 calories a day, but with our reasonable training program and attention to fuel, we kept our fluids and calories up. We drank Exceed both times."

"Because of my biking, I don't play much tennis now," Bill said. "However, I could probably resume competitive play with fewer knee problems because biking has improved my knees."

FITNESS REGIMEN

"Like most people," Bill explained, "there has been a marked shift in my diet from a traditional midwestern fare, maybe 12 years ago, to the last ten years during which I've had an absolute conviction to move away from fat for a couple reasons. One, a lot of fats contain cholesterol. I have a very low cholesterol, in the 130 to 145 range. I'll eat meat, but I avoid things like french fries that don't taste so good to me now. A second reason for avoiding fats is calories. You pick up nine calories per gram rather than the four calories per gram that you get with carbohydrate and protein. There has been a big change in my diet to more carbohydrates, cereals, breads, fruits, vegetables, rice, and potatoes, and there is less emphasis on high protein and high fat. I still do sweets like cookies, but I avoid the high sucrose stuff. I don't eat pies and things like that, and I don't eat much candy."

Bill discussed a problem that endurance athletes must confront. "When you are exercising and burning up as many calories a day as I do, you have to replace those calories and that's sometimes a problem. If you get too much fiber and carbohydrates, you may have bowel trouble. There seems to be a fine line between your intestinal tract and your body needs."

"Assuming you have a balanced diet and watch your cholesterol and lipids, the key thing is to maintain your body weight once you have your ideal level. I monitor my weight; if it's dropping, I increase my caloric load, and if it's going up, I back off. I'm never fighting a problem of more than a couple pounds and my weight fluctuates in a narrow range. I weigh myself about every other day. The time of the day is important, and it should be the same each time you weigh yourself."

"The basis for my exercise regimen is cycling," Bill said. "I belong to an informal cycling club, and the members help to push each other. I keep good records of my indoor and outdoor cycling, and the number of miles I ride each year has increased from 2000 in 1986 to 6000 in 1989. I do about 45% of my cycling indoors, so weather is not a factor. I average an hour a day cycling on weekdays and one-and-a-half or two hours per day on weekends. During the outdoor season, I may ride four to five hours a day Saturdays and Sundays. I ride 120 to 150 miles a week year-round, accomplishing this by keeping a good pace of 18–21 miles per hour so it does not take as much time as one might think. The indoor miles are pleasurable because I read or watch TV while I cycle. My outdoor rides often include friends, and we cycle in beautiful areas or do something competitive. I supplement this aerobic work with some cross-country skiing."

Bill said, "I lift weights about three times a week. I use the Nautilus program a couple days, usually on weekends, and I do a dumbbell workout. The weight work has been a maintenance program the last several years. I want to maintain my strength rather than gain bulk."

"My supplemental exercise includes walks with my wife," Bill said. "I've been avoiding the stops and starts in racquet games because of my knee problems. I hope to do something significant physically when I'm 80 or 90, and to do this I want to have a fairly good set of knee joints. By keeping joints in good shape and by exercising regularly, it's amazing what can be done past age 70."

Mental Attitude about Health and Fitness

"The benefits of exercise go beyond the number of trophies won," Bill said. "For example, exercise can improve our work performance and appearance, make us feel better, help us avoid drowsiness in the afternoon, and control our weight. These are clear-cut benefits. Another nice thing about exercise is that it makes you monitor how you spend your time. People should think about these benefits more than medals and trophies."

"In my early years, I viewed exercise as something that was a by-product of playing a sport. Now I view exercise as an important element of my daily life. Without a healthy body, I may not achieve my goals and aspirations. As I get older, I expect to have more discretionary time and financial assets. It would be unfortunate to be caught in the dilemma that would preclude me from using my time and assets because my body could not participate in the ventures I would like to do."

"Exercise is both enjoyable and a means to help accomplish my goals at an older age," Bill said. "It will enable me to get away from the retirement mentality because I don't want to retire. I might change careers and I might change the way I spend my time, but I don't plan on retiring. If some things I do make money, fine; if they don't, fine. We need challenges, goals, and mountains to climb, and we need to contribute to other people's welfare. By doing all these things, we can feel good about the time we are spending. In regard to helping others, I believe the balance has to be there for a complete picture. If we're going to help others, we have to be in shape to do it. We've got to have the spiritual, physical, and emotional resources to help effectively, and exercise can build these resources."

"A training regimen should not add stress to already stressful work and home environments," Bill stated. "Stress can be added if you have to make sure your training regimen is adequate so you can compete in weekend activities. However, if you view your regimen as a means to accomplish other things, it has a different format and can be fun. Jay Lehr has expressed this to me several times. Jay competes in events that aren't really pleasurable to him. He says he isn't a competitor, but I think he says that to make his point. He enjoys training, and he gets more benefits from exercise than from the competitive events which wane in comparison."

PERSONAL FITNESS GOALS

"My personal fitness goal might be unrealistic," Bill said. "I want to get into better physical shape as I get older, which is the opposite of what everybody thinks happens with aging. I envision having more time to exercise and to do things without reneging on family and work responsibilities. I want to commit more time to training, but I don't want to overtrain or let training become too big a part of my life. I want to explore more things in terms of exercise, beginning with unusual things on the bike. I derive so much pleasure from exercise that I hope my goal is not a selfish thing; I think it will have a positive impact on others."

"In regard to specific events, I have talked with others about biking across the country at a pretty good pace but not doing 350 miles a day like the Ramride. For another event, Jay Lehr and I have talked about biking 300 miles from Akron to Cincinnati in one day. I may try competitive cycling if I can find a safe circuit."

RECOMMENDATIONS FOR IMPROVED FITNESS OF PEOPLE OVER 40

"First," Bill recommends, "understand the reasons for physical fitness because there's a need to be convinced and committed. Then, three words I use to describe any new venture apply here:

1. **Vision** — Visualize the goal to be accomplished.
2. **Implementation** — Implement a habit-forming scheme. Do something enjoyable at a certain time each day to form the basis of your regimen; the other things you do will supplement your basic program.
3. **Enthusiasm** — Get positive feedback from this venture; if

you are not enthusiastic about your sport or activity, do something else. Look for different ways to approach it."

"These three things need to be going on simultaneously. In terms of implementation, put your goals in writing and record your daily accomplishment so you can see whether you are measuring up."

5

LET'S TALK ABOUT FITNESS

I want to draw you a road map of a fitness program I have developed that will work for you. I'll explain why fitness is for everyone and why I care so much about the subject. I'm going to tell you some things that you may have already read or heard, but I'll also offer information that will surprise you. I will include some instructive information about fitness on everything from diet to your actual exercise program. I'll offer basic tips that will interest you, and then discuss how you can mentally internalize them in ways that can change your life.

I have become an expert on physical fitness by studying and practicing the subject for most of my 54 years, during which I have pursued a dual career. People in the ground water industry who learn that I'm off in Hawaii doing the Ironman, or out running somewhere at 5 o'clock in the morning, or hear of my other exploits as an athlete (sky diving, ice hockey, gymnastics) wonder why the National Water Well Association is paying me to be their executive director. Where do I get time to run this 20,000-member organization with a staff of 80? The fact is that due to the level of my fitness, I require very little sleep. I can get 19 very productive hours out of every day, which is enough to pursue two separate careers. I spend a great deal of time at my job on airplanes, flying mostly at night and working during the flights. If I weren't fit and weren't an athlete, I don't think I could even do the job required of me by the National Water Well Association. I don't suggest that you pursue two careers, but I insist that you'll enhance both your work and personal life when you become more fit.

I especially enjoy lecturing and writing about fitness because it isn't my job. I often go into health clubs across the nation and see a bunch of gorilla-like people telling others what to do to get fit. I guess they know what they're talking about, but I prefer to talk to people who are integrating fitness into their lives and not doing it as a profession. Perhaps, because this is the case in my situation, you will listen to me more closely than you would to a hired fitness professional.

Society's Fitness Profile

Those of you reading this book probably range from the very fit to the not fit at all. I'll describe you to yourselves.

Ten percent of you are incredibly healthy. You do virtually no exercise and are getting on in years, yet you have boundless energy and follow no prescribed fitness program. You probably do all of the wrong things, and yet you're in good shape and feel great. The reason for this is that you inherited great genes. You're just lucky. You inherited genes that are doing the job for you, and you don't need to pay attention to anything I say. You know who you are because your dad, mom, and your grandparents are the same way. Read on, but you don't need my help.

Another ten percent of you are also in good shape. You don't do much exercise, or at least you don't follow a prescribed plan. You're in great shape because you have a correct lifestyle. You have the right job and the right jobbies; you live in the right place; you breathe the right air; you eat the right food. You simply have good lifestyle habits. You're in good shape, and you don't think about an exercise regimen or fitness program.

Twenty percent of you do think about exercise and fitness, and you are already following some kind of program that's meaningful to you. You know that you're feeling better than you did when you weren't exercising. You know that it pays to be in good shape.

The remaining sixty percent of you have problems. If you could ask me questions, you would give me a litany of things that bother you through your daily and weekly life. It could be tiredness or an aching back. You might have problems eating or problems sleeping. All of these are a result of the fact that you are not fit. You may be overweight; you may be underweight; but you are not fit. A significant number of you, perhaps a third of that sixty percent, are going to learn something in this book that may change your life. You will finish reading this book and a year from now, you might write us or tell others that this book changed your life. Conversely, some of you will lay down this book and ignore everything you read. The rest of you are going to give it a lot of thought. Some will say "I'd like to give it a try but I don't think I have the wherewithal." A few of you may get moving for awhile and then fall back; a few of you may think about it but never get moving. I hope you are one of the individuals who will use the knowledge you are about to learn.

REASONS TO BE FIT

There are a lot of reasons to be fit. An obvious one is personal vanity. It is not the best reason, but it is the greatest incentive to get yourself to get fit. But I care far less how a person looks than how he feels. I'm less interested in reshaping your body just so it looks good in the mirror than I am concerned about how you are going to feel about yourself every day, and how much more you are going to get done, and how much you are going to enjoy all the days of your life. Vanity is just an incentive to get people going.

There are advantages, I suppose, in being trim. I know that your clothes can be less expensive if you are a smaller size. My wife tells me that there is a real economic advantage in not having to buy special sizes. But let's talk about those aspects of fitness that play a major role in your life. Many of you are aware that women have a calcium deficiency called osteoporosis which increases with age. We know beyond a shadow of a doubt that exercise, particularly strenuous weight-lifting exercises, dramatically retards if not eliminates osteoporosis.

Your entire arterial system declines as you get older. Exercise keeps the capillaries open; it keeps the whole plumbing system moving. You're just a walking plumbing system, and you all know what happens to pipes when you don't care for them. As they age, they get clogged with chemicals and precipitates and you have to clean them or change the pipes. The human body is the same way. You are born, you go uphill for awhile, and then you begin to self-destruct. The genetic code is unraveling and you're all self-destructing; you're all going downhill, but you **CAN** do something about it. In fact, your blood, you capillaries, your entire arterial system begins degrading and you've **GOT** to do something about it. Doing nothing about it is just accepting the shortest, least-quality lifespan available to you. Exercise **will** improve the entire plumbing system which carries the blood which carries the oxygen and nutrients throughout your body.

If you are over fifty years of age and you have never had a backache, you should be very proud. Most people have back problems because of the disuse of muscles and imbalance in muscles. We know today that the way to treat backaches is with exercise. It isn't bed rest, although if your pain is so bad that you can't walk you may have to start off with a day or so of bed rest. The primary cure for backache is not manipulation by chiropractors, although there are occasions when you are in such bad shape that this is the best thing to do. Ultimately it's the strengthening of the muscles that keeps you upright. That is done with exercise. We all experience general muscle strains throughout every-day life. If you're doing something, you're straining something. When you are fit, these pains will decrease dramatically. Exercise improves the quality of every-day life and allows you, if you're late for a meeting, to run 100 yards to catch up with yourself. If the driveway is full of snow and you have got to get out of the driveway, fitness allows you to shovel quickly without wrenching your back or risking a heart attack. Exercise allows you to change your pace of life, radically, through the day or through the week, without suffering the consequences of this change.

A five-year experiment was completed with about 200 men over sixty years of age. The study consisted of two groups: one group had five years of aerobic training and the other group led a sedentary life. At the end of the five years, it was shown that a dramatic difference in mental acuity (I.Q.) existed in men in their sixties who exercised vs. men who didn't.

If you think about it, it makes sense. What does the brain need to function? It needs oxygen. When your blood system starts to slow down, not enough oxygen is getting to your brain. You all know people who get older and begin to lose their mental faculties. I'm not talking about Alzheimer's disease or becoming totally mentally incompetent. I'm just talking about becoming a little less sharp. How many of you have said about someone, "he or she is not as sharp as they used to be." It's little more than the inability of the body to carry oxygen to the brain.

Your physical attributes and mental attributes tie together. We are not talking about vanity. We are not talking about how you look. We are not talking about being overweight, although weight is a factor. We are talking about the quality of your life.

Those of you who are thirty or more are already on some level of decline. Do you want to accept that decline, or do you want to fight it? I believe you can fight it more effectively than you ever dreamed. You don't have to give in to it. I am not talking about not wanting to get old. I am speaking of the battle against the degradation of the body.

Do you move into a brand new house, furnish it, and then sit down and watch that house degrade for the next 20 years? Or, do you give it an occasional paint job? Do you fix the plumbing after five years? Do you fix and clean your furniture? Do you have your carpets cleaned? Of course you do. You don't let your house degrade because if you do, you know that in time you won't be able to live in it.

I'm not sure I can help you extend your life. But I virtually guarantee that you will be healthier the day you die. I know that sounds crazy. If you're healthy, why would you die? Well, you'll die from some other reason, not from a general physical decline. One out of five people dies from cancer. Some people will die of congenital heart disease because their hearts just aren't genetically suited to last too many years. But while I am not sure we can significantly alter our lifespan, we can extend the lives of people who would die of general unhealthiness. Recent studies clearly indicate a difference in life expectancy between individuals in good physical shape and those in terrible shape.

Our lifespan primarily relates to our genes. My father and mother died at 75. I feel fairly confident, if my parachute continues to open, I will last until 75. I don't have any delusions that I can extend my life much past that age. If I do, that's great, but if I don't, it doesn't matter. What really matters is how I feel today, tomorrow and next year.

Now let's consider what the degradation cycle looks like so you can spot your position in it. You know who doesn't need to exercise and yet does most of it — people under 25. They've got everything going for them. It doesn't really matter what they do; their bodies are still going to look pretty decent. Right around 30, we're entering that twilight zone where we should start to get serious about fitness. While the decline begins in the 30s, even then we recognize only moderate changes that most of us can live with. You won't have a serious decline in your 30s unless you contribute to it with exceptionally poor health habits, but at 40 the decline of a physical system that is not cared for can be dramatic. It gets steeper in the 50s, and if you've done nothing into your 60s — if you're not living that great lifestyle I've described — and you don't have those great genes, you can become unnecessarily old and decrepit. But it can be arrested.

A young person, in his or her early 20s, going into a significant program of weight training and aerobic exercise, will experience, over a 12-week period of training, a ten percent improvement in strength. That exact same program, when done by an individual who is 50 years old, will yield a fifty percent increase in strength. Because the decline by age 50 has been so dramatic, you can experience five times the improvement of a 20-year-old.

Weight lifting will be the new path for the older generation. I'm not talking about big barbells and a sweaty gym — but a weight-lifting program for people of advanced years will be the coming thing. The results will be absolutely amazing.

Diet and Exercise

Now let's get to the specifics of diet and exercise. I want to touch on three things. I'm going to talk about diet, then I'm going to talk about aerobic exercise, and then I'm going to talk about weight lifting — in that order.

Most of the diets people go on are kind of crazy. They subject themselves to more hardships than are required. There's only one food that you have to worry about not eating, and there's only one number you have to count. Don't eat fat; it's that simple. Fat is what kills you. Fat's the stuff that clogs up the whole plumbing system. Eat anything you want as long as you don't eat things with fat in them. Now you can't really avoid fat completely. If you try to eat no fat at all, you'll eat all the fat you need to be healthy. I guarantee it. But avoid the things that are mostly fat. There's only one book you'll need and it's a book you can get at any local bookstore; it's called *The Fat Counter*. The book is a listing of how many grams of fat are in any food on the face of the earth. Read it and find out what to avoid. You already know the worst ones. Margarine and butter have no redeeming qualities. Don't eat fried foods. Don't use oil-laden salad dressings. No magic here. Fat has no redeeming qualities, and you can replace it with better things. If you are really trying to lose weight, you can make a salad dressing with lemon and herbs and make that salad taste very good. You can steam your vegetables and put herbs on them and they taste even better than with butter. Of course, you can't totally avoid fat, but you can limit yourself to 22 grams of fat a day. That's all you have to do.

If you need to lose more weight, the other thing you can do is count calories. If you want to go on a diet, eat 1000 calories a day. Anyone can get by on a 1000 calories of the right foods.

I happen to eat 5000, but I exercise for almost four hours a day.

People ask me what I think about while I exercise. Only one thing. Food. I earn my food. I don't eat it if I haven't earned it. Other than fat, I eat everything. People are amazed at what and how much I eat. I just make sure that my calories match my exercise.

Drink plenty of fluids. People don't drink enough water. Part of the function of the plumbing system is washing stuff out of you. You have to drink a lot of water. Some people say not to drink any diet sodas, but I don't mind a diet soda. Just wash a lot of fluids through your body.

Take vitamins. I'm a believer in vitamins. I don't think any of us eats such a healthy, well-balanced diet that we can ignore vitamins. So, I take a multivitamin every day. I'm also a vitamin C freak. I've read all of Linus Pauling's books and I really believe that a megadose of vitamin C reduces the number of colds you get. If you do get a cold, an even bigger megadose reduces the symptoms that make you feel rotten. I won't go into that; read a book by Linus Pauling. He's written about five of them on vitamin C, and they're all interesting.

Another pair of vitamins/nutrients I strongly recommend are potassium and choline. If you tend to get muscle strains and muscle cramps, you are probably low in potassium. I recomend taking at least two potassium tablets a day containing 99 mg each of potassium, which is the equivalent of about three bananas a day. I also eat a banana every morning. I find it especially useful in curing tight back problems. Potassium does work as a muscle relaxer. The other thing that I eat all the time is something you have probably never heard of — it's called choline. It looks like a kind of rubbery sand, and it is available in health food stores. It does two wonderful things: it improves your mental acuity and allows your body to burn fat a little bit faster. Nothing dramatic. You're not going to lose weight with it, but it is an assist. It reduces my tension level and increases mental acuity, especially if you're sitting in a lot of meetings and spending a lot of time getting frustrated with people. I have found that everybody who eats a couple of teaspoons of choline a day can see the difference.

I can personally prove the value of choline beyond a shadow of doubt. My wife will tell you I am not an easy person to live with. I have no temper and don't get mad; nor do I ever complain. The problem is that I never get tired. I keep asking her if she wants to go to a movie or take a bike ride or go out somewhere even if she's told me four times already that she doesn't want to go. I claim it's not nagging. I just want to be absolutely sure I got the answer right. But she claims that it's normal to get upset with me from time to time. After she started taking choline, she went five months without uttering a harsh word to me.

Can you imagine going five months without uttering a harsh word to your husband or wife? I rest my case.

AEROBIC TRAINING — MORNINGS

Now, let's talk about aerobic training. I believe that every human being on the face of the earth should have one hour of aerobic exercise a day. Most books will say a half-hour, or three or four sessions of 20 minutes a week, but I think that it should be every day. If you really want major results, if you want to be really fit, we are talking about an hour a day. I'll show you how you can get that hour a day to work for you. I'll find you the hour that you didn't know you had.

I can hear you saying that you don't have an hour to exercise; that you can't get done what you do now. But you do have the time. First of all, you sleep too long. I don't care how long you sleep, get up 30 minutes earlier. Get yourself an exercise bicycle — any kind of exercise bicycle. If you have other ways you want to do this — fine. But if you're doing nothing now, I guarantee that the exercise bicycle is the easiest approach because you can do it indoors. Riding a bike outdoors is great, but we want something you can do all of the time. So go out and get an inexpensive exercise bike. It can be cheap, but it must be comfortable.

The most important thing about riding a bike is that the seat height has to be correct so you don't hurt your knees. When sitting squarely on a bike, one leg should extend so that your heel reaches the pedal at its fullest extension with your knee bent about 5 degrees. If your seat is such that your knee is bent much more or much less than that, you are going to experience discomfort in your knees.

An excellent biking program is as follows. Get an exercise bike and start biking every day. If necessary, get up half an hour early to do it. You won't need the extra sleep once you get the exercise. You can be almost still asleep and get on an exercise bike. I do it every day. I crawl down to the basement not really awake, get on the bike and start moving my legs. At first, it's like slow motion. After a few minutes, the pace picks up. Start off the first week with only five minutes a day. Five minutes, no more. At the end of the first week, add two minutes for a total of seven. You may think you can get on the bike and ride for 15 or 20 minutes right away, but don't do it. Five minutes is all you're allowed. I kid you not. **FIVE MINUTES!** When you get off that bike, I want you to hunger to get back on. Your reward at the end of the week is to add two minutes and then you're up to seven. At the end of two weeks, you can add two more minutes and thus ride for nine. You must

NOT alter this. You'll add two minutes every week until you get to 30 minutes and that will occur in the 14th week. I want you to take 14 weeks to get to 30 minutes because my goal is not to make a biker out of you; my goal is to create such a habit that to get out of bed and not get on that exercise bike will drive you nuts.

Now here's what has happened. Five minutes of sitting on an exercise bike is so easy that it's not a problem. So you do it for a week. What a silly thing; this is so easy. So is seven minutes, then so is nine minutes. You're going to get to 30 minutes without having suffered for one split second. You're creating a habit.

Habit is what matters in fitness. It's ingraining some desire in your body for a good thing that is then hard to break. Most of you could get on the bike and ride for 20 minutes and that'll be okay for a few days. But then you'll notice that 20 minutes was pretty tiring and you pulled a muscle or there's something else you'd rather do this morning. You don't want to do the 20 minutes and you don't do it and you haven't formed the habit. But once you've done this for a few weeks, you will have developed a habit and you'll find it hard to break.

After 14 weeks, you'll be riding for 30 minutes. Now look what I will have done for you in that 30 minutes. You will recognize long before you reach 30 minutes that your whole day is going better. You're starting your day with your blood racing through your system. You've warmed up your body. You've jump-started yourself. Sure, you lost a little sleep, but you will see that your performance through the day is better than it used to be. So, eventually, you sleep 30 minutes less each day in exchange for a greater efficiency in whatever you are doing. Biking indoors is warm, and you can do it in your pajamas. I don't care what kind of exercise bike you get, most of them are pretty decent. You don't have to spend a lot of money. If you already have a bike, you can buy a stand and put your own bike in the stand. Okay, that's half of your hour a day.

Aerobic Training — Evenings

The other half is going to be a little tougher, but it's going to do even more for you. The other half is walking fast and perhaps eventually running. It's done at night right before your evening meal. This is a little tougher to do with the mix of things that are going on in your day. You should try to do it outdoors before your evening meal. I don't care what the weather is, although if it is really bad you can get a walking machine and do it indoors. Inside or out, you must walk very fast for five minutes every day for a week. Again, you add two minutes at the end of each week. Again, it takes 14 weeks to get to 30 minutes. The object here is to continue increasing the speed of your walk as well as the distance. If you ever get to the point where you can't walk fast enough, you may decide to jog. That's fine. When fast walking gets uncomfortable, jogging actually becomes easier. If you already jog or know you have the capability of jogging, jog five minutes. Add two minutes a week until you get to 30 minutes of jogging. I don't care about the speed as long as you consider it "brisk." I care primarily about the time. It is important that we are talking about fast walking or easy jogging, and I'll tell you why.

It does a number of things for you at the end of the day. Number one, it is the greatest stress-reliever in the world. Everybody builds up tremendous stress by the end of an average day. I don't care whether you're dealing with household problems or business problems. Nobody has much energy left. People say, "I can't walk at night; I'm pooped." But when you finish doing this, you won't be pooped. Exercise doesn't take away energy; it gives you energy. This may not seem logical to you, but it's true. It's a scientific fact. You will definitely increase the quality of your evening.

If I tell you that you're going to improve the quality of your day by biking in the morning, the impact on your evening is going to be double what the biking does in the morning. In the morning you didn't have stress, but by night, you do. You're going to remove stress. You're going to rebuild your whole energy system and you're going to do it, hopefully, before dinner.

You can walk after dinner if your dinner wasn't too heavy. If you just can't work it in and you have already had your dinner, wait 30 minutes and walk then. When you finish, I guarantee you will have three quality hours left in your day for whatever you want to do. The pounding of your feet really does shake out what we call "stress" in your body. So, jog or walk in the evening. You will build another habit until you actually resist eating dinner without having done your evening exercise. It's going to take you a while to get there, but you will build the habit. Don't be concerned about speed. If you feel sub-par, go a bit slower but still move briskly. Everyone knows what brisk is for him or herself. It is a funny word, but we intuitively know that it describes a state of activity that is clearly not laid back.

My theory about exercise is counter to many others. You have heard of "no pain, no gain." I believe in "never any pain." If it hurts, don't do it. If you're not comfortable, slow down until you are comfortable, but stay on the edge of brisk. Young kids can suffer pain, but adults don't need to. We shouldn't subject ourselves to something that's unpleasant and uncomfortable for any length of time. We certainly can't develop a habit of doing something that hurts. So, if you feel badly, just do it more slowly. I really don't care how slowly you actually bike or how slowly you walk, but there are no excuses for not doing both. If the weather is rotten, put on extra clothing. Don't tell me you can't go outside because it's too cold. Add enough layers of sweaters and jackets to keep you warm, which isn't much if you are moving fast enough to generate some of your own body heat.

WEIGHT LIFTING — BELIEVE IT

The third part of your program is the resistance exercise, and this is something you've probably never heard before. Three times a week you should spend 30 minutes lifting weights. The weight lifting that everybody in the world needs is very simple. It's done with dumbbells, not barbells. A dumbbell, of course, is not your child or spouse; it is a small hand-weight with a hand-grip in the middle and two balls of metal on the ends. They can be purchased from one pound on up. I do 14 different dumbbell exercises that cover every part of the upper body. We're not going to worry about the lower body because you're running and biking — but every upper body muscle can be easily exercised with dumbbells. You can do them while you're watching television. Put the weights in your family room and spend part of your evening lifting weights and watching television. You can still be a couch potato, but just sit on a bench or sit on the floor instead of the couch and pump iron while you're at it.

I recommend that women buy a set of dumbbells ranging from 3 pounds to 15 or 20 pounds, which includes a 5, an 8, a 10, and 12 in between. Men should probably go up to 25 pounds. They can fit on a rack four feet long which stands on the floor. I recommend that some people buy chrome dumbbells so they can put them in their living room. They are four times more expensive than plain iron dumbbells, but they look nice and literally beg to be used. My wife has chrome dumbbells and she loves them. They cost about $2.00 a pound. You can buy regular dumbbells for 50 cents a pound and can get a stand for between $100 and $150. Put it in your entertainment room and it's furniture. When you're watching TV, you do your exercises. There is no need to describe a detailed program here since you can buy a book that outlines a program at any weight-lifting store in the country where you can buy the dumbbells. Nearly all the books are good. One of the best is Rachel

McLish's *Perfect Parts*. There are more than 14 excellent dumbbell exercises. You wouldn't usually do all 14 at once, but rather between 5 and 7 exercises in a session. This will take you less than 30 minutes. Work on different parts of your body each day. Alternate between one set of exercises one day and another set a couple of days later. In three sessions a week, of about 30 minutes each, you will realize a dramatic health improvement.

Men will build moderate musclature. Women will not so much develop muscle as tone their upper body. Both men and women will get significantly stronger. Muscles do become stronger without increasing in size. Men's muscles tend to get bigger, but women's don't. The women you see with big muscles take steroids. Before women started taking steroids, the most muscular girl had small feminine muscles. Rachel McLish, who was one of the early women body-builders, has a gorgeous body with attractive muscles.

You will develop a more attractive physique and like what you see, but the program we're talking about is not intended to build muscles; it's purpose is to do resistance work to improve your bloodflow, lower your cholesterol, strengthen your bones, and improve your physical strength and skeletal balance. Weight lifting also has benefits similar to aerobic exercise. It burns just about the same amount of calories and you continue to burn an increased number of calories for several hours after your weight-lifting session.

You begin each exercise with 15 repetitions with a light-weight set of dumbbells. Then you put them down and take the next heavier set of dumbbells and do the same exercise 12 times. Then put them down and use the next heavier set 8 times. For most of the exercises, you won't need more than 15 pounds, maybe 20. You might start at three pounds or you might start at eight. So for most of the sets you might use 5, 8, and 10; or 8, 10, and 12; or 10, 12, and 15, depending upon how strong you are and what the exercise is.

An old friend of mine does a trick with his weights. He leaves his dumbbells all over the house. When his phone rings there's bound to be a dumbbell right there. He picks up the phone, then he picks up a dumbbell. While he's talking, he's working out and instead of having one formal workout he integrates it into his daily routine. It's an interesting approach, and it works for him.

If you don't require your body to do resistance exercise, your body's muscles cannot maintain fitness. They will degrade rapidly with advancing age. You can reduce the decline due to aging by eighty percent with exercise and weight lifting.

I'm 54 and I'm getting better at everything I'm doing. I'm not even close to my potential. Of course, I have an advantage — I was not very good at anything when I was a kid. I had no where to go but up. I am still improving as a swimmer, as a biker, and as a runner. I'm working at it. So, this whole mindset about getting old and declining physically is not necessarily so. I admit that I must work harder at it than a 25-year-old trying to accomplish the same things. He'll get where he's going quicker than I will, but that's not too big a price to pay as far as I'm concerned.

JOINTS, LIGAMENTS, AND SPEED

Allow me to provide you with a potpourri of ideas as we move toward a conclusion of this discussion. You must have good shoes. Throw away your old sneakers, go to a good running store, and get the newest technology in walking or running shoes. I don't care what they are; you must have good shoes or you're in serious trouble. I personally wear running shoes with my three-piece suits. I'm not ruining my knees, my ankles, my day, or my back by wearing dress shoes when I have to walk a lot. If I just have to sit down somewhere and get up for a few minutes, I'll wear dress shoes. But I try to avoid them. You must have good shoes to protect your ankles, knees, and feet. They'll last you a very long time. Find an athletic store where the salespeople know what they are talking about. NIKE has given me free shoes to race in. They make good shoes with air-cushion soles. My knees and ankles, my whole skeleton has loved these shoes. But a lot of companies make good shoes, so be sure you choose some.

If you're having problems with your legs while walking or jogging, I can solve 60 percent of them by telling you to go to a running store and buy heel lifts — soft rubber heel lifts called Sorbethane. It's a jelly-like rubber that never hardens. Good running shoe stores sell them. They are rather expensive at $10.00 for a set of two. Put them in your shoes, and they will change the mechanics of your stride. A majority of your leg problems will be eliminated just by wearing heel lifts in your shoes. By simply starting your stride from a quarter-of-an-inch higher, everything in the mechanics of walking and running is different, so whatever was rubbing before, it's rubbing differently now. You could develop new problems from the new mechanics, but few people do. If you do, take the lifts out. It's a simple trick and works for almost everyone.

Stretching — If you're going to exercise, should you stretch? Maybe. Why would I say "maybe?" Why would I be so cavalier about stretching? The reason is that I'm not advocating anything very strenuous. I didn't tell you to go out and run many miles or bicycle very fast. I'm advocating starting out slow with everything, so you may not need to stretch.

You do need to stretch (cool down) when you're finished. If you get to where you're biking fast or running fast, you'll see that things will tighten up. Stretch whatever tightens up. Stretch your back a little bit; lean over and stretch the back of your legs. When you're finished exercising is when stretching is important, and you'll know what you need to stretch when you see what tightens up. We're going to start everything so slowly that you probably won't need it before you start. I think there's too much emphasis on stretching and, in fact, if you over-stretch before you start while you're cold, you can pull muscles and create unnecessary injuries.

If anything bothers you, just put ice on it for 20 minutes. If it keeps bothering you, put ice on it every hour or two for 20 minutes. Ice is the greatest muscle-problem curative. It does several things. First, it is an anesthetic; second, it eliminates bleeding of any little capillaries in the area; and last, after it finishes shrinking everything and you take the ice off, blood vessels expand, allowing an increased bloodflow without the possible damage from heat. Heat is okay if you're sure you don't have any internal bleeding. I'm never sure, so I never use heat. Of course, you might consider it inconvenient to walk around with an ice bag strapped to some part of your body, but the rapid improvement experienced from treatment with ice will make you such a strong believer that you will become less self-conscious.

Don't use a watch to time your speed during aerobic exercise. Use it only to determine the length of your exercise period. I don't care how fast you bike or how fast you run, a watch is a terrible thing. I have ranked among the top ten Ironman triathletes in my age group in the world and I never use a watch. I don't want to know how fast or how slow I am. I know whether I'm going fast or slow for me. I don't want to intimidate myself by worrying about my speed.

I have two more points to make. The first is about flexibility. The most important thing in my whole program is listening to my body and being flexible with my game plan. They are one and the same thing. I never tell myself what I am going to do tomorrow in specific terms. I tell myself that I will do so many hours of exercise, but I don't know what it will be. I do only what my body feels like doing. I have never had a bad training day in my entire life, because if I decide to go out and run, I never decide in advance how fast I'm going to run, which would then make me disappointed if I could not run that fast. I say, okay, body, let's go out and run. You do whatever you feel like. If you want to go slowly, fine. If you want to slow down in the middle of the run, that's okay, too. If you feel good and want to speed up, that's fine. Whatever my body wants to do, that's what I let it do. You probably know that if you want to get good you have got to do some fast running or cycling. During a two-week period, my body wants to run fast often enough. I may not have improved dramatically over the years, but most of the people who started working out with me have retired long ago. I'm still at it. I'm a turtle. not a hare. I make progress slowly. You can too, so don't intimidate yourself with a watch. I personally do one big speed workout a week. Recently, I went out to a college track at six o'clock in the morning, and I did ten quarter-mile sprints with ten slow quarter-mile jogs in the middle. You might say, "How fast were your sprints?" I have no idea. I didn't have a watch. I just ran fast. I knew it was faster than I normally run, so it was fast for me. It was hard. It wasn't too hard because I don't do anything that's too hard. I don't want to suffer. But it was harder than normal so, for me, it was a speed workout. If I had a watch on and had seen how slow it was, I might have said, "That's depressing, I thought I was running faster." Then I might say, "I'm going to go out faster next time." Then next week I wouldn't want to go out because it hurt too much. Don't suffer pain. Don't use a watch. You know what your body tells you; do whatever it feels like doing.

There's only one thing you cannot allow your body to decide. You can't allow it to tell you not to do anything. Make it do something. Let it have its way, but don't let it tell you to forget your bike ride in the morning or your run in the evening or whatever program you select. If you want to replace the bike ride with a rowing machine or you want to take an aerobic class in the evening, that's up to you. I guarantee you, however, that my way works.

Finally, a little trick about getting any of these things done. I know that one third of the 60 percent of the people who are not in good shape are going to finish this book and be different people. You're really going to get going. But the rest of you aren't so sure. I have a couple of simple tricks that can work for you. Frank Zane, a former world champion body builder, who really got me going in weight lifting, has a technique he calls "positive affirmation." When he very much wants to do something that's important to him, he describes it to himself in a very short phrase and then says it over and over, internally, hundreds of times a day. That is, when he's not doing anything that requires his mental attention, he is repeating the phrase over and over and over again, hundreds of times a day, thousands of times a week. It has an amazing ability to get you to do it. I gave up sweets that way. I developed an affirmation that "I would eat no sweets." It sounded like "I will drink no wine before it's time." I repeated it over and over again. I couldn't stand the ringing in my head. I didn't want to hear that stupid phrase anymore. I think I gave up sweets in defense of having to say it over and over again. I cheat a little on occasion, but that's okay. You can decide what it is you can't get yourself to do, make up a little phrase, and say it over and over again: it's simple, but it works. Habit, habit, is what we are talking about. You must make exercise a compulsive habit from which you cannot escape. Then, fitness will be yours!

In the following chapter, you will find the answers to everything you ever wanted to know about fitness and even more that you would never have thought to ask. It's written in dictionary form but can be entertainingly read straight through from A to Z. It is not dry textbook knowledge, but rather knowledge learned from a lifetime of trial and error, with every thought verified within the community of individuals who are fit beyond their years. Read it, enjoy it, and use it.

6

An Encyclopedic Discourse on Physical Fitness

Abdominal muscles (Abs): These are invariably the weakest portion of our physique once we reach maturity. For most women, childbirth spells the end of a firm stomach. For men, the sag usually begins sometime between 25 and 35. This is a shame because anyone in his or her youth who decides to maintain a firm abdomen throughout life could do so in six to eight minutes a day. In fact, that's all it takes at any age, but once the tone of the abdominal muscles is lost, it will take up to two years of serious effort to regain them. While two years may seem like a long time, only twelve minutes a day, five days a week will do the trick. We won't go into the specifics of the abdominal exercise routine here, but will simply urge you to obtain the best routine available entitled "SynerAbs" from Health For Life. It was developed at Stanford University. The booklet is fully illustrated and has twelve separate phases of development. A firm stomach, especially if it is not hidden by excessive fat, can be a source of great joy and satisfaction to mature men and women. Furthermore, firm abdominal muscles will go a long way toward eliminating back pain so prevalent among older people. Back muscles and abdominal muscles oppose each other and, thus, both must be strong. It's worth two years of effort. After all, we are not training for an event next Saturday but a

211

healthier, fuller life. There really isn't too much hurry. When you're ready, send for "SynerAbs." You won't be sorry.

Ability: The power we all have to be in better physical condition than we are now.

Abstain: A word that must be applied to the use of excessive quantities of alcohol, smoking, and the eating of fatty foods.

Abuse: What we do to our bodies when we don't abstain from fat, alcohol, and cigarettes.

Accelerate: To increase one's speed; not commonly necessary in a mature fitness program.

Accentuate: Something we do to positive aspects of our life, while eliminating the negatives.

Accessible: Where exercise equipment and routines should be so that you trip over them amidst your daily goings and comings.

Accommodate: Something you should do to any partner who is willing to exercise with you. Exercise is good at any speed, and friends in search of fitness are hard to find.

Accuracy: It denotes precision, something an exercise program need not be. Stay loose, stay flexible.

Aches: A physical annoyance that comes from using a part of the body not frequently activated. They increase with age as your circulatory system loses its capacity to carry healing warmth and oxygen throughout the body and then carry away dead cells. They can be dramatically decreased through regular exercise, although you must remember that the initiation of all new activities will exacerbate aches for a reasonable period of time. You can figure out the difference between an ache and a pain by recognizing that most of us continually accommodate some aches, but few of us can easily live with pain (see *Pain*). You can continue to exercise through aches; in fact, while exercise may exacerbate the ache in the short term, it will heal the ache in the long term. This is not the case with pain.

Achilles tendon: The large tendon running from the heel bone to the calf muscle. Injury to the tendon will quickly immobilize an individual, making exercise all but impossible. This tendon may be the most important part of the body to stretch prior to exercise. If you tend to be tight below the calf muscle, simply stretch it before activity by leaning up against a wall from a distance of a few feet. The ultimate Achilles tendon injury is the severing of it, requiring surgery and a lengthy period in a cast. A word to the wise — stretch it before use, especially if it is tight.

Tendons have very little blood supply and thus stiffen and age more rapidly than other elements of the body. What a shame when a 30-second stretch each day can prevent it. Simply stand 3 to 4 feet from a wall with your legs straight, lock your knees, and extend your hands to the wall slowly, allowing your body to approach the wall as you bend your elbows. The Achilles tendon will be felt to stretch. Hold the position for 30 seconds and then get on with your day.

Action: In the 18th century, Isaac Newton developed four laws of motion. One of particular importance to a person's body can be paraphrased as follows: "it is much easier to keep a body in motion than it is to start a body moving." Unfortunately, after our youth, too many of us essentially park our bodies. It does them as much good as keeping an automobile in a garage for a year without starting it. The automobile needs to have its lubricants flowing through its system just as the human body, as a result of exercise, needs its hydraulic system of blood and other fluids coursing rapidly through it on a regular basis. A small percentage of people (perhaps 10 percent) live a long and active life with little exercise, as a result of exceptional genes. Don't count on having them.

Activity: In the context of physical fitness, it is absolutely any event which will have a positive benefit to the body. Aerobic activities, such as swimming, cycling, rowing, and running, require rapid movements to exercise the heart. The slower activities, such as resistance training with weights or Nautilus equipment, exercise the muscular and skeletal system but do not have aerobic benefit.

Acupuncture: An Oriental method of treatment involving the insertion of needles into the skin at precisely determined points. There is some indication that it can be successful, but it should probably only be considered as a last resort in therapy. Beware of any therapy that claims to heal anything. Acupuncture is one such therapy.

Acupuncture and other placebos: When age increases our physical pains, we tend to buy our way out of them with any eccentric techniques that come to our attention. In fact, exercise which will reduce or eliminate most physical discomfort is usually a last resort. While acupunc-

ture has undoubtedly, on occasion, had some beneficial results for some people, most will be better off saving a considerable amount of money by avoiding it. Its placebo effect will carry a patient back for many useless repeat visits until it becomes clear that little permanent improvement is being achieved by the technique. It is probably best left to the Chinese and Russians who, indeed, have very successfully used it in place of anesthetics during surgery.

Adapt: Something one must do when beginning an exercise program until it becomes a natural part of everyday life.

Addiction: Exercise and fitness will, eventually, become an addiction if you develop your program correctly. Building up by small increments (as described under *Incremental training*) will make it difficult to miss a day of exercise — at which time you can be said to be addicted. Exercise is a positive addiction.

Adhesion: When muscle fibers become bound together. The micro fibers generate in muscles when they become traumatized by some type of an injury. They rob the body of both flexibility and strength but can be lessened in impact by deep body massage.

Adipose tissue: Synonomous with fatty tissue. Approximately 25 percent of female body tissue and 15 percent of male body tissue is adipose. A fit, athletic female can approach 15 percent, while a fit male can approach 10 percent or lower.

Adrenalin: A chemical substance generated within the body to increase the heart rate under conditions of excitement or sudden stress. Virtually everyone has felt it under circumstances of fear or impending danger. Athletes experience it regularly when faced with an extraordinary challenge. Individuals embarking on a fitness program will find that they get frequent adrenalin rushes as the result of instantaneous enthusiasm for an exercise they may be undertaking. This is not to be confused with the runners' high. Adrenalin rushes are encountered much more frequently and do not create the feeling of euphoria of endorphins. When resulting from athletic activity, however, adrenalin rushes produce positive experiences.

Aerobic training: The type of exercise that forces the pulse rate to a high enough level to strengthen the heart and improve the cardiovascular system. It must be continued for a minimum period of 20 minutes to achieve beneficial results.

Aerobics/jazzercize: Many people perform exercise better in the company of others. For this reason, aerobic and jazzercise classes have prospered throughout the country. They are fun and effective, but a regular schedule must be maintained if this is one's primary aerobic exercise. Particular care must be taken to avoid high-impact classes which place too much stress on older joints. Too much jumping around is counterproductive. Most classes are now classified as high and low impact. Stay with a low impact.

Affirmation: The mind is a wondrous thing, and it can be trained to control the body. Positive mental affirmations can be the base for the development of will-power, of which few people believe they are capable.

A positive affirmation is the creation of a short phrase describing what you desire to do or achieve. This phrase should be repeated to yourself in every spare moment — possibly over a hundred repetitions a day. The affirmation must be feasible, although it need not be insignificant. From a training perspective, it could be as simple as this statement: "I shall perform aerobic exercises one hour each day." If weight is a problem, your affirmation could be: "I will eat no sweets." It seems simple, but it works. It took me only three days, at 300 repetitions per day, to change from an addicted dessert-eater to someone who laughs at offerings of empty calories.

If you are just starting out, adjust your affirmation down to say, "I will run 10 minutes each day," or "I'll eat only one sweet per day." Then, change it with time as your goals need adjustment to higher plateaus. I get through long training runs with the simple affirmation: "Just keep on keepin on."

How does a senior athlete develop good training habits after years of a sedentary existence? There are two secrets to this. The first is a positive affirmation of your goal. The second is a realistic goal.

From a training standpoint, having the proper mental attitude involves a sincere desire to achieve fitness as well as the ability to visualize a goal you want to achieve in a reasonable period of time. That reasonable period can well be a number of years. Rome wasn't built in a day, and you can't change your internal and external physical structure in a short period of time. But with the right attitude, the fact that you can change it is no longer in question.

Age groups: Many athletic activities

that offer competition today offer age-group participation. 10K races, marathons, triathlons, bicycle races, swimming, and track-and-field contests are frequently held not only for youth but for masters' level competitions (generally over age 40). Prizes are awarded in categories encompassing either five- or ten-year age groups. This allows individuals of advancing years who care about competition to compete against those who have reached roughly the same level of aging. This has been a wonderful boon to competitive people but should not, in any way, dissuade those among us who have no competitive instincts from exercising strictly for the fun and health of it. Quite frankly, the authors of this book are ranked among the latter group. We could care less if we ever beat anybody or where we stand in a group. It's quite exciting enough just to get out and do it; enjoy the activity, and sense those very real feelings of increased aliveness that comes with being fit.

Aggravate: What you can do to a physical injury by continuing to exercise it. Although exercising an injury can assist in the healing process, it can be difficult to tell if one is overdoing it and aggravating the early injury. All that can be said, if full mobility is possible, is that pain should be your guide. If it hurts too much, don't do it.

Aging: A general process of physical decline that comes with advancing years beyond a probable mid-point of improving physical capability that exists at least to the age of 30. The aging process is clearly a genetic unwinding, so to speak, of the human spring which results in a loss of flexi-

bility, a decline of lean muscle mass, a reduction in the immune system, a loss of endurance, and a number of other factors. Scientists have discovered beyond a shadow of a doubt in recent years that the aging process can be reduced through aerobic exercise and resistance training so that few of the negative aspects of aging need impact the daily health of an individual well toward becoming an octogenarian. Aging will eventually do us in, but we need not feel badly as we approach the end of what can, in most cases, be a very wonderful life.

Agony: Something all athletes feel when they overextend themselves and encounter oxygen debt or, so to speak, hit the wall. This state should never be encountered by individuals engaging in a fitness program at the age of 50 or over. Such a negative experience will quickly dissuade one from further fitness activities.

Aiming low: The destroyer of old athletes is unrealistic, short-term goals. Set your heart on achieving any particular time in any particular activity that's a little tough to reach and you are setting yourself up for disappointment and failure. Our parents made a big mistake when they told us, as children, to hitch our wagon to a star. One day we all woke up and realized that we couldn't all be number one; we couldn't all be champions; but most of us could, indeed, be failures. You may find it hard to believe, but we haven't failed in achieving a goal in many, many years; not because we're particularly good at anything, but because we set goals so low that they are easily achievable. There's always time to raise your sights when you get to your first milestone. However, there's nothing worse than the demoralization that comes with failure. Often in the company of really great athletes when we describe our goals, people snicker. But we don't mind, because we learned long ago that the race doesn't go to the swift of foot — it goes to the ones who keep on running. If there's anything we do well, it's continuing to run. We've left many a champion behind.

Airplanes: If you travel a great deal by air, you already know that it is physically debilitating. It is not your imagination. It is a result of major changes in altitude and, subsequently, atmospheric pressure which literally puts your body through a wringer. As a result, your joints will swell and your body stiffen. It's easy to reduce the impact, however, in two ways. First, always take an anti-inflammatory pill before departure. This can be an over-the-counter formula such as aspirin or Excedrin or an anti-arthritic prescription you may already be taking from time to time. Second, during your flight get up and stretch all parts of your body in any area of the cabin where there is a little extra room. Simply stretch everything that feels tight so that when you get where you're going, you'll feel more like the living than the dead.

Alcohol: Everything and anything is okay in moderation. It's a proven fact that a little alcohol has a positive effect on the aging human body. A single mixed drink or a couple of beers will not hurt you if you can stand the calories. Becoming inebriated, on the other hand, has no redeeming qualities and, in fact, does irreparable damage to the body. That's right, irreparable! Obviously,

you can survive a bout of inebriation once in a while, but if you do it more than three times a year, your body will have internal scars that are unnecessarily difficult to overcome. Enjoy a drink at social functions; it's relaxing and encourages open social interaction. If you can't stop at two, stop at none.

Alibis: There are no acceptable ones for regularly missing or dropping out of an exercise program.

Alternate: What you should do with your various aerobic exercise opportunities in order not to lose interest, get bored, go stale, or burn out. Rowing, cycling, running, cross-country ski machines, swimming, and aerobics can all be rotated into a fitness program to serve your needs and keep the regimen refreshing.

Altitude: If you live high on a mountain or in Denver, Albuquerque, or Cheyenne, exercising there or anywhere is easy because your body is adjusted to the thin air that carries your blood throughout your system. You probably feel exceptionally fit when you come down from the mountain. But, if you live near sea-level, altitude will take its toll and no amount of exercise over the short duration of a week or two will change that. It will simply further debilitate you. Take it easy at high altitudes. It has never been proven that athletes truly benefit by training at altitudes except that it teaches them to deal with increased pain. For the older person used to some fitness routine, cut back 20 percent for every 2000 feet of altitude you encounter on a short business trip or vacation. If you move to a high altitude, you can completely adjust to a normal routine in two or three months.

Altruism: A state of total unselfishness which tends to cause individuals to spend all their time contributing to others and not enough to themselves. Fitness programs will always steal time from other activities and, in fact, a certain amount of vanity is required to continue the pursuit of a fitness program as other incentives may be inadequate. Vanity is antithetical to altruism. But remember, you can better help others when you feel good about yourself, not to mention your capacity to better serve others when you are more energetic and in better health.

Amateur: What we all (over 50) are at everything, so we should never be intimidated by others at any level of expertise or excellence.

Ambulatory: The only requirement necessary to be able to exercise. Actually, many physically impaired people who are not ambulatory are becoming fitness fanatics, such as wheelchair racers (WOW! are they fit). Now, what's your excuse.

Amino acids: Twenty organic nitrogen-containing compounds form the building blocks of protein. A balanced diet contains all of the necessary amino acids. Body-builders virtually all take supplemental amino acids in order to enhance their capacity to build muscle. The supplements are generally thought to be effective.

Anaerobic: This is activity that takes place in the absence of oxygen. It is normally a technical term used to describe arduous physical activity at a rate beyond the capacity of the body to supply needed oxygen. Swimmers, runners, and cyclists toward the end of a short, fast sprint-type of race will go into what is called an oxygen debt which is, in fact, anaerobic activity.

Ankle weights: It is not uncommon to see people in aerobic classes wearing ankle weights. They can be beneficial in adding resistance in a variety of slow, static, calisthenic movements to improve muscle tone of the legs. They should be avoided when actually locomoting the body. They put increased stress on the back, just as hand weights do, and we strongly oppose this. If your goal, however, deals with improving the tone of your legs and buttocks, ankle weights can be useful. If you try them, start with extremely light ones of one pound and build up in weight very slowly. Rarely will you ever want or need to exceed three pounds. We recommend against using them in aerobic classes unless the class is an extremely low-impact one.

Anorexia: A loss of appetite resulting from strict dieting and fear of being obese. It results in depression, anxiety, and sometimes death. It is almost always accompanied by, if not directly linked to, psychological problems.

Anticipate: Something we have to do on a short-term basis, to be sure we get our hour of aerobic exercise each day. Don't let your schedule crowd you out; anticipate your day in advance.

Arch supports: Shoe inserts that improve support and stabilization. A high-tech form of arch supports is called orthotics. These are normally custom-made by foot specialists. They are an extremely good idea for individuals having consistent problems with their ankles and knees following extensive walking or jogging.

Arms: Next to our abdomens, we are most likely to let our arm strength deteriorate with age. Conversely, if we use our arms effectively, our entire upper body will benefit. A certain amount of resistance exercise is a must for the arms. See the extensive exercises under *Weight lifting*.

Arteries: The vessels that distribute your blood and its oxygen throughout the body. These pathways can become clogged with fatty tissue or other restrictions as a result of poor diet and disuse.

Arthritis: Rheumatoid arthritis is a disease requiring medical attention. Exercise will definitely help, but it won't cure it. But the arthritis that comes of age and injury befalls nearly all of us. Exercise can reduce its effects dramatically. It is a result of calcium deposits forming ever so slowly in the joints due to age or in response to jarring injuries. Just as a rolling stone gathers no moss, joints which are constantly articulating do not allow the easy precipitation and solidification of calcium. There has commonly been a false belief that the onset of this calcification we now call osteoarthritis should lead a person to lower his or her physical activity level. If anything, the reverse should be true. We should avoid jarring impacts as they do exacerbate the problem. But the easy and continuous motion of walking, jogging, cycling, or swimming definitely retards the stiffness that we all experience with age. The key is motion without stress or weight on the joints. Run slowly, cycle in easy gears, swim slowly but, if anything, increase your activity to fight arthritis — don't reduce it. As always, check with a sports physician before beginning any new program.

Aspire: To be fit, and you will be, with a minimum of will power and a reasonable amount of time.

Associative thinking: When a person exercises, he or she will either think about what they are doing or purposely avoid this and let their minds wander. The former is called associative thinking and the latter, dissociative thinking.

Normally, when we walk, jog, or run, we like to let our minds wander. Unless you are racing the clock, which should be avoided anyway, dissociative thinking is desirable. It's relaxing when your mind wanders and productive if you allow yourself to ponder problems of the day. The same is true for swimming, but less so for bicycling, when a bit more concentration is required to stay upright and out of the path of motor vehicles. If, on rare occasions, you wish to time an activity or even enter a race, then the most effective way is to focus on every movement for the duration of the activity.

Athlete: Not what this book is about. We just want plain folks to experience a higher quality of life through exercise. Whoever participates in sports is considered to have natural talent. This book was not written for today's athlete but will be very useful for all those who may once have been athletes and lost sight of the path of physical fitness. Being a natural athlete is too often a double-edged sword. The athlete who does not have to work exceptionally hard to obtain high levels of competence in his or her youth tends to do even less with progressing age and falls totally out of shape. A surprising number of very fit gray panthers were never natural athletes in their youths. Thus, do not think for a moment that because you never were, you can't be.

ATP (adenosine triphosphate): A complex, chemical compound formed as a result of energy released from food. It is an immediate, usable form of chemical energy stored in muscle cells. Some pharmaceutical companies have attempted to isolate it as a form of instant, nutrient energy. None have yet succeeded, but it could happen one day.

Atrophy: A wasting away as a result of inactivity. This applies to every part of the body. Inactivity is far and away the worst crime we commit against the human body. Nothing facilitates aging or atrophy more rapidly than disuse. This is a lesson that older generations were, sadly, never taught.

Attitude: The saying that "it's seventy-five percent of everything we do" is not far from the truth. It certainly is the most important ingredient toward becoming a fit, mature individual. Without a positive attitude of enthusiasm toward remaining an active, energetic person in our advanced years, there is little hope of achieving it.

Babies — training with: While this book is definitely intended for mature individuals who are less likely to be saddled with babies or small children, you may be having a second family or experiencing the joys of grandchildren. Minding children need not curtail periods of exercise, as there are on the market today a number of outstanding baby strollers made to be pushed ahead by a runner. They have amazingly comfortable seats for children and large,

well-aligned wheels for effortless motion. Similarly, the technology of bicycle seats for infants has moved to the point where one need not worry about the comfort or safety of the children on bicycles. If you spend a significant amount of time minding small children, these devices are an excellent investment and will allow you to enjoy this period of time while still following some of your exercise desires.

Backs: With over 50 percent of all people over 50 having backaches from time to time, it has taken the medical profession the better part of the 20th century to learn that rest and other forms of immobilization were, in fact, counterproductive to the care of such problems. We now know that the crux of supporting the spine and sacral portions of the lower back, in the vast majority of cases, is having strong lower back muscles gained through exercise. A smaller percentage are indeed caused by ruptured discs and sciatic nerve damage. But if medical investigations turn up neither of these, then exercise is the solution. First, the same exercises that will eventually strengthen the abdomen will also benefit the back. It is not the intent of this book to offer precise exercises for each body part because this information can be accurately found in many excellent books available in your library, bookstore, or sporting equipment shop. My personal favorite is *The Athlete Within,* a comprehensive, extremely well-illustrated text written by two physicians who really know their stuff (Little, Brown, 1987).

Bacteria: One-celled plants which

infect our bodies and cause disease. Personal hygiene will eliminate most bacteria that can prosper on moist bodies. We must be cautious of athlete's foot and swimmer's ear.

Bad knees: Why do all of our athletic friends over 50 complain of failing eyesight and bad knees? If you're over 50 and your eyes and knees are fine, check your birth certificate. You may not be as old as you think. Or more likely, you may think you can see and walk comfortably, but don't know a good thing when you see and feel it. The process of aging reduces flexibility in eye muscles, leading to myopia almost 100 percent of the time. If you are not wearing some form of eyeglasses, you probably are not seeing as well as you could. Similarly, aging reduces joint flexibility and concurrently joint strength. If your knees feel great, you either don't remember how great they felt in your youth or you never stress them. But fear not! Be you a fibber or an honest person, your knees can make a comeback at almost any age if the arthritic damage is not yet irreversible, which it obviously isn't if you do not know you have a problem. The answer to weakness in knees is the ultimate mechanical advantage offered by Nautilus leg extension and leg curl machines. There are also Nautilus clones such as David and Eagle. These machines need to be used to strengthen the hamstring muscle (by curl) and the quadricep muscle (by extension) so you can support the knees. Then work your knees with light weights and high repetitions through just 15 degrees of movement from straight to bent and back. Concentrate on perfect form, no super-

heavy lifts. Remember, at 50 the saying "no pain, no gain" is tantamount to athletic suicide. Our slogan is: "If it hurts, stop. If it's not fun, avoid it."

If you don't do Nautilus now but do free weights at home, you might not think it worth joining a Nautilus club just for two machines. But it is. Do three sets of light-weighted, 15-degree moves on the leg extension, one leg at a time; then do five sets of full extensions with both legs on each machine, graduating from light to your heaviest weight on each succeeding set. It will make the visit worthwhile and your knees and legs sturdier than you believed they ever could be again.

Additionally, if biking is one of your sports (if it isn't, it should be), spend a few hours a week and pump an indoor bike or the real thing out on the roads at high RPM, in low gears, which doesn't stress the knee joint. In time, this improves knee articulation. It doesn't all happen overnight but, who's in a hurry? Fifteen years ago, Jay Lehr was a hopeless arthritic with heavy braces on each knee, requiring crutches 40 percent of the time. His 1987 3:39 Columbus Marathon and 12:08 Ironman Triathlon seem to indicate that one can recover from bad knees.

Badminton (see also *Tennis*): Everything we explain under the entry for Tennis goes equally for badminton, and even more so. It is possible to become quite a good badminton player and move very little around the court. If you have good timing, good positioning, and a good swing, you can be a killer on a badminton court without being a runner. Come to think of it, maybe badminton is better exercise if you're not very good at it.

Balance: It is quite interesting to note how we tend to lose our balance with age. Much of this is our inability to adequately control our skeleton with our muscular system. Quick movements easily lead the unfit person to lose his or her balance. An exciting by-product of fitness, almost totally unrecognized, is the maintenance of exceptionally good physical balance through fitness.

Balanced diets: The simplest way to put it is that, by definition, every fad diet is unbalanced and thus unproductive. Nutrionists have learned over the years that all human beings need a diet of carbohydrates, protein, and a small amount of fat. Most of us should eat around 60 percent carbohydrates, 25 percent protein, and 15 percent fat. Learn to read labels and you can balance your own diet with foods you enjoy.

Balistic stretching: Stretching exercises that are performed rapidly to the complete limit of possible movement. They result in muscle pulls and are considered inappropriate for essentially all training programs.

Ballet: An excellent exercise routine which contributes outstandingly to aerobic fitness. Women give it up way too early in life. Today, many professional athletes are taking up ballet because of the balance and fitness it provides. It may be too late for most older men to start ballet, but it may not be too late for older women to resume their training.

Banana: A wonderfully healthy fruit that contains a significant quantity of potassium which is extremely impor-

tant in keeping older muscles limber. If your stomach can handle it, as many as three bananas a day makes for healthy carbohydrate calories and an amount of potassium that will noticeably reduce stiffness in muscles.

Baseball: A wholesome, relaxed game for spectators but one that virtually no one over 50 can effectively participate in because of the natural reduction in physical reflexes.

Basement: A fantastic place to put exercise equipment which you can visit regularly. However, keep the TV down there so you don't get bored!

Basketball (see *Baseball*)

Beans: Near perfect food. High in carbohydrate and low in fat. Add them to your diet.

Beat: In a competitive sense, something we need never consider in relation to others. Competing against ourselves is enough.

Beds: A common source of back trouble. When your tires wear out, you can tell by the loss of tread, but it is harder to tell if your bed is worn. If you have chronic back pain, suspect your bed and see a good bed-supplier for information on new and improved beds to support backs. If your bed is over eight years old, you may be pushing its effective life. Generally, firm beds are the healthiest for the body, but a nice soft covering over the mattress can add a good deal of comfort without reducing the benfits of firm internal springs.

Belts: If you lift free weights, and you should (unless you are over 114 years of age), wear a weight belt. Not a leather one, but the new nylon variety that form-fit to your waist and fasten with Velcro. They correct your posture and protect your lower back from strain.

Bench: A place where many of us spent our high school and collegiate athletic careers. It should not dissuade us from doing better in our later years.

Benches: Everyone should have one that, preferably, can be inclined. All weight stores sell them at a reasonable price. It is the only piece of equipment a person over 50 needs to complement a set of dumbbells, the presence of which should be mandatory in every senior citizen's household (see *Weight lifting*).

Benefits: More than you can count, as a result of physical fitness.

Beta-endorphin: A natural chemical released by the body during strenuous exercise that may cause feelings of euphoria and generally associated with the runner's high. Nearly everyone who exercises regularly will experience this phenomenon from time to time, but by no means regularly. There is likely a psychological aspect that relates to the onset of such a "high" during exercise.

Biceps: The main, arm muscle everyone can find. It is probably the easiest muscle to develop, although commonly amounts to little on mature bodies. Its development brings enhancement to the entire chest as well. While every-day lifting chores retain it in some semblance of a muscle shape, such chores are invariably inadequate once you are no longer working as a longshoreman or ditch-digger.

Bicycle fit: It is crucial that a bicycle fit you properly. If it does not, you will experience back and knee problems. By all means, buy from the very best bicycle shop where experts know how to fit you. If they don't know that the seat should be adjusted such that when your heel is on the top of the pedal with your leg at full extension your knee joint should make approximately a 5-degree angle between your upper and lower leg, go elsewhere. The distance between the seat and handlebars and the handlebar height and width are also important. Professionals know this; amateur salespeople do not.

Bicycle shoes: Anyone who is going to bicycle as a form of exercise should learn to use toe clips on their pedals to hold their feet firmly in place and allow the cycling motion to gain power both on the upstroke and the downstroke. Experienced cyclists use cleated shoes that fit firmly and stationarily onto the bicycle pedal. Advanced bicycle shoes lock into the pedal system much the way ski boots lock into a ski binding. An excellent compromise, however, is bicycle-touring shoes. These have grooves cut into a hard rubber bottom that comfortably engage the pedal but can be effortlessly removed when one comes to a sudden stop. Some form of bicycle shoe is always recommended over a common sneaker or running shoe because they all have a very firm, inflexible sole which allows a greater amount of the energy of the leg motion to be translated to the pedal and ultimately the wheels, rather than dissipating some of that power into the bending of a shoe.

Bicycle tires: If you are currently or plan to become a bicyclist for purposes of gaining aerobic exercise, you will likely be confronted with a question at your local bicycle shop as to whether you prefer sew-up tires or clincher tires. The latter are the standard tires you have known all of your life, which are made up of a tire and a rubber innertube. When it goes flat, you have to take off the tire, take out the tube, and either patch the tube or replace it with a new tube. This is a tedious but inexpensive process. Today, one has the option of a less tedious but more expensive alternative using the sew-up tires. These tires have the tube sewn into the tire and when they go flat, one normally simply tears them off or peels them off the rim and places a new tire onto the rim in a fraction of the time it takes to replace a clincher tire. Such tires require a different rim than the one utilized for the foundation of the clincher tire. If funds are short and time is long, stick with clinchers. If you have a few extra discretionary dollars, aren't terribly good with your hands, and want to enjoy bike rides without fear of flats, talk to your local bicycle shop about sew-up tires. We, personally, wouldn't be without them.

Bicycle types: If you plan on biking outdoors, buy a good 10- to 14-speed bike with racing tires in the $300 to $600 range. The more expensive bikes will be lighter in weight and provide less frictional resistance, which makes riding easier, but since exercise not speed is our goal, it does not make much difference.

Mountain bikes with nobby tires are now also popular for outdoors, but they cannot be used indoors on riding stands, so I don't recommend them. No matter where you live, you'll get more daily riding done indoors than out.

If you buy a bicycle stand, be sure it's the magnetic resistance variety because they make the least noise.

If you buy an exercycle, buy a simple inexpensive one, though not the cheapest. The ones with lots of bells and whistles are a waste of money and often intimidating.

Bicycling: This is the best all-around form of exercise for the mature individual. It can be done inside or out with little or no stress on the budget. The indoor exercise bike, or bicycle set on a training stand, will provide excellent aerobic training at any pace while enabling one to read or watch TV. We firmly believe that each day should begin on an exercise bike for 30 minutes, but the initial effort should be five minutes per day, adding two minutes a day each week until reaching 30 minutes in the 14th week. Cut back your sleep time by setting the alarm clock the same number of minutes you will ride the bike, and riding half asleep. No warm-up is necessary. You will get your blood pumping almost effortlessly while catching the morning news, via TV or newspaper. Reading stands attach readily to most types of bikes. Pedal at high revolutions per minute (cadence) with little resistance. The primary purpose is to achieve aerobic benefit rather than muscle strength. The latter will follow automatically as your aerobic and pedaling efficiency improve with practice.

A morning cycling program will enhance your day far more than the additional sleep would. On weekends when the weather is good, venture out and enjoy the benefits of the cycling skill you will have obtained.

Biochemistry: The interaction of inert chemicals and living organisms, generally referring to the interaction of bacteria and chemicals which combine to form products different than those which result from interaction of chemicals alone. While chemistry of the human body is an important aspect of health, natural bacteria which reside in the body play a significant role in processing everything that we injest.

Bite: The set of your jaw has an effect on muscle contraction. A bad bite between upper and lower teeth scrambles electric impulses from the brain. Lift with your mouth open. If you clench your jaw and find you are a bit weaker, you have a bad bite. See a dentist who specializes in bite problems.

Bladder: Something that will need even more frequent emptying if you pursue a fitness program and drink the copious quantities of fluid that are required. Be not concerned with the frequency; it simply comes with age. While you may have to empty the bladder a few times even during sleep, it will no longer be an annoyance because you will sleep so well when you are fit, you'll be delighted to wake up for the joy of so easily going back to sleep.

Blood flow: One of the most critical aspects of human health for those of advancing years. If we cannot maintain a vigorous flow of blood through our body, we cannot supply all the parts of our body with adequate oxygen and nutrients. One of the most important aspects of aerobic activity is to enhance blood flow. Many of the common ailments that aging individuals are heir to are the result of dramatically declining blood flow in later years. There is absolutely no reason that this situation should occur if an individual will take part in a reasonable schedule of weekly aerobic activity.

Blood pressure: In general, high blood pressure is considered negative and low blood pressure is considered positive. High blood pressure is often a result of obstructions in the arterial system of the human body that do not allow blood flow in adequate quantities unless the pressure supplied by the heart is increased to move the blood through restricted areas. Thus, high blood pressure is generally indicative of potential blood-flow problems. It can be lowered by exercise and improved diet that minimizes the cholesterol and fat that are thought to clog the arterial system. Someone who operates on lower blood pressure is operating with a heart that does not have to work as hard. People, however, with very low blood pressure can be prone to dizziness if the pressure is not enough to keep blood flowing up to the brain when an individual embarks on a sudden, rapid vertical movement such as standing up quickly from the sitting or prone position.

Body building: SURPRISE! A must for all older people. You either build the body or it falls apart. You need not look far to see it happen. Mature people need to lift weights far more than young people to slow the body's genetic unraveling. We now know that a person can build muscle at any age, but it does take more time as you get older. Weight training dramatically strengthens the bones of aging people and retards the onset of osteoporosis among women. For complete explanations of a weight-training program, see *Weight lifting.*

Body fat: The percentage by weight of

your body which consists of fat. A fit percentage of fat for men is in the 17 to 18 percent range; for women, 22 to 23 percent range. The very fit fat percent drops below these ranges for both men and women. An exceptionally fit male will approach 12 percent body fat and females 14 to 15 percent. Essentially, only competitive athletes will pierce the 10 percent fat barrier for either men or women. Below a seven percent body-fat content is considered, by many, to be unhealthy. Body fat is, perhaps, the best single measure of a person's correct physical weight and fitness proportions, but it is not easy to measure. The most accurate system is generally done by weighing one's body in and out of a container of water to determine density and calculate the percentage of weight that is fat. It is now also done by electric resistance examinations which place a slight current through the body. The simplest but least accurate method is a pinch test which can, under skilled supervision, approach a few percentage points of accuracy. It is worth having one's body fat tested at a time when you are considering beginning a fitness program, as it will be a very good indicator of progress three to six months later.

Bones: Our bones definitely get more brittle with age, but this degeneration can be slowed or arrested with weight-resistance training.

Boring: Exercise is not boring unless you are boring. You do, after all, have your mind to occupy you while you are running, swimming, or biking. Solve a problem, real or imaginary; write a paper, story, or report on the tablets of your mind; or, from time to time, study your every move. When

you cycle indoors, read or watch TV. When you weight train, watch TV or listen to music. When you cycle outdoors, enjoy nature. If you're bored, you're not doing it right.

Bottles: Things to be filled with water or energy drinks and set beside your indoor stationary bike for continued use **or** set behind a tree or bush on a circular jogging course so that continued fluid ingestion can be achieved.

Bounding: A little-known running technique which allows a faster runner or jogger to keep pace with a slower companion. It involves pushing off one's calf muscle so that you accentuate the up-and-down motion a little more than the forward motion. It utilizes excess energy while strengthening the calf muscle without increasing speed; thus two runners of widely differing capabilities can enjoy running or jogging together.

Boundless energy: A feeling that can be acquired as a result of a proper diet and exercise program. It is often considered to be antisocial behavior, but if you've got it, flaunt it.

Bowling: A sport allowing moderate exercise if your body is already in shape to handle the various arm, leg, and back stresses.

Brace: Many joints and muscles will, from time to time, require bracing. Sore muscles dramatically benefit from firm wrapping with 6-inch wide elastic bandages to give additional support and reduce discomfort while all but eliminating the opportunity for further injury. Wobbly joints may need bracing with more sophisticated devices that can be recommended by a sport orthopedic specialist.

Breakfast: A meal that everybody in

the nation now knows is of the utmost importance to good health and energy.

Brisk: A nice word to describe the pace at which all exercise should be undertaken. If it feels brisk, it is brisk.

Bruise: Superficial injuries which may produce subcutaneous bleeding, resulting in black-and-blue marks. As we age, we tend to bruise more easily partially as a result of poor circulation. The pursuit of fitness-forming exercise will, from time to time, result in some bruising, but as we achieve fitness, those bruises will become less of an annoyance.

Burn: A feeling one recognizes in the muscles from doing continued and difficult physical exercises that can run the gamut of aerobic dancing, difficult calisthenics, stretching, or even continuous activities such as skiing. It occurs when a heavy load is placed on a muscle and the muscle begins to generate lactic acid, which is not quickly absorbed; it remains in the muscle, creating a burning sensation. The burn is something that many people feel they should strive for in an exercise program from time to time to enusre that they are pushing themselves far enough to achieve significant results. We have no reluctance to see people carry activities to a burn, but we stand by our primary philosophy that if it hurts, don't do it. Exercise should be fun. No one should feel that in order to become fit one has to experience discomfort such as the burn. We will be the first to admit that when one is exercising rigorously and feels a burn, there can be a tremendous mental satisfaction in the accomplishment that outweighs the brief physical discomfort, which can always be eliminated by simply stopping the exercise.

Caffeine: A drug which does increase alertness and improve short-term athletic performance by a small percentage. When taken continu-ously, however, it simply robs Peter to pay Paul by allowing the expenditure of excessive near-term energy, while likely extracting the price of being excessively tired later.

Calf: The primary leg muscle below the knee. It is necessary to maintain tone in the Achilles tendon, with which it is connected to the heel. The muscle is usually small and limp in older people, but can readily be seen as a sign of increased fitness from running and cycling as the muscle takes form again. Cycling and hill running, walking, or jogging provide them with a good workout. They deteriorate much the way the bicep does and need focused exercise. If you can keep your calf muscle toned, the rest of your leg will automatically benefit. Periodic bounding, while jogging, is an outstanding way to condition calves.

Calisthenics: Aerobic exercises that have largely been replaced by continuous exercise sessions set to music, sometimes called Jazzercize. Still performed extensively by athletic teams but rarely by individuals on their own, unless set to music.

Calorie: A unit of energy derived from food which, when not burned, creates weight on the human body. 3500 calories make up 1 pound. The human body easily metabolizes carbohydrate and then protein into caloric energy but does not as easily metabolize or burn calories from fat. Remember from this day forward — all calories are not the same. Calories from fat should be kept to a bare minimum.

Cancer: The term for a variety of diseases involving the uncontrolled multiplying of body cells which can destroy healthy cells and produce tumors. They are the cause of death of 20 percent of our population. Recent evidence points to a lessening of the risk of cancer with improved diet and exercise programs.

Canoeing: A delightfully pleasant exercise for the few that have access to it. Fewer still can do enough to make it part of a fitness program.

Can't: A word which should be eliminated from the average vocabulary.

Carbohydrate loading: A consumption of excessive quantities of carbohydrate-laden foods and liquids prior to an exercise event that requires endurance. Such a diet maximizes the storage of glycogen in the muscles which can be called upon for use for as much as four to six hours of activity. Such a dietary program should be undertaken in moderation over a two- to three-day period. Short-term, dramatic changes in food intake both with regard to quantity and type can have deleterious effects if the stomach is not accustomed to them. Loading usually consists of concentrating on eating solid food such as rice, pasta, bread, and potatoes or liquid supplements such as EXCEED, highcarb formula.

Carbohydrates: The primary food molecule that is converted to energy by the human body. A healthy diet should contain 50 to 70 percent complex carbohydrate which includes most pastas, fruits, and grains. Pure forms of sugar are simple carbohy-drates that provide only short-term energy, converting quickly to fat in the body.

Carriage: In our case, it deals with the way we carry our bodies; thus, it relates to posture. When you're fit, you have the musculature to carry your body in an upright position, signifying good posture. Lack of fitness almost always goes hand-in-hand with the inability to carry the head erect, hold the shoulders back, and hold the abdominal muscles in. Concurrently, the stride is usually short and uneven. All of the aforementioned attributes work with a negative impact on the physical system. Proper posture evenly distributes the load and allows for the the best aerobic and oxygen distribution throughout the body. Thus, poor carriage reflects a lack of fitness and in turn contributes further to the decline of fitness.

Cars: Vehicles which provide an excellent opportunity for isotopic exercises, sometimes referred to as dynamic tension, where muscle contraction can be purposefully experienced while no motion or physical work takes place. Desks provide similar opportunities.

Cassettes: Audio tapes which can provide excellent accompaniment on a walk, run, or bike ride in low traffic areas, allowing either entertainment or education.

Celibacy: No studies have ever shown that sexual activity has a negative impact on fitness. There are some, however, who believe that celibacy may have a negative impact. We believe the latter.

Cellulite: This is a word manufactured by people selling things that claim to reduce the fatty tissue primarily on the outside of women's thighs. It's simply another word for fat, and there is no magic way to spot-reduce or remove it. Diet removes fat equally throughout the body and exercise tones the muscles and skin where the fat has been removed. The word is so ad-agency oriented that you may want to beware of any product that addresses itself to the elimination of cellulite. Somewhere involved in the product exists an individual who cannot be totally trusted.

Challenge: Life without challenge is exceedingly dull. Most people in one or another phase of their lives enjoy tackling a challenge, which can be defined as a task that cannot be readily accomplished under average or normal circumstances. That is to say, it requires some extraordinary effort on the part of a particular individual to accomplish whatever that individual perceives as a challenge worth undertaking. In the area of fitness, challenges are good but are not absolutely necessary. We stress over and over again that if one places too large a challenge in front of himself, a challenge that is unrealistic, it is more likely that the effort will be discontinued and the challenge never conquered. We believe in incremental or very small challenges to succeed in the long term. In essence, anything that we do which is more than we have done before is a challenge. Its achievement should yield a considerable amount of personal satisfaction as well as progress toward one's overall goal such as fitness. Probably the most significant challenge everyone should face is that of becoming fit. On the way to accomplishing that feat, there will be many

mountains to climb — small hills that can be perceived as acceptable challenges.

Champion: An accolade deserved by all gray panthers who achieve and maintain physical fitness throughout their advancing age. Today, society recognizes that everybody who completes a marathon run is a winner. Older, fit people are now held with the same esteem.

Chiropractic: A system of therapy involving manipulation of the spinal column and other skeletal segments. It can be very effective when activity or muscle imbalances pull the skeletal frame out of its neutral position. Beware of chiropractors claiming the ability to cure a diverse number of ills, or those who market their services on a too-frequent basis. If your body is physically out of whack due to a sudden movement or excessive activity, it is very possible that chiropractic will be the quickest, surest, and most economical solution to the problem.

Chlorine: A swimming pool disinfectant that makes swimming goggles a must and an antichlorine shampoo desirable to avoid green hair and split ends.

Cholesterol: This refers to an organic substance that promotes the collection of fatty tissue in the arterial system, which ultimately contributes to the clogging of arteries. We now know it to be a major contributor to what we have thought of as "heart disease" which, in fact, is simply the clogging of our personal plumbing system. While some individuals have genetically high or low cholesterol levels, they are largely controlled by diet and, with rare exception, can be placed in a healthy range by avoiding high cholesterol foods as well as by focusing on healthier foods and regular exercise. It's one of those words no one ever heard of a few years ago and no one can escape today.

Choline: An unusual nutrient which has two endearing qualities and can be found in any health-food store. First, to a minor extent, it is a fat burner that tends to have a minimal, positive impact on neutralizing some fat intake. Its greatest quality, however, is its ability to generate the growth of neural transmitters in the body that improve mental acuity and thus tend to reduce frustration levels brought about by brain lock. It is particularly effective for those who have to sit in meetings for long periods of time and for anyone who simply wants a clearer head. It's a granular, rubbery, tasteless substance that can be readily swallowed with water. A tablespoon a day of the highest concentration granular variety available is a surprisingly inocuous but useful nutrient.

Choosing friends: If good physical and mental health is to be achieved, one must begin to separate one's self from negative people who focus on problems and complaints instead of opportunities and benefits. Excess energy is required to deal with negative people and returns little in satisfactory personal relationship. Try to alter and improve their state but, failing in the effort, distance yourself from them because you have but one life to live and you really can't afford to waste it.

Cigarettes: While the Centers for Disease Control has not found a negative effect from less than 5 cigarettes per day, at the same time no beneficial qualities have been as-

signed to them. As the risk of heart disease and lung cancer increases exponentially with their use, to put it mildly, one would be far better off without them.

Circuit training: A series of exercises performed one after the other with minimal rest in between each exercise. The program can be with weight machines or calisthenic apparatus and promotes both aerobic training and muscle development. Such programs are commonly set up at health clubs and have the advantage of moving large numbers of people through a program in a relatively short period of time. There may, however, be a significant waiting period before one can begin the program because everyone has to start at the same activity or apparatus. If time is a problem, and you can build your own home gym, a circuit training program can be an excellent idea.

Clocks: The enemy of all fitness programs when used to measure speed, but perfectly good to measure duration. Try to avoid dividing time into distance which gives speed because we don't really care. The object is to get the job done. Improvement in quality or speed will accrue naturally without measuring. Measurements are intimidating because we too often set unreasonable goals that are not easily met. Give them to your kids and let them worry about time.

Clothes: For exercise, they should be comfortable, loose-fitting, and make you feel good. If you're into clothes, tight clothes are fun if you are weight-lifting; warm clothes are a must outdoors (always wear multiple layers rather than thick bulky clothes); old clothes are great but much of the new athletic wear makes sense and is worth the money for factors such as light-weight moisture absorbency, warmth, and flexibility. It's worth visiting a professional triathlon shop for a look at advances in athletic clothes.

Coaching: Many people require continued direction over their fitness program. This can be accomplished by joining groups and classes. All communities have aerobics classes. Most have masters' swimming groups and a few have running clubs. If you like groups, join them. If not, go it alone but seek advice from local experts such as the types organizing and directing groups.

Additionally, excellent advice is available from specific books on every imaginable type of exercise. Most books are a good value. Read a few on each area of your interest and choose the coaching advice you like best. That may sound like the old joke about asking a lawyer how much two and two is and the lawyer responds, "What do you want it to be?", but it really isn't.

You see, you can't force yourself to perform any physical regimen unless it makes sense and is feasible and pleasant. If you read enough different ideas, you will become informed enough to make proper value judgments.

In short, though, one way or another you should obtain expert direction if for no other reason than to insure the efficiency of your time and the significance of your results. You will find many specific tips in this book, but very likely not all the information you desire or need.

Coffee: Everyone recognizes that a dependence on coffee or, in other words, caffeine is a habit no longer considered healthy. A reasonable amount of daily coffee such as a cup or two in the morning and a cup or two in the evening is not, however, going to have a negative impact on one's health. If you're dependent on coffee to keep you full of energy throughout the day, then you do have a problem. A limited amount of caffeine, 200 to 300 milligrams per day (one cup of coffee contains approximately 100 milligrams), has been shown to have no deleterious effects. In fact, a limited amount of caffeine can have a beneficial effect on fat consumption in the body. As with all things, coffee can be a wonderful enjoyment and modest stimulant when taken in moderation, but when overdone it resides on a long list of substances that reduce one's chances to be fit. If you must have caffeine at times to stay alert, a No-Doz type product is very efficient.

Coke: A soft drink with sugar and caffeine that increases energy and alertness, but not the best way to do either. Soft drinks in moderation will do little harm but can be replaced with more beneficial products. High-carbohydrate energy drinks or fruit juices are more healthy.

Cold: A temperature that significantly affects outdoor activity. Don't swim in water below 70 degrees if you can avoid it. It simply is not fun and thus deprives you of the joy of exercise. Don't bicycle at temperatures below 55°F unless you have exceptionally good, cold-weather bicycle gears. You can walk, jog, or run safely outdoors down to 20°F if the wind is not strong and you are dressed for it. Cold, however, should never be an excuse not to exercise. Make indoor activities available through a health club or, preferably, activities in your home such as an exercise bike, electric treadmill (running machine), or free weights (dumbbells).

Never allow yourself to be excessively cold when exercising. Obviously, it's not healthy, but, worse, it leaves a bad taste in your mouth for future exercise — something one should never do.

Color of your hair: The grayer the better, when you are in shape. The better shape you are in, the more you like people to know your age. Once your body doesn't show it, you need the gray hair to be tell-tale.

Comfort zone: The singularly most important concept in being fit over 50 is one's "comfort zone." This is the zone in which any and all activity is enjoyable. we are primarily referring to the speed at which one proceeds with the activity. If we are to continue with any exercise program, it must be relatively enjoyable. If it is not, as sure as night follows day, we will eventually abandon it.

We are, unfortunately, brought up on the inaccurate proposition that where there is no pain, there is no gain. While there is a modicum of truth in this for young athletes striving to excel, there is no application to the senior individual desiring to maintain fitness for life. If one maintains an activity without pain or, in other words, within our comfort zone, progress and improvement still occur but more slowly. Eventually, we will perform at higher activity levels which will increase benefits. These same increased activity levels or speeds encountered too soon would only serve to discourage us as a result of the discomfort they bring. Activity

out of the comfort zone is often referred to as speed work or interval training, both of which are addressed in this book and are considered by the authors often to be counterproductive. A far better alternative is "incremental" training, described elsewhere.

Compete/competition: While many individuals enjoy competition, or use competition as a way to achieve a goal, as we pass our first half-century we're all competing with Father Time, the aging process, and our own basic instincts of laziness. Thus we can all win the latter competition by convincing ourselves that we can overcome perhaps 70 to 80 percent of the deterioration we recognize as aging and maintain a higher level of fitness into our advancing years than we may ever have achieved in our youth. In general, there is too much stress on competition with our peers, and though many enjoy it on a regular basis, it intimidates many more. The eternal chase for fitness is competition enough for us.

Complacency: A synonym for self-satisfaction which so many of us achieve by personal tomfoolery. That is to say, we convince ourselves that we are not so bad off by comparing ourselves to those who are worse off — a truly terrible trick we play on ourselves. We step out of the shower, avoiding a glance into the mirror at our naked body in a candid and unflattering position. Men hold in their guts, and women wear girdles and flattering clothes to achieve complacency. Choose better role models and your satisfaction will quickly melt away. Then realize that with few exceptions, those role models did not get where they are as couch potatoes.

There is virtually nothing that you can fail to achieve in regard to fitness if you give yourself two years to accomplish it. Saying that to a youth could be totally depressing, but to those of us who understand time a little better, with age comes patience and the ability to deal with a long-term project. Of course, if you don't plan on living more than another two years, maybe it's not worth the effort.

Compulsive runner: An individual who runs daily, allowing no obstacles to stay his course. While we promote daily exercise without planned rest, a shortage of time, periodic injury, or severely inclement weather are excellent excuses to take a rest. Unwillingness or inability to do so are signs of compulsive behavior, which can also result in depression, anxiety, and anorexia when exercise is made impossible. We think a healthy desire to maintain an exercise schedule is admirable, but there is a limiting point this side of sanity.

Condition: The state of your fitness. You are in either poor, fair, or good condition. It is also synonymous with shape, i.e., being in good shape. In time it wouldn't hurt to begin using some of that athletic vernacular even if you have no intentions of being an athlete.

Consistency: Next to the comfort zone, consistency ranks second in a fitness program. Whatever you do, do it regularly. The key is to assign a part of every day to fitness-producing activity. It makes little difference what the activity is, when you do it, or how fast you do it. It is the inbred habit of consistency that will pay off without exception. When exercise becomes as regular as eating and sleeping, you will be assured of a greater sense of well-being for all of your life.

Convenience: An exercise program must be convenient or it won't become a habit. If you have to climb a mountain or cross a river to get to an activity, forget it. Make it easy on yourself or you won't make it at all. Do what you can at home. If you walk, jog, or run, try and start from your front door because your front door is a convenient place to start from. A nearby park, track, or health club may not be. If you join a club, it better be close by. If you are going to lift weights, don't put them in your garage — put them in your TV viewing room. Get the picture?

Cooking: Obviously, nutrition is an important part of fitness. The cooking guidelines are easy. Simply eat no fried foods. Steam your vegetables and eat lots of them. Use little or no butter or fat in your cooking. Attempt to make 50 to 65 percent of your diet completely carbohydrates, like pasta, rice, beans, and other vegetables. Try to reduce fat in your diet to 15 percent but no more than 25 percent. If you avoid all fat, you will still get enough fat in your diet because you can't avoid it.

Cool down: Gentle exercises performed at the end of a workout to prevent too rapid cooling of the body. Such exercises also dissipate buildup of lactic acid in the muscles. It is an excellent idea to always cool down slowly after a rigorous exercise program rather than to stop suddenly. Cooling down is more important than warming up, because warming up can be built into any exercise program by simply beginning as slowly as is extremely comfortable. Something as simple as walking around or swinging the arms can serve as an effective cool-down program.

Cooling (see *Ice*)

Coordination: The ability to move different parts of the body in an organized manner so as to achieve efficient and rapid movement. Individuals lacking such ability rarely succeed as athletes, as coordination is generally necessary to excel at most sports. It is common that an innate lack of coordination, recognized at an early age, keeps individuals off of playing fields all over the world. Then, in later life, these individuals resign themselves to a life without adequate physical exercise. What a terrible mistake that is, because coordination, while nice and useful, is generally unnecessary in the quest for fitness. One might take a little longer and look less rhythmic in his or her movements, but the effects and importance of exercise are in no way diminished by a lack of coordination.

Cross-country running: Normally considered to be running on natural grass and dirt surfaces over hither and yon. It's an excellent activity for younger people but is not conducive to the older body because of the very uneven surfaces provided by grass and dirt. Any problems with ankle, knee, and hip joints will be exacerbated on such surfaces. We recommend jogging, running, or even walking on smooth, graded surfaces, hopefully, those with some resilience. As an example, macadam road surfaces are considerably more elastic than cement. Running a significant distance on cement will make itself known to the skeleton the following day, if not before, as compared to a run on a macadam or asphalt surface. Rubberized running tracks

at high school or college athletic fields are devoutly to be wished, but rarely to be found. All running machines have adequate resilience.

Cross-country skiing: The skiing equivalent of cross-country running, which is very comfortable for the aging body. The snow provides a smooth surface, the equipment is light, and it can essentially be a form of graceful hiking in the woods or on open terrain which provides outstanding aerobic training capacity. It can be performed at any speed, and as long as the terrain does not require steep ascents or descents, no great skill is required to obtain the training effect.

Cups: Half-full, half-empty! A positive attitude will contribute to fitness. Take pride in small achievements and view a half-cup as half-full instead of half-empty. Be happy with what you get done, not upset over what you fail to do. Some days are difficult. Be pleased with whatever you accomplish on those days.

Cybernetics: The study of communication and control. The term has been used in a variety of books which have, in recent years, conned people into thinking they could be whatever they want to be without paying a fair price. Basically, it's a sophisticated approach to the power of positive thinking which can indeed contribute marvelously to a healthly life if you are willing to move the body as well as the mind.

Dabbling: One of the major problems in developing exercise programs for adults is the tendency to dabble at them; that is to say, to do a little bit today, do a little bit next week, do one thing here and another thing there. You are just fooling yourself if you dabble at an exercise program. While we fully admit that any exercise is better than no exercise, unless you develop a regimen, a routine, and a consistency, you are not going to achieve enough in the way of fitness to give you the incentive to maintain a program. Eventually, you will decide that the exercise does you little good when, in fact, it wasn't the exercise but the periodicity and manner in which you approached it.

Dairy foods: A major source of strength and health in our youth, but of less value in our advancing years. Milk, eggs, cheese, and butter have less value to us in our second half-century. They either contain too much fat or too much cholesterol and need to be held to a minimum.

Dandruff: Some who have it believe it declines with improved fitness: could be!

Dark: You can walk, jog, or run after dark but always wear a light-reflecting vest for safety. If you are afraid of dogs, carry a small stick. Small flashlights, which attach to your arm by a Velcro strap, are also excellent.

Darling: A nice word to apply to your spouse on a regular basis when he or she is supportive of your fitness effort. They might even be encouraged to join you.

Darwin: A famous scientist who, a century ago, described the survival of the fittest. Somehow the message got lost on a lot of people. Don't let it get lost on you.

Daylight: Use it all. Get in the habit of rising at dawn. As the days get longer, you'll get more done and have lots of extra time to spare. You can always ride an indoor bicycle in the morning before dawn but sometimes,

for a change of pace, an early morning run is nice. On a regular basis, a late-day run will be more beneficial because your body is warm and it relieves the stress of the day.

Days off: Don't plan days off—just let them happen. When your entire exercise program is aimed at your enjoyment within the comfort zone, days off are not necessary, but one a week is fine. Once in a while your body craves a day off, so take it. You can exercise an hour a day for the rest of your life with no ill effects.

Death: Everyone will eventually experience it. Don't live in fear of it. The more fit you are, the less it will scare you. Being fit may extend your life and it will most certainly guarantee that you are healthier when you die. That may sound a bit ambiguous, but it's not. You will likely die of a disease relatively unrelated to your level of fitness and can thus feel healthy right up to the time your body breaks down and dies.

Debilitating: Anything that weakens us: poor diet, lack of sleep, lack of exercise, and bacterial infections are common causes of debilitation. Many unfit people are in a permanent state of debilitation.

Dedicate: …Yourself to fitness.

Deep breathing: Most people breathe off the top of their lungs, which is not very beneficial. Get in the habit of deep breathing, especially during exercise, but don't overdo it to the point of hyperventilation, which can cause dizziness.

Defeatist: One who admits that he can't achieve his or her goal. He or she is always correct.

Dehydration: Excessive loss of body fluid caused by sweating. It leads to reduced performance, then illness, and eventually death. Drink! Drink! Drink!

Depression: A state of mental despair which we now know emphatically responds positively to exercise. Psychologists have had amazingly consistent results in treating many forms of mental illness with increased exercise programs along with other accompanying therapies. We all but guarantee that periods of psychological lows can be dramatically improved immediately with periods of exercise and long-term physical fitness. The same can generally be achieved when combatting low-level physical illness such as mild infections which reduce one's capacity to perform but do not fully incapacitate one.

Deteriorate: What occurs to your body more from disuse than abuse or aging. It's almost incredible that years ago we recommended that old people slow down in order to preserve their remaining years when, in fact, we were sentencing them to reduce their capability to live full lives.

Determination: An ingredient without which there is no hope of becoming fit. As Cher once said about fitness, if it came in a bottle, everyone would have it. Fitness is not something achieved without a certain degree of mental toughness, best defined by the word "determination."

Develop: There is no reason to fool anyone into thinking that you can develop a fitness attitude and a fit body quickly. You can't. While it isn't hard, fitness takes an investment of time and requires patience. However, certain mileposts like feeling better and having more energy are so quickly evident that they should be incentive enough to continue to develop a program.

Diarrhea: Many older people have a problem with regularity. This is clearly a result of an improper diet and lack of activity. When you begin to exercise regularly and eat correctly, you are more likely to encounter loose bowel movements rather than none at all. While diarrhea is not the result of good eating, many older people think that they are experiencing this when, in fact, they are experiencing a very easy movement. This will be a result of exercise and a high-carbohydrate diet including a great deal of fruit and grains.

Diary: We are opposed to requiring a regimented schedule that can be intimidating if we are unable to follow it to the letter at all times. However, it is a very good idea in the early months of a fitness program to retain a diary of all of the activities that contribute to your fitness program. The reason for this is that a periodic perusal of your diary will be an enriching experience and give you the satisfaction that comes with a job well done. That leads to the healthy incentive to continue on your very rewarding course.

Diet: As we state continuously, diet has to be combined with exercise in order to achieve fitness. In short, your diet should consist of between 60 and 65 percent carbohydrates, 20 to 25 percent protein, and no more than 15 percent fat. As we get older, we need considerably less protein than younger people, although if you're going to move into a weight-lifting program you will need protein to build new muscle fiber, which you are very definitely capable of doing. No one needs much fat, though a limited amount is required for bodily processes. However, if you try to avoid eating any fat, the odds are you'll get all the fat you need because there is so much fat in the normal foods we eat on a regular basis. Your carbohydrates should be fruits, cereals, pasta, rice, and vegetables. Avoid simple carbohydrates such as sugar. Beware of labels on food that show foods to be high in carbohydrates if, in fact, you know that those carbohydrates are sugar. This is true of many of the morning cereals aimed at the youth market. If you avoid fat and sugar, you may never need to "diet" again because your body can handle most of the other foods that you enjoy eating in the quantities that you are capable of eating. Exercise will not necessarily increase your appetite, so you need not worry about that. Your net caloric burn may surpass your caloric intake, offering you a very simple, though slow, weight loss during the initiation of a fitness program. Vitamin supplements to any diet are a wise choice. Any multivitamin supplement is probably advisable to ensure a proper balance of nutrients as well as 1- to 3 grams of vitamin C a day and 100 to 300 milligrams of potassium a day.

Dietician: Wonderful people to visit if your uncontrollable appetite for poor quality food has created a weight problem. Believe it or not, it is possible to eat large quantities of great-tasting food and not have to fight fat. The trick is truly knowing the sinful foods and why they are so terrible and, conversely, what is both good and good for you. We all have a general idea of this, but not the depth of knowledge required to convince our minds to change our eating patterns. A good dietician can educate us to voluntarily recognize the importance of eliminating poor foods from our diet. If you choose to visit a dietician, insist that he/she spend a few hours with you and your spouse or signficant other in a supermarket, where a lecture on food quality comes to life as a "touchy-feely" experience. You will benefit from handling food packages and reading their labels which contain the clear evidence of exactly what your body will be getting in the bargain with each food. An entire morning, afternoon, or evening spent with your dietician, methodically moving up and down the aisles of a supermarket discussing every single food you might consider purchasing, will be the best time and money you will ever spend toward health education. The concept may be new to your dietician of choice, but insist on it or locate a more agreeable expert.

Dieting: By now, everybody has read at least two dozen fad diets and learned that they all work for a while, and in the end ninety percent of all the people embarking on the diet end up gaining back all the weight, now common enough to be called the "yo-yo syndrome." At the same time, we are seeing an explosion of celebrities on television advertising a variety of weight-loss systems, most of which involve the purchasing of specially packaged foods or food substitutes that definitely work and will take weight off which, of course, is far less than the problem of keeping weight off. The latter is only the result of changing one's eating habits, which can only be done by changing one's thought processes. You simply must develop a case of vanity, meaning that you care enough about how you look to eliminate fatty foods from your diet, which includes all fried foods plus nuts, cheese, cream sauces, butter, fatty meats, sweets, cream soups, fast-food hamburgers, hot dogs, potato chips, corn chips, guacamole dip, avocado, whole milk, and not a whole lot more. When you come right down to it, dieting isn't something one does for a few months to get to an ideal weight. Dieting is something one does permanently to retain an ideal weight. The most important basic rules are to try to eat three reasonably sized meals a day. Never eat to the point of feeling uncomfortable. Eat slowly because your mind only finds out that your stomach is full twenty minutes after it becomes full. Eliminate sugar from your diet. Try to reduce or eliminate your food intake during your last three waking hours of the day, because this is a period in which you do not metabolize your food as well and there is more likelihood of fat intake truly becoming permanent. Our best advice is to make this diet your last diet. That is to say, embark on it and stay on it permanently.

Digest: The way we eat our food can, at times, be as important as what we eat. Eat slowly in a relaxed state. Eat small portions and tend to eat more often during the day. Try to avoid the one or two big-meal syndrome that so many of us experience. Your body does not process food nearly as well in large quantities, so it is well-known now that we are better off eating 4 to 5 small meals a day rather than a couple of large ones. It is difficult to exercise immediately after eating because the digestion process draws blood and oxygen that is needed for exercise. However, it is better to exercise immediately after eating than not to exercise at all.

Dinner: Defined by most as the evening meal, though by a few as the mid-day meal. We will focus here on the evening meal and point out that more important than what the meal consists of is when the meal is eaten. Late night meals within two hours of retiring for the night charge the body with a digestive challenge at a time when it wants to be at rest. A regular habit of late eating will tend to yield a poor metabolic rate and a greater storehouse of fat in the body. Your evening meal is best taken at least three hours before bedtime and should, as with all meals, be a balanced diet, with the majority of calories consumed being carbohydrates, lesser amounts of protein, and minimal amounts of fat. It is generally now believed that fruits as a source of carbohydrate should not be eaten as much in the evening as earlier in the day for beneficial digestive purposes. As with all meals, dinner should be eaten slowly, which benefits both the digestive system and the utilization of the injested calories. More importantly, it triggers the awareness of the brain that fullness is reached which, unfortunately, is a message that requires 20 minutes to arrive from the stomach. The slower you eat, the less likely you are to overeat.

Discomfort (see also *Aches; Pain*): A feeling that you are likely to encounter when making the transition from poor fitness to enhanced fitness. As your lungs and your muscles become stressed beyond their previous norms, they will tell you about it. Most discomfort resulting from aches from unused parts of the body will disappear with time. If the discomfort does not disappear, it becomes a medical problem that requires the attention of a physician. As cautious as we are about making the road to fitness a slow, orderly, and enjoyable process, we would be other than honest not to be abundantly clear about the fact that it will entail some discomfort from time to time. Any discomfort, however, will be abundantly outweighed by the mental and physical benefits achieved from climbing the fitness ladder. Another type of discomfort that you will encounter which can and should be fully eliminated deals with ill-fitting clothing, poorly fitted shoes, improper positioning on exercise bikes, stair-climbing machines, and rowing machines. Invariably, if you are not comfortable on any exercise equipment you choose, it is because the equipment does not mechanically fit your body. Almost all equipment has a degree of adjustment or proper method that allows its use effectively without discomfort. If any of these outside aspects of a fitness program creates discomfort, seek assistance from experts in the clothing, shoe, or equipment field who can explain how to correct the problem.

Disease: A form of illness generally produced by some type of damaged or poorly formed genes in the human body which impair the performance of a vital function. Physicians, in recent decades, have conquered many previously incurable diseases and extended the life and viability for individuals with many other diseases that are yet incurable. One surprising fact that is now all but unanimously agreed upon is that physical fitness is one of the greatest defenses against nearly every known disease. The onset of disease can be stalled by fitness, while the maintenance of an acceptable lifestyle with an existing disease can frequently be improved through exercise and fitness. We by no means want to say that exercise and fitness have miraculous benefits or that they cure everything that ails you; on the other hand, we don't want to say a great deal less than that either.

Dissociative thinking: When you are exercising and choose to think about something other than what you are doing, that is called dissociative thinking. It makes time pass and can be very enjoyable while running and swimming. If you think about what you are doing, that is associative thinking and it is good when you wish to focus on improving what you are doing.

Distance: How far you swim, bike, run, row, etc. is a matter of personal preference. All aerobic activity should last a minimum of 20 minutes so you should calculate a minimum distance based on that. Either exercise a set distance that will require over 20 minutes, or simply exercise for a set period of time. We will repeat over and over again that you should *not* force yourself into a particular speed mode on a regular basis. Try to do everything at a brisk but enjoyable pace. Let your body be your guide, ensuring at all times that your mind is enjoying the experience. A mile swim is a very good long-term goal, but may take a year or more to achieve. A ten-mile walk, jog, or run is another excellent long-term goal that may take two years to achieve. A 20-mile bike ride is easily achievable within six months of preparation time.

Diuretic: A substance that tends to dehydrate the body. Beware of foods, drugs, or vitamins that increase urination and drain fluid from the body. Women are inclined to take diuretic substances in order to avoid fluid retention. Be aware, however, that part of the result is dehydration, which will have a significantly negative impact on all exercise performed.

Doctors: If you exercise regularly, there will no doubt be some exercise-related injuries from time to time. Average doctors are not experienced in dealing with such injuries. Find a doctor or clinic that specializes in sports medicine for the best, briefest, and most effective treatment.

Do something: It's almost always better than doing nothing when it comes to fitness. We often establish an exercise plan for an hour or a day. If for one reason or another we find that we cannot fulfill our plan because we can't go as far, as fast or as long as we planned, don't cancel the whole plan. Do something — a half-full cup is better than an empty cup.

Often a very fit individual who maintains a very active schedule intimidates those around him or her because they feel that they could not do what the fit person does. They fail to realize that a journey of a thousand miles begins with the first step. The fit person, in the beginning, could not do what he does now either. Start **somewhere** and do **something**.

Doughnuts and holes: Some see the doughnut, others see the hole. If the "glass half-full, half-empty" saying to describe attitudes and personalities doesn't strike you as meaningful, you

might enjoy the aforementioned phrase. We do.

Down-time: There will be periods of illness in which we cannot accomplish our fitness program.

Dread: Don't do anything you dread. You can't do it for long, so why bother doing it at all? We are all too old to challenge ourselves with activities we don't enjoy. If there is an element of dread in any activity, cancel the activity and find something you enjoy. You may have to cast about for awhile, but there are few exceptions to the rule that everyone can find an enjoyable, aerobic exercise activity. The only absolute, mandatory requirement that may, for some, cause the experience of non-fun sensations is getting up off the couch and doing something and, eventually, doing that something for a sum total of seven hours of aerobic exercise a week. Of course that's only if you desire to become "fit, firm and 50."

Dry: A term with many meanings for the fitness enthusiast. It is a state that can't be achieved when exercising, because a good sweat is an excellent indicator of a useful workout. Dry is a state somewhat desirable when running in cold weather, which is achieved by light-layered clothing rather than heavy, bulky clothing. A dry state indicates the absence of significant amounts of alcohol, which is surely desirable for fitness.

Dry heat (see *Sauna*):

Dumbbells: Individual hand-held weights used for body-building fitness exercises. They have the advantage of being easy, inexpensive, and extremely safe such that injuries are rarely associated with their use compared to the excessive strain sometimes encountered with barbells. They can be stored in plain view anywhere in one's house for easy accessibility and convenience for use. All body parts can be exercised with simple techniques clearly described in a multitude of manuals on body-building (see Bibliography).

Dunlops disease: A tongue-in-cheek description of robust individuals involved in athletic coaching whose bellys "dun lop" over their belts, making the feet ever more difficult to see and their credibility as coaches ever more difficult to believe.

Dynamic: A state of activity readily achievable by fit people who find that the more they exercise, the more energy they have and the more dynamic they are perceived to be. It is a feeling you will definitely experience when you're fit.

Early: The key word in an excellent fitness program. It is the time at which one should arise for the day in order to get a jump start. Most people will explain that they have no fitness program because they have no time. Many are correct that their day is, indeed, very full. This is why the best program starts early, possibly before your normal rising time such that you sleep a little less. Most people can cut 30 minutes from their sleep, use it for exercise, and end up much healthier.

Ears: Keep them clean. Exercise will create perspiration that can lead to bacterial growth. A word to the wise should be sufficient.

Ears (swimming): Swimming is a wonderful recreation and exercise but it frequently leaves water in the ears, which eventually can spawn bacterial growth and infection. Always be sure to shake out or swab out residual water. If the problem is continuous, earplugs or lambs' wool placed in the ears during swimming may be helpful and bactericidal ear drops after swimming should be considered.

Easy: While nothing really worthwhile is easy, physical exercise should be undertaken at a relaxed pace or eventually it won't be undertaken at all.

Easy days: Days of exercise planned to be less strenuous than the norm. Most exercise programs alternate between easy and hard days. We don't believe one needs to plan that in advance but prefer, simply, to listen to one's body each day in terms of the distance and effort that will be put forth. The body will automatically balance easy and hard days.

Eating: A joyous event for most of us but, if not undertaken with appropriate care, will foil all efforts toward fitness. The rules are simple. Eat slowly in order to give your brain a chance to learn that you are full before you overeat. Avoid eating foods with high fat content — read labels. Make carbohydrates the largest part of your diet, followed by protein, then fat. Two tablespoons of chocolate syrup is better for you than two tablespoons of fatty salad dressing, and they both have the same number of calories. Eat a lot of fruit and green vegetables and avoid stupid snacks. The best, by far, of the common munchies are pretzels and air-popped popcorn. Crisp toast like bread and cracker products are also good. Eat lean meat, and watch out for cheese.

Chinese food is great, but cut out the spareribs, fried eggrolls, and fried rice. Repeat 100 times a day that you will not eat fats or sweets and even though you will cheat, you will improve your diet seventy percent.

Eccentricity: When your exercise program becomes an obsession, your friends and acquaintances will begin to view you as eccentric. Enjoy it!

Eight-minute Abs: A good abdominal (Abs) workout can be accomplished in eight minutes a day. A simple series of leg-lifts and abbreviated sit-ups, when performed in rapid-order fashion, will tighten and flatten most abdominal muscles within two years (that's right, you read correctly — **two years!**). Abdominal muscles decline rapidly after youth and are resuscitated only with great difficulty. It takes very little time per day to achieve abdominal fitness, but it will be many days before the change is evident. The best Ab workout is illustrated in *SynerAbs: 6 Minutes to a Flatter Stomach,* Second Edition, from Health for Life.

Elasticity: A measure of muscle and joint fitness, the lack of which is the surest sign of aging and physical decline. Retention of body elasticity through exercise and stretching is perhaps the most rewarding benefit of a fitness program. It is not difficult to achieve.

Elbow: A joint tightly tied to tendons which can become easily inflamed by tendonitis, which results in various problems referred to as tennis elbow, although the cause can vary from tennis to weight lifting to bicycling. It can be avoided with proper warm-up before activity and application of ice following activity. Simple straps worn above or below the elbow reduce tendon vibration, much like a strap on guitar strings which changes their tone.

Elbow tendonitis (see *Tennis elbow*)

Elderly: A word referring to a state of mind. It can be accurately or inaccurately applied at almost any age and, surprisingly, is used more often to describe people whose physical capacity is considered decrepit more so than as an indication of age. We all know elderly people in their late 60s and early 70s, but no one would call Ronald Reagan elderly.

Elevate: If you injure any part of your body where you suspect swelling may occur, be sure to elevate that portion of your body be it an ankle, knee, elbow, hand, etc. Elevation is one part of the four-part program for the healing of injuries known by the acronym "RICE" — rest, ice, compression, and elevation. Obviously, you cannot keep a body part elevated for a continued period of time other than during sleep. However, especially in the first 24 hours and productively even for 48 hours, whenever it is convenient, elevate.

Elevation: Activity at high elevations (above 2000 feet above sea-level) will commonly be impeded by the reduction of oxygen in the air, which results in a shortness of breath. Above 5000 feet, activity is seriously encumbered and at over 8000 is all but impossible for older individuals. The difficulty tends to decline and nearly disappears once the body becomes acclimated to the reduced oxygen in the air. This invariably occurs when one moves permanently to a higher elevation, but may take weeks or even months. Individuals visiting high altitudes should reduce their physical activity or even eliminate it for short stays. Exercise will be less fun, and we should always remember that if it is not fun, we should not do it.

Eliminate the negative: Physical fitness invariably has an element of mental health which can be enhanced by the elimination of negative factors in one's life. These factors are best represented by individuals in your circle of friends and acquaintances who look consistently at the gloomier side of all issues, real or imagined. You should think positively, seeing glasses half-full rather than half-empty and skies partly sunny rather than partly cloudy. Then, put these negative people outside your circle. They may bring others down, but not you.

A theme song for fitness seekers could well be the old song, "Accentuate the Positive" which goes on to say "eliminate the negative and don't mess with Mr. in-between." Ignore those who put down your effort to be fit as a useless exercise in immaturity. A positive mental attitude is the enemy of mediocrity and vice versa. Don't balance your life with positive and negative attitudes, acts, or people. Life is too short to dwell on negatives or allow negative people to occupy your time and space.

Endurance: The ability to continue an activity for an extended period of time without a dramatic reduction in energy level. There are physiological differences in people involving the make-up of their muscle fibers which make some people good for the long run and others good for the short run: slow twitch fibers for the latter and long-twitch fibers for the former. Some people are blessed with greater endurance than others, but a considerable amount of endurance can be developed by all individuals. Endur-

ance is built up over a considerable length of time and will not improve as rapidly, for instance, as muscle strength will as a result of resistance exercise. In Chapter 5, we recommend a 14-week program to merely get to 30 minutes of continuous activity, whether it be running, cycling, or another aerobic exercise of your choice. It is interesting to note, however, that once a reasonable level of endurance is achieved, the incremental time that will advance one to an hour is considerably shorter than it took to get to 30 minutes. Consistent with that fact, one who is truly interested in endurance activity can advance from one hour of continuous exercise to an hour-and-a-half or two hours in an amazingly short period. A good rule of thumb is never to extend an activity more than five percent in any given week as one pushes toward greater endurance capability. We break the five percent rule in our 14 weeks to 30 minutes of continuous exercise program because we are beginning with so very few minutes of activity. Once past an hour of activity, the five percent rule is a very safe bet to continue fitness improvement without encountering injuries.

Energy: One of the amazing things about exercise is that instead of depriving you of energy, it will make you more energetic. Most people fail to exercise because they lack energy. They sadly do not realize that exercising will renew their energy sources. Exercise in the morning will make you more energetic to tackle your day. Exercise in the evening will reawaken you dramatically, improving the quality of your evening hours prior to retiring. There's a simple, common-sense reason for this. A far greater benefit of exercise than the burning of calories is the oxygenation of your blood, which properly distributes the nutrients and fuel to your entire physical being, allowing you to operate once again in an energetic fashion. Thus, for the normal person, while exercise burns calories, there is a net gain rather than a loss of energy. You will not find a single fit and active individual who will disagree with that statement.

Enjoyment: The feeling that should be encountered during most physical activity. If it isn't enjoyable, you are probably going at it too hard, too long, or wrong. This rule hasn't won many athletes many trophies, but it has gotten countless thousands of people fit. Just as one gets more enjoyment from a meal eaten slowly with small bites, one will travel a distance of a thousand miles taking many small steps just as effectively as taking fewer large steps. But the short steps are easier and enjoyment is your partner. All fitness activity should be synonymous with your own idea of enjoyment or it will not effectively come to pass. It will be slow but it will be steady, and at our age most of us relate far better to the turtle than the hare.

Enthusiasm: A philosophical fuel that makes all activities easier and more fun. Loss of enthusiasm for one's activities has the very same effect on humans as running out of gas has on an automobile. The capacity to be enthusiastic as one grows older is commonly looked upon suspiciously. Simply ignore such negative behavior. It has been said that the attitude which is synonomous with enthusiasm is 75 percent of becoming successful. That may, in fact, be a low estimate. Enthusiasm can be like a nuclear power plant — it leads to a chain of positive reactions which propel one forward. At an advanced age, few around you will support your contrary effort to achieve or maintain fitness, but with adequate enthusiasm you can fly right by this human obstacle course.

Enthusiasm is often a direct result of energy. When you have more energy from being fit, you will be more enthusiastic. People's personalities vary and their level of enthusiasm varies accordingly. But within the range of their personality type, their enthusiasm will ebb and flow with their level of fitness and energy. In general, extremely fit people have a great deal of enthusiasm. There are, of course, exceptions to that rule with whom we are all familiar.

Environment: There are two aspects of environment. First, we want to be concerned with the environment from a health standpoint. We want to breathe clean air; we want to have adequate lighting; we want to experience a minimum of loud noises; we want a healthy water supply and litter-free surroundings. All of these lead us to a greater sense of well-being. The second aspect of environment relates to the actual locations at which we exercise. Biking in rural areas makes for a good environment. Running in suburban residential areas makes for a good environment. Swimming in uncrowded, clean pools makes for a good environment. Any exercise we can do in and around our home is environmentally favorable. The more positive we can make our environment, the more likely we are to perform in a satisfactory and pleasing manner.

Erosion: The wearing away of things like the earth, equipment, and the human body. It occurs to all things at rest in the inhospitable climate offered by most environments. It is overcome by a planned maintenance program. In the human example, activity and exercise can pragmatically forestall erosion.

Estimates: Of what a person can achieve physically are almost always incorrect. When your spirits are low, you will invariably underestimate your capability. When they are high and you are not fit, you will overestimate. Simply don't estimate; just do it and thus know what you can do.

EXCEED: A sports-energy drink, in liquid form, which somewhat revolutionized the capacity to gain usable energy for exercise. Its primary breakthrough is related to its high carbohydrate source product for strenuous endurance efforts. This breakthrough was made possible by the development of a long-chain carbohydrate molecule which passes easily through the lining of the stomach. Many companies now offer brands of carbohydrate source drinks, useful before and during exercise. They should be strongly considered for use by serious physical fitness devotees, as they are generally far superior to the normal fluid products created to satisfy the thirst of the general public.

Exercise: Is obviously what this book is all about. It should become your hobby, your recreation, your diversion, your oasis, your escape, and your ladder to any fitness plateau or health peak. To most, it is a chore to avoid. When its rewards are proven, it becomes a creamy, delicious dessert consisting of negative calories.

Exercise at home: Exercise away from home is a luxury; exercising at home is a must. No one can consistently get to a health club for necessary workouts. At home, the opportunity is always there and the weather is always fine. A program beginning or ending in the home will succeed.

Extra exercise: There are many daily opportunities for unscheduled exercise. There is an old fitness adage that says, "Never lie when you can sit; never sit when you can stand; never stand when you can walk; never walk when you can run." Here is how to apply it to get a little extra exercise.

Walk whenever you have a chance. When driving, don't always look for the closest parking place — walk a distance. Avoid escalators and elevators. Walk up the steps instead. Stand while you're talking on the phone and do some stretching at the same time. Stretch in the shower. Stretch while you're talking to good friends. Suck in your abdomen numerous times during the day.

Extreme: This book is not about extremes. We all read about people whose fitness or diet programs go to extremes. They become compulsive about whatever they do. One thing is certain. They never keep doing whatever they, obsessively and compulsively, are doing for very long. They will tire of it, burn out, or become physically ill from it. We are not talking about extreme. We are talking about a healthier, better lifestyle for the remainder of our years on the planet. Seven hours of aerobic activity a week and an hour-and-a-half of weight resistance activity is not an extreme but an optimum amount that will achieve exemplary fitness within two years, with mileposts at frequent intervals.

Eyes: One of the most sensitive parts of your body. Protect them with glare-proof and wind-proof glasses when you exercise out of doors and, always, with goggles when swimming. When exercising, it is important to see properly where you are going. If you are over 40, the chances are nine out of ten that your vision needs correction with eyeglasses. You can check this situation by yourself at your local discount store which now sells magnifying glasses for gray panthers. It is difficult to feel fit if you can't see clearly. Fuzzy vision often precedes fuzzy thinking.

Failure: There are no failures over 50. Trying in itself is success. While Star Wars' Yoda said, "Do or no do, no try." he was, remember, talking to young warriors — not the over-the-hill gang. For us, trying is succeeding and only quitting is failure.

Falling: Something all individuals involved in aerobic activities will do from time to time. Practice it occasionally so that the ground or floor will not seem so unfriendly.

Fanny pack: A specially designed bag worn around the waist, sitting up above the buttocks, which can carry a variety of nutritional aids, extra clothing, or fluid during extended periods of exercise away from home base.

Fartlek: A method of running training that involves varying one's speed for different distances along a run in a random manner to suit one's mood. It could apply, as well, to biking or swimming. It promotes the very kind of nonchalance and spontaneity that we have tried to stress throughout this book.

Fatigue: We all experience fatigue. It is the result of an inadequate amount of fuel to match the body's energy output. It is possible to be fatigued without doing much exercise because we are not eating right. Lack of exercise itself brings on fatigue because the arteries bringing the body's nutrients, blood flow, and oxygen are not open to proper circulation. When most of us think of fatigue, we think of over-work and over-exercise.

Surprisingly, fatigue is much less common as a result of those aspects and more common as a result of lack of fitness to take on a normal day's effort and lack of appropriate diet to fuel that effort. Whatever the fatigue you are experiencing, a reduction in normal and regular fatigue will be one of the earliest positive feedbacks of a fitness program.

Feeble: A physical state you need never experience if you become fit. It may sound strange, but nowadays it is possible to be fit until the day you die. Obviously, being fit won't preclude your ultimate demise. Something in your physical system will eventually break down and end it all, but it really is possible to be a healthy-looking corpse rather than a feeble-looking one. You may think that's morbid, but if the thought of it gets you disturbed enough to do something about it, all the better.

Feet: Two of the most overlooked treasures of the human body. Treat them with the best sport shoes money can buy. Don't stand on them too long when it can be avoided. Ice them down when they are sore and tired. Cut the toenails regularly and keep corns and callouses under control.

Firm: Partly what this book is all about. Firm is an adjective given to the human body when it has relatively little fat on it and when its muscles are relatively tight and capable of quick and efficient physical movement.

Firmness is one of the goals of a fitness program. It requires a strong focus on a weight/resistance exercise program. Many aerobically fit individuals do not have a firm body because they do not exercise the muscles that are not engaged in their aerobic activity. As an example, runners and cyclists might have excellent legs but have very poor upper body development, wherein these body muscles are not firm. Weight-resistant exercises are necessary to achieve that firmness and, in fact, muscle growth will be a likely result regardless of one's age. A weight-lifting program for mature people should consist of three 30-minute sessions a week of simple, hand-held dumbbell exercises. Descriptions of such programs are available in any store that sells weight-lifting equipment as well as from the authors of this book.

Fitness philosophy: It's a lot like a religion but it does not concern itself with yesterday or tomorrow. You work to be fit today for the feel of it and the look of it. Vanity and health are its focal points. Until the individual develops a fitness philosophy, i.e., religion, the road to successful achievement will be filled with potholes.

We'll even challenge the well-accepted rules of alternating hard days and easy days. Our body frequently wants to put two or three hard days together and at other times two or three easy days together. Most of us are not shooting for the moon — we simply strive to be as good as we can be and a damn sight better than the average guy or gal on the street who still isn't in what most of us would call good physical condition.

Flabby: A state in which, if you are in, you want to get out of, and once you get fit you'll never get back into. Excess weight and flab put stress on the heart and add nothing useful to the body's regimen. It develops as a result of too much caloric intake and too little caloric burn via exercise. A fitness program that combines proper exercise and nutrition will eliminate it, but not overnight as is suggested by so many fad diets.

Flexibility: The range of possible movement around a joint. Flexibility may be specific to each joint rather than general to the whole body. Find out which joints in your body have the least flexibility and work on them an extra amount in order to increase your range of motion. Gentle movement in the directions that movement is difficult will, over time, improve flexibility of that joint in that direction. The aging body suffers approximately a 1 percent loss in flexibility per year beyond the age of 30. This can be reduced with flexibility exercises, since it is commonly increased by the total disuse of joints. The mature individual with significant flexibility experiences great satisfaction from that capacity when he or she compares himself to his or her peers. The decline in flexibility becomes obvious with age.

Flexible training: We have found it to be a wonderful feeling not to look too far ahead in our training program. Normally, we do look toward tomorrow and think about our time schedule and what events might fit in best. We begin to psyche ourselves on the eve of each day. But if the day brings a different physical or mental feeling or weather conditions that don't fit our plan, we simply change the plan to fit the situation. With rare exceptions, therefore, each day we perform exactly what we want to do, not what we have to do, and that is where the true relaxation of exercise enters the picture.

Fluid replacement (see *EXCEED; Water*)

Food: A synonym for fuel. Think how your car would run on a mixture of sugary drinks and fatty foods; just about as well as your body does — not well at all. It is not possible to be fit on improper or inadequate food. The day will come when our collective life expectancy will increase radically as knowledge of proper diet is fully uncovered. In the meantime, you set the pace by increasing your intake of complex carbohydrates and reducing or eliminating your intake of fat. Try for 65% carbs, 20% protein, and 15% fat. Eat more rice, pasta, and potatoes plus green vegetables; eat frozen yogurt instead of ice cream, sugar substitutes instead of sugar, forget what cookies taste like, and never eat butter or fried food.

Frail: The state of being too thin and without muscle development. Most people as they grow old tend to lose not only excess weight but too much weight. Older people are far more commonly frail than overweight. In fact, overweight people don't generally get to be very old because the heart can't carry them very far through life against such an excessive load. Excessive weight loss in older people which leads to frailty is almost as undesirable as excess weight. Exercise will awaken the appetite and allow one to engage in a more balanced and nutritious diet that will yield appropriate weight maintenance and, hopefully, a healthy weight increase as the body becomes toned and firm.

Free: The approximate cost of fitness. Shoe leather, bicycle tires, and dumbbell weights, when amortized over their useful life, won't show up on anyone's budget. Healthy foods cost less too.

Free weights: A term used for weights not connected to a machine such as barbells or dumbbells.

Frequency: The number of times per week an exercise routine is performed. We recommend that most regular activities be performed at least three times a week and that some activity be performed each and every day. Try not to plan things too specifically, however, as the less regimen we promote in our programs, the more enjoyable the programs will continue to be. Never plan a day off. They happen on their own.

Friendly conversation: Something you can always engage in during exercise if you have a partner. You need never go so fast or so hard that you can't talk while exercising.

Friends: Surround yourself only with positive, optimistic friends. Negative, pessimistic people will wear you down and serve as an impediment or obstacle to being a fit and healthy person. Generally, negative people will undermine your efforts in addition to causing you physical stress that is an unnecessary part of your life. Postive and supportive friends will enhance your capability to achieve and maintain fitness in advancing years.

Fruit: Among the most important carbohydrate sources we can find. Everyone should eat a great deal of fruit, and as we grow older, its importance increases. If you avoid the normal snack food of potato chips, dips, and sweets and switch to a piece of fruit when you get hungry, you will be doing yourself a tremendous favor while still satisfying your hunger cravings.

Fun (see *Enjoyment*)

Gains: As we get older, improvements or gains in physical fitness will come more slowly. Don't be hard on yourself but, rather, look for small improvements over reasonable periods of time. They will be there. Take pleasure in them all. Don't demand too much of yourself. Remember, you're not trying to improve yourself for a dance or a game or activity next weekend, but rather to maximize enjoyment for the rest of your life. Gains can be in the form of being able to exercise faster or maintain more comfortable breathing while exercising, or moderate weight losses, better fit of clothes, improved muscle tone, greater energy through the day, and an overall improved sense of well-being.

Gait: Gait describes the length and frequency of one's stride when walking and running. Virtually everybody should include in their fitness program a period of fast walking or slow jogging. The key to an effective and comfortable gait is preliminary stretching of the quadricep (thigh) muscles and the hamstring muscles behind the leg and the area of the groin where the legs attach to the body, so that you can have a comfortable stride without stretching stiff muscles. Gait is a personal thing.

Some people tend to have a longer stride than others. Some have a faster paced step than others. What matters most is that your gait is comfortable for you, individually, and thus contributes to the enjoyment of your walk or run.

Games: There is an unfortunate misunderstanding with regard to the place of games in the promotion of physical fitness among people of mature or advanced ages. Normally, games are not played to get into physical condition. Rather, one gets into physical condition so that he or she can play games. Few people play games actively enough in a week or a month to maintain conditioning from those games alone. Secondarily, the quick starting and stopping that one encounters in most games can be extremely damaging to the body if the body is not initially fit. Thus we see huge numbers of injuries on the part of people who play softball, basketball, tennis, racquet ball, and the like periodically. They will play and enjoy these games far more if they are involved in a fitness program that brings them to the court or playing area physically prepared to take on the effort. Some games have very little value whatsoever in the realm of physical fitness but are often thought of as promoting same. Golf and bowling, to name but two, fall into this category. While many sports require hand/eye coordination and are strenuous to certain muscle groups within the body, they do not contribute in any significant way to physical fitness. Conversely, however, they do contribute significantly to physical ailments encountered by people of advancing age who pull back muscles and strain elbow and arm muscles from engaging in these sports without being physically prepared.

Garage: A place where one should not store exercise equipment. Out of sight, out of mind is a very true axiom. Thus, exercise equipment stored in garages does not get used. This would include stationary bicycles, exercise machinery, or hand weights such as dumbbells. While some people allot a certain space in their garage for physical exercise, they are few and far between. The exercise equipment should be stored in the house where it is constantly viewed and results in an incentive to be used. Garages, on the other hand, are a good place for storing outdoor bicycles which, by the way, should always be hung from hooks in the ceiling rather than allowed to set on their tires throughout the non-use period during most of the year. Storage on the tires will result in the destruction of the tire and continuous flatting. Small bicycle shops sell ceiling hooks for the very easy, out-of-the-way storage of bikes hanging upside down by the tires, one hook for each tire.

Glory: Young athletes compete for the glory of victory; older athletes and physical fitness buffs perform for the glory of competing in a race or event, but more often for the glory of well-being that each day brings.

Glycogen: The chemical that is produced from the processing of carbohydrate foods in the body. It is stored in the muscles, providing a reserve of energy. It is the glycogen store that is increased through carbohydrate loading (see *Carbohydrate loading*). It is vital for all endurance activities.

Goals: Everyone has to have some

goals in life — targets to drive them forward. The problem is that most people's goals are unreasonable — dreams that can never be reached. Goals are best set at realistic levels that can be achieved in reasonable periods of time and which bring on exceptional feelings of well-being. Once reaching a goal, one can lift his or her sights and move forward to another easily obtainable goal. Goals can and should be the incentive that carry us all forward in our quest for physical fitness, but unfortunately, too often, they become the source of our disillusionment and disappointment which causes us to give up that quest.

Golf: A delightful sport often maximizing social interchange but minimizing physical activity. Many have described it as a way to ruin a perfectly good walk in the woods. Golf can be a good way to eliminate stress. It can also be an even better way to increase stress. It is a great hobby for many men and women, but should never be considered as making a contribution to physical fitness, unless you are walking each and every one of the 18 holes on the golf course carrying your golf bag. In this day and age, few people do that and, in fact, few courses today even allow that. If you do walk the course, measure its length and you can factor it into an effective weekly exercise schedule, which should consist of no less than 12 miles per week, if walking is your primary aerobic activity.

Gorging: A word describing what many people do, on occasion, at meals so as to maximize the enjoyment of eating for the short-term. Unfortunately, the habit dramatically expands the period of ill-feeling following eating. It has always been a source of wonder that even with the miracle of the human body, it takes 20 minutes for a message that the stomach is full to reach the brain. Thus, we all tend to overeat on occasion and suffer the uncomfortable consequences afterwards. The excess calories and eventual fat are with us for a long period of time. The way to eliminate being full is to eat slowly, thus allowing adequate time for the fullness message to reach the brain before the stomach is distended and the body reaches the point of discomfort. Overeating is frequently a direct result of this poor communication system within the body. It is also negatively affected by periods of stress for many people. Two important simple dietary rules that relate directly or indirectly to gorging are never to overeat when you are hungry and never eat at all when you're not hungry. To avoid overeating at special social events, eat a small snack before leaving home. A small can of tuna fish packed in water with a few crackers will go a long way toward reducing the monstrous appetite we commonly arrive with at a party.

Gorp: A strange word describing a mixture of dried fruit and nuts carried by hikers and athletes for quick energy during endurance exercise activities. It can be purchased at outdoor stores or put together at home according to individual tastes.

Gortex: A fabric that allows moisture or water vapor to escape from the body to the outside air while keeping heat in. It has allowed for the manufacture of light-weight, warm athletic gear. Many other manufacturers have been able to duplicate the effect of Gortex with other tight-weave fabrics that achieve the same results. Anyone who plans a regular walking or running exercise program throughout the year in a temperate or cold climate should invest in a good light-weight, warm, Gortex running suit. It is money well spent and it will offer many years of wear and enjoyment.

Gravity boot: A padded boot that allows an individual to hang upside down from a bar, once thought to be very beneficial to circulation. While still used sparingly, resulting discomfort to knee joints has put this faddish program into decline.

Groin: The area of the body where the legs meet the pelvis. The abductor and aductor muscles emanating from the groin into the thigh are among the most common muscles to be pulled by mature adults. They require significant stretching for three or four minutes a day before performing aerobic activites. All manuals on stretching will contain numerous effective exercises for maintaining flexibility in the groin area. A significant amount of the rigid ambulation seen in old people is a result of tightness and loss of flexibility in the groin. If you maintain a stretching regimen in this area, while you may never be able to perform a dancer's split, you will enjoy ambulatory movement with great enthusiasm throughout your life.

Group training: Many people enjoy training with a partner or a group. No one can question the added enjoyment of the comraderie when training with others. You're fortunate if you have a friend or a spouse who can accommodate the times at which you are available to exercise. If you can find a group that works out on a schedule that you can meet, this is also advantageous. Having said this, however, most people will find that groups and regular partners are not readily available and even when available, for reasons of their and your schedule, will be inconsistent. Thus, it is absolutely imperative that you have the capacity and the initiative to train on an independent schedule of your own which is not allowed to vary dramatically by inconsistencies in the ability to train with others. Thus, we strongly recommend an independent training schedule which will make activities with a friend or a group an enjoyable luxury when possible.

Gyms: A gym is the place we all remember exercising in during our formal school days. Many of us still go to gyms or athletic clubs to perform our exercises since it is pleasant to go to a place where friends and acquaintances are engaged in similar activity. It is a mistake, however, to rely on such locations for exercise activity because they are not always conveniently located. To whatever extent one has to move oneself from point A to point B to get into an exercise mode, inconvenienced by travel, traffic, and weather, that exercise program will suffer. Gym activity can be very positive, but it must be a supplement to an exercise program that is not dependent on locating oneself in the gym. Small effective programs should be centered around the home, with activities at other locations serving as enjoyable supplements rather than the core of the program. Few of us have enough time to invest in travel and waiting in line to engage in an effective regular fitness

activity. Health clubs are flourishing as much for social reasons as workout accommodations. For every person who maintains an effective fitness regimen at a health club, we will show you four persons with health-club memberships who think that the possession of a membership card contributes to some form of physical fitness.

Habit: What exercise must become if fitness is to be possible.

Hair: If you're going to be an athlete or an exercising person on a regular basis, you might as well get used to wearing your hair short. It saves an awful lot of time in washing and drying it after strenuous exercise. Running and biking during warm parts of the year causes a great deal of perspiration from the scalp and thus will require frequent hair washing following exercise. But only the individual involved with swimming as an aerobic activity needs to be cautious about the treatment of his or her hair. Most individuals swim in a pool loaded with chlorine, which does chemical damage to the hair and at times will give it a greenish tint. The answer to this potential problem is the use of special shampoos on a regular basis.

Hamstring: The large muscle behind the thigh or quadricep muscle which makes running or jogging possible and gets additional use in bicycling. It needs to be as strong as the quadricep because they are opposing muscles which need balance. Nautilus-style, leg-curl machines shape them up quickly.

Hand grips: Devices that can be used at any time to strengthen one's hands, wrists, or forearms by the action of squeezing them. They can be as simple as a small rubber ball such as a handball or a special device made of a medium-hard rubber that fits into the palm of the hand with indentations for the four fingers for easy gripping and squeezing. They are rather fun to use because you can carry them with you and squeeze them any time benefitting the hand, wrist, and forearm, along with a little mental stimulation from the recognition that you are getting the most out of your time.

Hand weights: The light weights carried in the hands, primarily by runners while exercising, to further stress the cardiovascular system and exercise arms. While extremely light weights may have some minor advantage, increasing to any significant weight like three pounds in each arm is more likely to place undue stress on the back, which far outweighs any of its exercise benefit. We recommend against them. Do one thing at a time and focus on having a good time.

Hard days (see *Easy days*)

HDL/LDL: These terms refer to the two types of cholesterol in one's body. The medical profession has now proven that a high cholesterol level, which is the summation of the HDL and LDL cholesterol, is an indication that individuals may be prone to heart disease. Normally, a level above 240 is considered somewhat hazardous to one's health. A level below 200 is considered to be very safe and in the 200 to 240 range one should have moderate concern. It should be noted, however, that the LDL cholesterol has a positive impact on the body such that a high total cholesterol that consists of a high LDL and a moderate HDL is not

considered a cause for concern. It is now common for doctors to calculate both the sum of LDL and HDL and the ratio of HDL to LDL in assessing cardiovascular health.

Headache: Headaches can be a result of many malfunctions in the body, although the primary source is considered to be stress. We know that increased fitness goes hand-in-hand with decreasing physical stress. There is a measurable decline in headaches experienced by individuals who are considered fit and the decline continues as the level of fitness increases. This relates to improved blood flow in the arterial system that alleviates restrictions in blood vessels to the brain, which results in a high percentage of headaches. If you are an individual who experiences an extraordinary number of headaches in the course of a week or a month, you can optimistically look forward to a reduction in this type of discomfort as a result of a fitness program.

Health claims: Beware of the health claims made in all commercial advertising today. It would appear that we have become a health-conscious society. That may be less true with regard to what we actually do on the bottom line to preserve our fitness and health, but it is certainly true with regard to our being attracted to the purchase of anything that might improve our health. This relates to virtually all food producers who have gotten on a variety of bandwagons in recent years including "low cholesterol" and "oat bran." Commonly, advertisers tout the benefits of this and that when, in fact, the benefits of their product with regard to any special health impact are all but negligible. Certainly we want a high-fiber diet, but a little bran impregnated into this or that product has minimal health benefit. Certainly, we want a low-cholesterol diet, but we get that by eating foods that are low in cholesterol, not by one brand over another because of a slight dimunition of cholesterol. With few exceptions, health claims in the commercial food industry are blown so far out of proportion as to be meaningless. The same is true of devices of any kind for fitness and exercise which appear to offer the proverbial "free lunch." There are no short cuts. There are no easy ways, but there are, indeed, enjoyable and pleasant ways. These involve eating the right foods and finding the types of exercise that best suit your personality. Be a skeptic and you'll almost never be wrong.

Health club: A private club providing members with a wide variety of exercise-related activities. If you like working out around other people and have ample time to spend going, coming, and waiting, they can be an important element of a fitness program. The downside is that if you only exercise when you get to the health club, invariably you will not get to the health club enough. The best of all worlds is to have the discipline to exercise each and every day.

Heart monitoring devices: A current fad in exercise programs is the monitoring of one's heart beat through devices which commonly consist of a strap worn around the chest and a wrist-mounted readout that communicates by built-in radio transmitter with the chest strap. The wrist device can also be mounted on bicycle handlebars to give instant readings of the heartbeat rate. This allows one to know whether you are training at an effective level or over-training at too strenuous a level (see *Training effect*). Heart monitors are useful, cost-effective devices which can add knowledge and entertainment to those individuals embarking on a fitness program who like to keep track of their daily activity in a numerical manner. We don't think they are at all necessary, but recommend them for those inclined to get involved in the medical aspects of their program.

Heart rate (see *Recovery heart rate; Resting heart rate; Training effects*)

Heat prostration: Illness resulting from the body's inability to adjust to excessive heat. It generally includes weakness, dizziness, and nausea. This is not a problem to be dealt with lightly. It is best to stop moving, sit down, seek a cooler location, cool liquids, or compresses. Our capacity to deal with heat distinctly declines with age.

Heat stress: Excess loads placed upon the body by heat, making normal activites appear more difficult. Avoid exercising rigorously in excessively hot locations so as to reduce the potential for heat stress and over-exertion. Remember, exercise should be fun.

Helmet: Something you want to learn to wear when riding a bicycle so that falling off it will not be such a terrifying possibility. Bicycle helmets are now advised for all riders. They come in bright colors, weigh absolutely nothing, and adjust easily.

Hemorrhoids: Hemorrhoids plague many older people and can be especially uncomfortable for active older individuals. Running and, of course, biking can exacerbate the problem. The problem can be reduced significantly by wearing tight-fitting bicycle shorts when walking or running in order to reduce chafing. When biking, a very comfortable seat and/or seat cover should be used as well as padded bicycle pants. A dramatic reduction in hemorrhoidal discomfort can also be obtained by the use of Tucks or other pharmaceutical brand medicated pads to keep the area clean and sterile.

High: A feeling you will experience over and over again during exercise which will dramatically reduce your need to get high in more conventional manners.

Hiking: Cross-country walking; a wonderful activity, fulfilling both to the body and mind. Be sure to wear high-quality hiking boots or shoes.

Hips: The loss of flexibility in the hip area is common with age and must be attended to with special emphasis on stretching in the hip and groin area. The standard hip stretch requires one to lie flat on your back, leaving one leg extended, bring the other knee up, place the toe behind the knee of the opposing leg, and with the opposite hand pull the knee down toward the ground. This movement flexes the hip socket and the opposing muscles in the groin area. This will, if done regularly, dramatically reduce hip tightness which can lead to injury. At the same time, weakness in the hip joint will be strengthened by exercise and any resistance work done on the joint will reduce the proclivity toward osteoporosis that leads to so many fractured hips among older people.

Hobbies: Consider physical fitness, exercise, and sports as hobbies.

When considering whether or not you have enough time to get into good physical condition in order to have a fuller and richer later life, consider how much time you spend on passive hobbies. If your passive hobbies are the only place you can pick up some time, then you want to give a long hard look at how they contribute to your well-being and consider trading some of your more inactive hobbies for active ones. The best way to view the time spent being physically active and staying in physical shape is to view it as an active hobby.

Hockey: A game most commonly played on ice which allows men and, in a few cases, women to participate in a modified impact sport at an advanced age. Senior men's hockey leagues have sprouted up all over the United States. For those who were competent skaters in their youth, it can offer an unusual opportunity for physical activity.

Hotels: If you travel a good bit, you will find yourself in hotels with exercise rooms. Today, most have them. We find that individuals having some spare time on a trip will use the hotel's exercise room. This is a good thing, but this is where we really see the dabblers (see *Dabbling*). These are people who don't follow any kind of specific exercise regimen but finding themselves at the doorstep of an exercise room will take advantage of it for a short period of time, then go home and not keep it up. Again, any exercise is better than no exercise, but dropping in and out of exercise programs, periods, and places without consistency can't be expected to achieve much in the way of fitness.

Hot showers: A great comfort to the aging body. A hot shower prior to a physical workout, when the body feels stiff, is an excellent way to limber up. Hot showers, similarly, can be good following physical activity, but only if one has no chronic injuries that require icing before heating. For a hot shower to be of any value in limbering the body, it should last at least five minutes. While taking a hot shower, worthwhile stretching exercises can be performed primarily in the order of leaning over, locking one's knees, and letting your body hang until your hands touch your toes or the floor of the shower. This is among the most beneficial ways of stretching the lower back.

Hot tubs: A device more commonly used for socializing than for medicinal purposes, although the latter benefits are many. For people able to maintain a high level of physical fitness, hot tubs are an outstanding way of getting the soreness out and reducing tightness. They can be used the same way as the aforementioned hot showers and, of course, with even better results because of the ability to immerse the entire body in water. Water temperature of hot tubs is best set at 104 degrees for maximum and safe benefit. If you're capable of staying in the hot tub for more than 8 or 10 minutes at a time, then it is not hot enough to gain maximal advantage in limbering the body by increasing blood flow throughout the vascular system. Hot tubs with strong water jet action can be extremely useful in treating sore or bruised places on the body once ice has been applied for at least two days. After that time, directing the hot water jet onto an injured area will have the beneficial capacity of increasing movement of bruised cells out of the area bringing fresh healing blood into the area. The same is achieved, however, on a continuing basis through periodic icing.

Hot weather training: What care should be taken by the masters' athlete with regard to hot weather training? As with all matters of health, individuals of advancing age need to take greater care when training under less favorable conditions. Hot weather training can and should be an excellent way to improve overall fitness and your body's capacity to adjust to less than ideal conditions. But, the following rules should be observed:

1. Hydrate to the point of urination prior to training and plan to drink up to 12 oz. of water or other fluid replacement every 20 to 30 minutes.

2. Train within your comfort zone, as pushing to exhaustion will significantly delay recovery in hot weather. Thus long, slow distances will be more comfortable than quality speedwork in the heat. This is strongly recommended.

3. Neither begin a workout quickly upon leaving a cold environment nor move quickly back into one afterwards. Warm up and warm down in the heat. Heat can be an enjoyable environment if you focus on the loose and fluid manner with which your body will respond to it.

Hurt: Something you will get if you exercise regularly. You'll fall, stumble, twist, and turn things in manners that will create hurt. It simply goes with the territory, but a fit body heals far more rapidly than an unfit body and, at an advancing age, a few battle scars can be worn as badges of courage. Get to know a good sport medicine therapy clinic in your community. They are proliferating with talented practitioners who know the importance of getting their patients back into their exercise routine. They contrast with the doctor of old who with few exceptions prescribed lengthy periods of rest — something we now know to have a compounding negative effect on some types of injuries. In most cases, in the vernacular of the professional athlete, you will be able to play "hurt."

Hyperglycemia: Abnormally high concentrations of sugar in the blood caused by the inability of the body to handle normal amounts of sugar or resulting from the excessive intake of sugar. It can result in diabetes. Pure sugar has no redeeming qualities in the diet other than a delightful taste in many compositions. The body can get all the sugar (glucose) it needs by the breakdown of complex carbohydrates such as bread, rice, pasta, and potatoes. Sugar, the simplest form of carbohydrates, burns too quickly to be of any value as a source of energy and should be minimized in the diet.

Hyperventilation: Excessive movement of air in and out of the lungs. This can be caused by dramatic increases in the frequency of breathing or the depth of each breath. It primarily results from the inability of the lungs to clear waste carbon dioxide. It can result from activities requiring intensive, short bursts of speed. This is nothing for us older folks to worry about since we want to avoid short, intensive bursts of speed anyway. It can also result, however, from over-excitement not related to exercise.

Hypoglycemia: Inadequate levels of sugar in the blood. The opposite of hyperglycemia which is a more common affliction (see *Hyperglycemia*).

Hypothermia: A reduction of body temperature below 98.6 resulting in the body's attempt to warm itself by opening up the skin's blood vessels. It can result from extended exercise in extremely cold weather. Avoid same, just as you would avoid the heat. Remember, exercise should be fun.

Hypoxia: A lack of adequate oxygen which normally occurs as a result of exercise at high altitudes. The capacity of our blood to carry oxygen declines about 3 percent for every 1000 feet in elevation as a result of reduced air pressure. Exercising above 5000 feet is normally a hardship on anyone not acclimated to it. Avoid excessive exercise at high altitudes until your body becomes slowly accustomed to it. This is, of course, why snow skiing appears to be so incredibly tiring when all you are really doing is sliding down a hill. In fact, you are working very hard to maintain your stability in an evironment which allows your blood to carry significantly less oxygen to your muscles. If a ski trip is to last a week, start slowly, increasing each day to maximize the amount of enjoyable skiing and exercise you'll get during the trip.

Ice is nice: If you are an active, aging athlete and have not yet discovered that ice is the elixir of uninterrupted, relatively pain-free physical activity, now is the time to learn. Ice should not only be used as a rehabilitative process following injury, but as a constant defense technique against the chronic, physical problems which nearly everyone over 40 has.

Ice is the best friend an athletic body can have. Heat is fine for an uninjured body to work out stiffness, like soaking in a hot tub to get the blood flowing before a workout or loosening up after a tough day, but be sure you have neither a new muscle pull, tendon insult, or joint aggravation before you hop in. Heat is the enemy of injury because of the increased blood flow and, thus, the inflammation it causes. You may have heard that after 24 hours of cold (ice), heat can then be applied. Don't believe it. Old bodies bleed longer and stay inflamed more than 24 hours. O.K. How about 48 hours? I still would not risk it, especially when ice will do the same job as heat with no risk of exacerbating the damage. How, you ask, can ice replace heat? It's simple. Heat increases blood flow, carrying away damaged cells from the injured area. Ice, when used 10 to 20 minutes an hour, will first constrict or shrink the injured area while anesthetizing it. Then, when the ice is removed and the body part warms up, blood flow increases significantly until the ice is again applied. This process yields a massage to the blood vessels which alternately reduces and increases blood flow, clearing the area of dead cells just as heat can, but in no way creating the possibility of increasing new bleeding and inflammation in the injured area.

The problem is that few people have the patience to apply ice regularly, ten to twenty minutes per hour for several days. They want an easier solution. There are none, so the injured area tends to remain inflamed for a long time.

Ice, applied for less than ten minutes, is of little value; more than thirty minutes is just a waste of time because you have already reduced blood flow and now want the positive effects of increasing it again.

The real continuous advantage of ice, however, is the one nearly everyone overlooks. This is its use on chronic injuries or problems that always plague an athlete — they never go away, but don't necessarily slow or eliminate physical activity — the sore knee, ankle, or Achilles tendon are cases in point.

If you're over 40, something is going to hurt if you train for fifteen hours a week or more. At nearly any age something annoys you on a regular basis. It need not; that is, if you are willing to accept a little inconvenience. If you can get into the habit of applying thirty minutes of ice immediately following your workout to any body part which experiences chronic difficulty, you will find that the continued annoyance, pain, or slowed athletic ability can be reduced by 80 percent on a permanent basis. What we are saying is simply to apply ice as a defensive maneuver and, thereby, all but eliminate the plague of continuous aches and pains.

Of course, there are two problems which immediately work against this all but fool-proof procedure. The chronically, problemed body part does not normally hurt after a workout because it is so warm; second, who wants to strap on some ice for thirty minutes. When the area starts to hurt and stiffen up hours later, or even the next day, it's too late. Then you are likely to be in for a 48-hour rehabilitation program when 30 minutes of ice applied immediately would have eliminated the problem with no reduction in body flexibility.

It can be a real annoyance walking around with an ice-bag strapped to a knee, ankle, hip or what-have-you in your house, enroute to work in the morning or at dinner at night, especially if those trips or activities overlap, but thirty minutes of ice, soon after the cessation of a workout, will work wonders. If in doubt, if any part of your body so much as hiccups or squeals, slap it with ice now and often. When you start waking up in the morning without an ache or pain, limber from head to toe, you'll know the efficacy of ice.

We used to joke that if we ever woke up in the morning without an ache or a pain, we would have to assume that we died during the night. Not so any more. Ice is more than nice. It is the elixir of our life.

If it's not fun, don't do it: The feat of becoming physically fit is to be involved in fitness-related activities that are fun. It may be possible to convince a young person to engage in an activity on a regular basis that is not fun in order to achieve some very important goal, but it is virtually impossible to do the same for a mature person. We've had too much experience with disappointment and discomfort to continue to suffer for a goal that, at best, appears illusory. Thus, the secret to all fitness programs is that it must be a pleasant experience whatever it is you are doing or you're not going to do it for very long. Therefore, whatever program you develop, be it aerobics, running, cycling, swimming, dancing, jazzercise, weight lifting, calisthenics, etc., the intensity, duration, and the location must be such that you view it as a pleasant and rewarding activity. If not, don't waste your time. The "no pain, no gain" syndrome is strictly for the young. "If it's not fun, don't do it" is a far better slogan for us folks. And rest assured,

it is indeed possible to gain expertise in sports and overall physical fitness improvement on a continuous basis while enjoying every bit of it. That isn't to say you're not in a state of stress from time to time or that the intensity, duration, and the location of various exercises are not difficult, but the level of difficulty and the satisfaction achieved are balanced to the point that it is still enjoyable.

Illness: It's no secret to most that mature individuals may see themselves as being more prone to illness. They may also be more inclined to give in to illness. While in no way do we intend, in this book, to practice medicine, we want to point out that there are not many illnesses during which it is not possible to continue with a physical fitness routine. There is a tendency for everyone who feels below par to eliminate physical activity with the thought that less activity will provide for improved healing. While this may be the case with very serious illnesses, it is not commonly considered true of lesser debilitating problems. In fact, you will find in discussing this issue with physically fit individuals that, invariably, exercise improves their feeling of well-being. Exercise enhances blood flow and thus oxygen flow and the overall cleansing of toxic chemicals in the body. Thus, in most cases, one can continue a physical fitness routine, whatever it may be, though perhaps modifying your program in intensity and duration during periods that you are feeling ill. We are not, of course, talking about illnesses that require confinement to one's bed but rather ambulatory illnesses. If you are under doctor's care, obviously you want to check with the doctor before continuing. A good piece of advice is that if you are determined to follow a physical fitness program, you might want to seek medical advice from doctors with either a background in sports medicine or a bent for significant physical activity themselves.

Imagining: If your exercise program is aimed at improving capability in some particular sports, whether it be a game like tennis or golf or an exercise like running or cycling, it has been well proven that one's performance can be improved by imagining your activity in your mind's eye during periods of rest and relaxation. By now we all know that the mind is indeed a powerful thing and that mental preparation goes hand-in-hand with physical preparation. Of course, the power of positive thinking has been around for nearly half-a-century, but the idea of it is as valid today as ever. Thinking about what you are going to do to get fit will enhance both the activity that you select and the outcome you desire.

Inactivity: Probably the single greatest crime in the vernacular of healthy fit individuals. The older we get the more critical it is that we remain active. Periods of inactivity steal our capacity to perform in the most healthy and enthusiastic manner. Excuses for inactivity are many and varied and you've heard them all — lack of time, lack of opportunity, lack of desire, and, finally, lack of energy. Of course it's the latter that creates the biggest problem and inactivity itself steals energy from the body. Energy is a renewable resource. Up to a reasonable point, the more you expend the more you have. There are no good excuses for inactivity, and there is no way to achieve a fit body and lifestyle without activity.

Incline board: A board allowing an individual to hook their feet at one end in a raised position above the head, allowing for the performance of sit-up type exercises or stomach crunches with bent knees so as to strengthen the abdominal muscles. It's an inexpensive and efficient exercise device that, with time, can have a dramatically positive impact on the flattening of a senior citizen's abdomen.

Inconsistency (see also *Dabbling*): A most important part of any exercise program is consistency. If you want to achieve long-range goals, you have to decide that you are going to start a program and keep at it. You can vary the time you put in daily. You can vary the exercise you perform. You can vary the time of day at which you perform it. You can vary the intensity with which you perform it. You cannot, however, vary whether or not you do perform it. You cannot be inconsistent. Consistency will get you along a path towards fitness, achievement, and self-satisfaction. Consistency is what gained the turtle a victory over the hare — keep that in mind!

Incremental improvement (versus the shooting star): One should never look for dramatic improvements in capabilities. Such an outlook only leads to disappointment. Rather, one should look for very small incremental improvements over a reasonable period of time. The key is not to set yourself up for disappointment. At an advanced age, improvement is not rapid, although the increased feeling of well-being is easily and quickly measurable. Individuals who demand too much of themselves in the way of performance improvement will burn out rapidly from the excessive and unrealistic effort required, and then from the ultimate disappointment that must come when the rate of improvement levels off, as it will. Thus, the secret is not to demand too much of oneself, but to be realistic and reasonably confident that the goal will be achieved. This attitude isn't going to make anyone fit anytime soon, but it's guaranteed to achieve results for a better and more active life within a time frame that will leave you years and years to enjoy it.

Incremental training: This is a concept we have derived that achieves exceptionally good results for mature individuals. It focuses on always starting an activity at a slow, relaxed pace and then increasing the pace in tiny increments. The object is to always stay in one's comfort zone but attempt to increase intensity so that you get more out of every minute of exercise. An example when walking or jogging on a treadmill or running machine that shows your speed would be as follows: start out at a pace of 4 miles per hour, and increase your pace by a tenth of a mile every 1 to 3 minutes during the duration of your walk or run. Such small increments are easy to achieve. They give you a satisfying and rewarding feeling that you are able to push yourself a little harder without suffering any discomfort. The same can be done on a bicycle ride with a speedometer — try to increase your average speed incrementally through the ride every few minutes. In a swimming pool, if you're swimming laps, make each lap in a series slightly faster than the lap

before for 3, 5, or 6 laps and then start the series all over again. This kind of stress within your comfort zone is very effective in increasing performance and overall health.

Index gears: A new innovation for bicycles which take the guesswork out of shifting a ten-speed and trying to land the chain clearly on a larger or smaller sprocket wheel. Index gearing systems provide for a positive click indicating that the gear lever has been moved properly to the next setting above or below the gear being changed. Gear changing on ten-speed bikes can be a problem and a mystery to many novice bikers. Index gear systems have dramatically altered that impediment to enjoyable cycling.

Indoor bike trainers: Perhaps the most important single tool capable of yielding easy and convenient exercise leading to fitness. There's nothing much easier than jumping on an exercise bike in your basement or living room. Available today, even simpler and less costly than an exercise bike, are bike stands that allow you to place your outdoor bike in a stand and adjust resistance or ride in a stationary position with a reading stand set on the handlebars. Whichever way you go, stationary biking in the comfort of your home is the easiest possible way to get in relaxed, convenient, non-stressful, aerobic exercise while doubling your time input through reading or enjoying a favorite television program. The indoor exercise bike is particularly well suited for beginning your day with a stint right out of bed onto the bike. You can start slowly, warm up easily in the comfort of your home, get your blood flowing, and really jump-start your day while catching up on the morning news on TV or reading the morning newspaper. You are actually better off sleeping a half-hour less and putting that extra time into a morning, indoor cycle period as you will get more out of it than you would the additional sleep.

Injuries: There is no doubt that anyone pursuing a physical fitness program is going to experience injuries from time to time. They may vary from doing something as silly as stepping into a hole while running, pulling a muscle because you weren't properly warmed up, or extending an exercise period too long and experiencing overstress. The primary injury will be a pulled muscle; second will be a joint inflammation. The standard therapy for most injuries follows the acronym "RICE" — "r" for rest, "i" for ice, "c" for compression, and "e" for elevation. It will not always be convenient to do those things. The most important is ice, described in detail elsewhere in this text; second is compression, which is wrapping an injury with an elastic bandage to offer external support. A day of rest from the activity that caused the injury is always a safe recommendation and, at times, multiple days may be necessary with the advice of your sports medicine trainer or your own experience. The most important advice, however, with regard to all injuries is to let pain be your guide.

Just as we recommend that in exercise "if it isn't fun, don't do it," the corollary to that is "if it hurts, don't do it." Thus, if you are injured and are able to continue a particular mode of exercise with only limited discomfort, then it is normally okay to pur-

sue that exercise if it doesn't bring on pain. People of advanced years are more likely to take too much time away from exercise as a result of an injury than exacerbate the injury as a result of going back to the activity too soon. It takes a long time for mature individuals to get in shape but, sadly, it doesn't take long to get out of shape. Thus, one doesn't want to remain inactive too long while waiting for an injury to heal. A certain amount of healing will occur while activity continues and a certain amount of activity will actually promote better healing. Again, let pain be your guide.

Injuries can be kept to a minimum if one remembers to warm up slowly, to avoid rapid movements of stiff body parts, to stop activity at the onset of significant discomfort, to keep your eyes open for anything in your path that may create loss of balance, and, finally, to remember that "haste makes waste" and quick, unplanned movements often lead to negative results.

Inspiration: When you are past 50 and you are fit, you will be remarkable to those around you. They will not hesitate to comment on how fit you are and how much better you look than the average person. This positive reinforcement will inspire many people to attempt to follow in your course. Admittedly, most will not follow, but the satisfaction of influencing even a few people is considerable. It is interesting to note that young people, certainly below the age of 35, are not prone to comment on each other's physical fitness. But, invariably, people over 50 will comment when they see someone who looks great. Of course, they are a little jealous of anyone that looks better than they do. Yet that very jealousy can be turned into a positive inspiration.

Instep: A common place where foot injuries occur as a result of jogging or exercising in inadequate shoes. Good running shoes with proper built-in arches have dramatically decreased injuries that were once so common to the instep. Foot injuries can be very debilitating but can be avoided by never spending any significant time walking on hard surfaces in bare feet and ensuring that one does not step on or run over stones. Injured insteps should be treated immediately with ice and compression.

Instruction: Just as the carpenter or mechanic becomes expert at his craft by learning the use of the right tools in the right manner, all of us engaging in any type of physical activity can benefit from instruction which enables us to use our bodies more effectively. On the other hand, exceptional skill in any physical activity is unnecessary when it comes to achieving fitness.

It becomes rather a matter of efficiency. You can run, cycle, and row yourself into good health with little knowledge and poor form. You can go it alone by reading manuals on any particular activity or learn from experts in your community. One advantage of health clubs is that they frequently have staff members who can assist you in your program whether it's weight lifting, running, cycling, swimming, etc. Similar free assistance and guidance can be found at the stores where you purchase your bicycle, running shoes, or equipment. There are also excellent videotapes on the market. The best buys would be the triathlon training tapes by the likes of Dave Scott, Scott Tinley, and Mark Allen, all of which offer exceptional visual instruction in swimming, cycling, and running. Let me emphasize, however, that we are not about becoming great athletes. We are only about becoming physically fit through exercise. Form and efficiency don't make a whole lot of difference — just do it and enjoy!

Interval training: This is the common athletic terminology for a training program that alternates slow and fast performance levels. It is a must for young athletes to achieve their optimum capability. It is probably a must for mature athletes to become champions. It is definitely not advised for regular, every-day people who want to optimize a fitness program for continuous activity and a long and healthy life. The reason for this negative assessment is simply that it is far too demanding on the body, will likely create injury, and will, without exception, cause one to leave one's comfort zone and eventually be turned off by the whole program. Incremental training and incremental gains described previously are the replacement program for interval training. Without exception, interval training will take an individual to the wall or to the limits of his or her capability and create a momentary terror which a normal person is not readily inclined to repeat. Thus, programs that include interval training lead to "workout dread" and dreading a workout eventually leads to the elimination of that workout. It may be sacriligeous in champion athletic circles to talk against interval training, but normal, every-day people trying to achieve an optimum level of fitness might do well to listen.

Intimidation: The average out-of-shape individual is intimidated by those around him who are in excellent physical condition. Recognizing that he cannot achieve the status of the conditioned athlete any time soon, the results of intimidation are not to set out on a course aimed at improving one's fitness. As with most things, a journey of a thousand miles begins with the first step. You must not allow yourself to be intimidated by those who have already achieved some very significant goals. Everyone must set his own pace, recognize that goals can be achieved within some period of time, and ignore outside influences that might be a deterrent.

Introverts: Many people who are quiet and have tendencies toward introverted personalities are uncomfortable making any kind of a spectacle of themselves and often have difficulty in developing a physical fitness program that requires them to be active in public places. They must either defend themselves against views of the outside world about what they are doing or perform their physical fitness program in the privacy of their own domain.

Irritants: Anything that bugs you while you're exercising. Chafing of the skin, a pebble in your shoe, tight shoes or clothes, you name it — if it bothers you, it's an irritant and is going to dramatically reduce the enjoyment you receive from exercise. Before you get started in any exercise activity, make sure your whole system — body and clothing — is comfortable and nothing serves as an irritant. Otherwise, it won't be fun.

Vaseline and properly fitting clothes are the two best friends to the athlete wanting to function without irritation.

Isokinetic exercise: A type of exercise in which resistance is provided by friction such as an exercise bicycle. Controlled velocity can impose continued maximum resistance on the exercising muscles.

Isometric exercise: Muscular contraction without movement, such as pushing against a fixed object. This was a faddish form of exercise in the late 50s, thought to enable you to gain fitness in a few minutes a day. A certain amount of muscle strength can be gained from isometric exercise, but it has given way to isotonic exercise (see *Isotonic exercise*).

Isotonic exercise: Muscular contraction in which tension is varied against the muscle while moving a constant load, such as in the use of free weights or exercise machines. It is far more psychologically satisfying to work against a moveable object in which progress of motion can be viewed. Thus, isotonic exercise is both the most popular and, in the long run, the most efficient. The latter is usually easier and also pleasant because individual exercise such as running and bicycling allows one to commune with one's own mind and thus lends itself most favorably to the introverted personality.

Jarring: Something you should not experience during exercise. All movements should be smooth and fluid. Jarring your body has no redeeming qualities once our contact sports days are over. Exercise should be relaxed and comfortable, not jarring.

Jaw: Few people recognize that the carriage of the jaw can reflect the attitude of your entire body. If your jaw is held in a tense position, your entire body will be tight and lack the capability of fluid movement. A relaxed jaw, on the other hand, leads to a relaxed body. Be aware of the manner in which you carry your jaw at all times in all activities. Keep it relaxed, and you will be relaxed. Only a small number of people with clenched teeth achieve efficient or optimal results in anything they do.

Jazzercize: A form of aerobic conditioning set to music. An excellent way to obtain aerobic exercise that conditions the musculature as well as the lung capacity. Normally done in a group, it can be reassuring to some people, but intimidating to others. Classes are now divided into low and high impact, as are most aerobic conditioning programs. Avoid high-impact programs.

Jogging: A generic term for all types of slow running. Some running experts have tried to define the difference between jogging and running as when motion changes from more vertical to horizontal. That is to say, when jogging, it is easy to see a body move significantly up and down with each step. When reaching the speed of running, the vertical motion becomes minimal, and the forward motion of each step is more obvious. Such a transition occurs at about the point where an individual becomes capable of running a 7 $\frac{1}{2}$-minute mile — some of us will, but most of us won't. You may need to, for macho reasons, call yourself a runner; it might be more honest to think of yourself as a jogger. If you jog slower than 8-minute miles, as most of us do, don't be ashamed of 12-minute miles.

Inexpensive treadmills offer a wonderful alternative to the great outdoors.

Jogging requires no particular skill. Almost everyone can run a little, and style is relatively unimportant. To swim you need a pool and to bike you need a machine and an open road, but to run you need only the inclination to get out and do it.

Despite the fact that running style is not a critical matter, it's good to adopt a comfortable, economical way of running. Here are some suggestions:

• Run in an upright position. Don't lean far forward or backward. Keep your back as straight as you can with comfort.

• Keep your head up. Don't look at your feet.

• Carry your arms slightly away from the body with the elbows bent in and the forearms roughly parallel with the ground. Don't be rigid and don't flap your arms or hands.

• Keep your stride relatively short.

• Breathe deeply with your mouth open and take deep breaths as often as necessary.

Johns: A polite name for toilet or bathroom, something you always want to know the location of when out and about on a run or bicycling trip. Make it a habit of going to the "john" just prior to an exercise activity so as to avoid the dreaded need to go far from home with no friendly location in sight. As a safety precaution, however, carry a little toilet paper in a plastic baggy flat against your thigh, under spandex running shorts.

Joints: It's almost impossible to pass 50 without experiencing inflammation in one joint or another. It can be the result of misuse, overuse, or disuse.

Aspirin and a variety of strong substitutes are quite capable of keeping joint inflammation in tow. Regular exercise of joints in a non-damaging way is the long-time best cure for the problem. Joint pain is almost always related to the weakening of the musculature around the joint that allows the joint to operate in an inefficient manner. The strengthening of small muscles around the joint will cause the joint to operate in a very even plane without wobble and, thus, will alleviate the inflammation that occurs as a result of the wobbling articulation of joints. Knee and shoulder problems are the most common among older folks, followed closely by ankles and elbows. Ice should be a constant companion to those plagued with joint irritation. Regular use of low dosages of anti-inflammatories can work wonders. Nautilus-style exercise equipment is particularly good for increasing joint strength, as it fixes the various portions of the skeleton in preparing for a particular movement, isolating the joint and eliminating the possibility of further damaging an already weak area.

Jumping: Avoid it, whether it be on the dance floor or out of bed. It's jarring and has no benefits, unless, of course, it's out of airplanes, in which case the landing is intended to be as soft as falling into a feather bed — not always, however.

Karate: One of the many forms of martial arts that have become so popular today. Karate, and Tai Kwon Do, are probably the most popular of the arts currently in practice. They teach disciplined body control, all focused on movements that allow optimal self-defense if one were to be physically attacked. While many study martial arts so that they are prepared to defend themselves, many more study martial arts for the discipline and physical exercise that is involved. There is absolutely no age limit for the beginning of a martial arts training program, nor is there any limit to how far an individual can pursue a course toward a black belt, the highest level of achievement. Time spent in active martial arts classes, like karate, can definitely be counted in a weekly aerobic activity program. However, because a great deal of time is spent in a resting position watching example moves and listening to instruction, one should never count an hour of martial arts training as more than 30 minutes of aerobic activity.

Keeping back with your friend/ spouse/squeeze: The major problem in exercising is finding a partner to go along with you, if you are socially inclined. However, when you find the people who want to go along, you rarely find those who want to go at your pace. People who are faster are not a problem. You simply can't keep up with them, so forget them. People who are slower are our concern. They are worth nurturing and slowing down for. More friends, spouses, and squeezes would go along with their physically active cohorts if they felt they were not too much of a drag and could operate at their own speed. The fact is you can always slow down and still get much benefit from the exercise. If you're cycling with a slower individual, just cycle in a much lower gear that requires you to turn more revolutions per minute to achieve a speed that you could easily achieve with less rpms in a higher gear. It's excellent exercise, and it causes you to go slower. If you're running and can't use up all your energy going straight ahead, bound somewhat, pushing off your toes straight up into the air, during each stride, until your stride achieves the same forward motion as your partner. This is very difficult, very demanding, and works the lower calf muscles exceptionally well. If you're skiing, slow down and enjoy the scenery with your partner. Make more turns. Concentrate on your form. Eventually, your partner will appreciate what you're doing and will work to move a little faster if that need is perceived. How often do you see husbands and wives running together, cycling together, or skiing together? The answer, of course, is not often. This is unfortunate and works to the detriment of everyone when the simple recommendations we have just made can solve the major portion of the problems.

Kinesiology: A branch of science primarily concerned with muscular movement. It is through this study that scientists have assisted athletes in perfecting their skills. There has been a minimal amount of translation of benefits to those of us primarily interested in fitness, but nothing significant. It has probably been more useful for game-playing in terms of improving the mechanics of tennis and golf.

Lactic acid: A chemical formed as a result of the incomplete breakdown of carbohydrate in the body. Retention of lactic acid in the muscles following exercise results in an aching feeling. Warming down from an activity with light exercise will tend to minimize lactic acid retention and thus the aching feeling following an endurance effort.

Large muscle groups: These consist of the thigh muscles such as the quadriceps and the hamstrings, the shoulder muscles, the chest muscles, and the back muscles. In performing a weight-lifting routine, the large muscle groups should be exercised first and the small muscle groups such as the forearms, biceps, triceps, and calves last. The reason for this is that in exercising the small muscle groups, you will also bring into play the large muscle groups, and if you fatigue them too much, you won't be able to get the full impact of your weight-lifting routine when you focus on them secondarily instead of primarily. Beginning also with the large muscle groups will more rapidly improve blood flow throughout the whole body, creating the necessary warm-up function which will enable you to maximize the exercising of the small muscle groups later in your workout.

Layering: A technique of keeping warm in the winter by wearing multiple layers of thin clothing rather than a few layers of heavy clothing. The reason for its effectiveness is that the air trapped between the thin layers of clothing becomes an insulation warmed rapidly by body heat and retaining that heat by being trapped between layers of clothing. The result is multi-layered insulation, which is far more effective than thick, weighty clothing. At the same time, it is more comfortable and allows much greater ease of movement.

Lazy: Something we all are at one time or another. Lazy is basically a state of mind which tries to avoid activity. We feel lazy in the face of many activity options which we don't consider to be much fun. Once you learn the joy of exercise, your own inherent laziness will not impede your performing your exercise routine because it will not be something you deem unpleasant and thereby wish to avoid. Many people think we are perpetual motion machines, the antithesis of lazy. But if you want to see lazy, watch us when we are asked to perform chores we find unexciting.

Lean body mass: The total weight of the body minus the weight of the fat content of the body is equal to the lean body mass. It is primarily composed of the skeleton, the muscle mass, and associated tendons. It is sometimes called a "fat-free" weight and is something too many of us have too little of.

Lecithin: A group of phosphatides said to lower blood cholesterol levels and prevent heart disease; by no means a proven quantity. It is the darling of health-food faddists and, who knows, they could be right.

Leisure: Most of us, as we reach an advanced age, have more leisure time. Thus, it should be far easier for us to find time for a 7-hour weekly aerobic program and an hour-and-a-half weekly weight-training program. When we're fit, we can enjoy the rest of our leisure time in the active pursuits of other games and sports that would not be open to us were we not fit. Thus fitness clearly makes it possible to maximize the enjoyment of our leisure time.

Lethargy: A common feeling describing a lack of energy. Feelings of lethargy are either dramatically reduced or entirely eliminated when one achieves physical fitness. Part of the reason, again, relates to the capacity of a fit person's circulatory system to carry oxygen throughout the body, giving it energy and thus eliminating lethargy.

Lightfoot running: Always run light on your feet. Try not to be ponderous. Running with a light step means you're relaxed and going at a comfortable speed. Try it! You'll like it! Obviously, you can't defy the law of gravity and your entire weight must, eventually, impact on your feet. But part of running is mental and you can lighten your load if you focus on it.

Limits: There are no limits to what an individual of advancing years can achieve in the area of physical fitness. We have sadly been programmed to believe in the steep decline of physical capability with aging when, in fact, this steep decline was largely the result of inactivity. It is possible, beyond the age of 50, to become a competitive body builder, to run a three-hour marathon, to bicycle across America, to swim the English Channel, and to row with an elite east coast rowing club in competitive regattas. Few of us have any desire to rise to such levels of athleticism, but others have done it. The point is, there is no limit to what we can achieve regardless of our starting point. It may take longer to arrive at our goal, but who's in a hurry? As with all things, the chase is easily as exciting, if not more so, than the catch.

Liver: A very healthy source of protein and iron as food. Eaten once a week by women, it will significantly reduce their inherent propensity toward iron deficiency. Your own liver is a filtering device for your blood which becomes neutralized by excess intake of alcohol.

Log book: Diaries used to record daily and weekly exercise programs. They should only be used by personalities who enjoy recording their activities. If at any point they become a labor, they have defeated their value. If you are an individual who likes to see what you have achieved over a period of time, keeping a record of that achievement is an excellent idea. For us, personally, we are not out to conquer the world this week or next month. but rather to embark on a life-long journey to fitness which includes a considerable amount of repetition that does not require detailed logging. A drawback to log books is that while gains in activity levels are great at the early portions of exercise programs, they are few and far between after one is engaged in a program for a long period of time. Thus, looking at a log book in the later stages provides little positive feedback for progress. So, beware of the early advantages of keeping track of what you are doing and the later disadvantages and do what fits your own personal needs.

Longevity: It has often been said that physical fitness and exercise will not necessarily increase your life span but will most assuredly make the time you live more enjoyable. Scientific evidence, up to a point, is now beginning to indicate that your prospects for longevity are enhanced by increasing your fitness and activity levels with age. Of course it makes sense that if you keep your plumbing system operating smoothly and un-clogged, it will function longer than if you let it close up from disuse. While genetics bears heavily on longevity, there appears to be a spread of years that can be gained by anyone who keeps their systems in active use. Many of us avoid risks in order to live longer, but ignore maintaining activity levels which are likely to achieve more certain results.

Loose skin: Our skin is an organ. Loose skin is an indication of the decline and lack of fitness of that organ. It looses resilience with age and no longer fits tightly around all parts of our body. But like all of our other organs, it will prosper through exercise, stretching, and overall physical fitness. It is possible to be an octogenarian without having loose skin; the possible exception is the face, which requires extraordinary care to maintain tightness. This too, however, can be achieved with a variety of facial exercises and mois-turizing creams. If you have reached a point where your skin is already very loose, you can look forward to improving the situation perhaps as much as 50 percent but will likely be unable to fully tighten it over the whole body. If, however, you have not yet reached the age where your skin is loosening or it is just beginning to loosen, you can reverse a minimal problem and avoid a future problem by maintaining physical fitness throughout the remainder of your life.

The situation is exacerbated if initi-ating a fitness program also means a significant weight loss. This will re-sult in loose skin. It can be partially alleviated by massage, exercise, and moisturizing creams throughout the weight loss period. If the weight loss is done properly over an extended period of time rather than a radical short period, skin looseness will be reduced.

Lower back: Few people over the age of 30 have not experienced some lower back pain. Most commonly, it is the result of the weakening of the back muscles which allow the spinal column to get out of alignment. Thus, exercise that improves muscle tone in the back will go a long way toward minimizing or eliminating back pain. Chronic lower back pain can be the result of an inequality in leg lengths, something that can be determined by an orthopedic specialist and remedied by the utilization of a heel pad inserted in the shoe of the shorter leg. There are three simple lower back exercises that can be used in combination. The first is hanging from the waist with locked knees allowing the body weight to stretch the lower back as the fingers and eventually hands proceed toward the floor. The second is the reverse flexibility movement, done like a half-pushup, lying on the ground, pushing your upper body up off the ground with your arms while your pelvis remains on the floor. The third is the same exercise recommended under the hip entry, which not only exercises the hip but also helps align the spine. In any case, lower back problems do respond to exercise.

Lows: Periods one experiences at different times regardless of how upbeat and enthusiastic a person you are. The most positive people will experience "lows" when many things go wrong within their lives or with events outside the realm of their influence. Virtually all exercise enthu-

siasts have learned that lows can be radically diminished by periods of intense exercise. The reasons are quite understandable.

1. Exercise allows you to refocus your attention away from those things that are depressing you.

2. Exercise relieves physical and emotional stress by improving blood, nutrient, and oxygen transmission to the brain.

3. Exercise taken to the limit may stimulate the production of endorphens in the brain which create a mental high. Exercise is neither magic nor myth. It really works to reduce the effects of periods of mental depression.

LSD vs. speed: LSD stands for long-slow-distance, not the other stuff of the 60s. Long-slow-distance is pooh-poohed as much by many champion athletes as interval training is embraced by those same athletes. Speed, of course, is what champions aim for at all times. Older people shouldn't care about speed. They should focus on enjoying activity so they will get proportionately more out of going farther, longer, and slower. The object is to enjoy what you're doing. It's easy to enjoy a relaxed run, bike ride, or swim when you're focusing on just getting there and not how fast you get there. In the long run, the mature person will burn more calories by continuing activity longer than by increasing the intensity for a shorter period of time. This is not necessarily true for younger people, who are capable of achieving higher intensities altogether. Long-slow-distance will not make you a champion, but that's not what this book is about.

Luck: We all have it; some of it is good

and some is bad. There's a very interesting expression that says "the harder I work, the luckier I get." It applies to nearly everything in life, including fitness. The harder you work, the luckier you'll get with regard to having good health, fewer periods of illness, and, generally, more good times.

Lunch: A meal in the middle of the day that should never be missed. Proper health and fitness requires many small meals through the day. People who skip breakfast and/or lunch are fooling themselves with regard to eliminating caloric intake while penalizing themselves in terms of available energy to function efficiently through the day. Lunch, however, should not be so heavy a meal as to induce sleep. Overeating is the primary cause of sleep inducement because it drains the body of blood and nutrients which have to be utilized in the stomach during digestion. Secondarily, excessive intake of certain proteins will also induce sleep. Lunch is a good time to focus on fruits and salads.

Malaise (see *Lows*)

Massage: A highly underrated and misunderstood therapy technique. More and more of the most elite athletes in the world are relying on massage to optimize their fitness. In our youth, massage was something usually afforded only by very old and very well-to-do individuals. While we don't recommend massage on a regular basis, purely for economic reasons, a good sport massage expert today can help a mature individual work out a lot of stiffness and soreness that will make physical activity more pleasant and more efficient. It is important to remember, however, that a very good massage will commonly involve suffering a certain amount of pain and discomfort. Gentle rubbing on the surface of the body has very limited value other than overall relaxation. Deep massage, which functionally assists in fitness therapy, requires very strong hands on the part of the massage therapist and a reasonably good pain tolerance on the part of the participant. Many professional athletes get a massage before every important event. Most of us don't have these types of events and, thus, don't require frequent massages. But if you find a good masseur with a strong reputation in sports massage, treating yourself to a massage once a month might be a very good investment in fitness.

Maximum heart rate: The fastest a human heart can beat. It varies with age and is normally equal to 220 minus one's age in years. If you are 50, your maximum heart rate is likely 170. Aerobic activities should force the heart rate up to 60 to 80 percent of its maximum rate in order to sustain efficient health benefits.

Maximum oxygen uptake (VO_2 max): The maximum amount of oxygen that can be metabolized in the blood and circulated throughout the body. The greater the maximum oxygen uptake, the more work or exercise an individual can do before experiencing fatigue. It is distinctly a measure of fitness. The fastest way to increase your VO_2 max is to reduce your fat content, which robs the circulating blood system of oxygen. All sport medicine clinics and many doctors have the capacity to measure the VO_2 max by measuring oxygen intake and carbon dioxide exhalation during exercise periods on treadmill-type devices. If you plan to undertake a long-range fitness program, a VO$_2$ max test every six months is an excellent way to find out if your body is truly improving, in addition to the more obvious wellness factors that you will experience psychologically.

Meals (see also *Breakfast; Dinner; Lunch*): Don't skip any.

Meditation (see also *Visualization*): This is a form of rehearsing performance by meditating upon it. Meditation relates to focusing on positive thoughts that will ultimately help performance while significantly relaxing the body. Most meditation techniques are extremely worthwhile and valuable. The mind is, indeed, a powerful mechanism that can have a tremendous positive impact on one's physical fitness. Weight lifters can definitely lift more weight when they focus properly upon it, and athletes can move faster with the same kind of impetus. A general meditation program which fits into the overall picture of the power of positive thinking will improve the efficiency and productivity of a fitness program. There are a variety of audio tapes on the market that assist in the meditation process. We highly recommend those available from Frank Zane, a former world body-building champion now turned psychologist. Tapes are available from Zane Haven, P.O. Box 2031, Palm Springs, CA 92263.

Mental attitude: It's an age-old saying that mental attitude is 75 percent of anything we do. That is certainly true when it comes to fitness. Physical exercise can simply not be performed on any kind of regular, continuing basis without the mental attitude focusing on its value toward achieving a goal throughout life. The population can really be divided into two groups — those who care about fitness and those who don't. The latter group dwarfs the former. If you want it mentally, you can have it. There isn't any hurry. You will get there. The song about the ant moving the rubber tree plant is very meaningful to man's capacity to obtain fitness. The achievement of the right mental attitude can be gained by studying the entry under *Affirmations*. Having the proper mental attitude first involves a sincere desire to achieve fitness; second, you must have the ability to visualize a goal you want to achieve in a reasonable period of time. That reasonable period can well be a number of years. Just as Rome wasn't built in a day, you can't change your internal and external physical structure in a short period of time. But with the right attitude, the fact that you can change it is not in doubt.

Mileage: People who swim, bike, and run for exercise are commonly concerned about how far they should travel. They see conditioned people going a long distance and become discouraged because they can't imagine traveling a long distance on foot, bicycle, or water. The secret, of course, is to start short and let the mileage add up in small increments. It is interesting to note that the body's ability to extend exercise distance is not arithmetic but exponential. That is to say, it increases in larger and larger increments as the exercise program continues. For example, it might take a month to be able to jog a mile, but the second mile could be added in a couple of weeks, and the third mile in even less time. While there's never any hurry to add distance to any exercise activity you're performing, it is nice to know that the ultimate ability to add that distance gets easier rather than more difficult. An optimal running program might consist of 12 to 20 miles a week. A biking program might be between 30 and 50 miles a week. A swimming program might vary between 1 and 3 miles per week. As people get further and further into satisfying and gratifying fitness programs, they add mileage not because it will make them more fit but because exercise becomes such a pleasant form of relaxation.

Moderation: Actually, a very overrated term. One cannot argue that most things are best in moderation, but some things are wonderful when taken to the extreme. We have no quarrel with anyone who does everything in moderation but, likewise, we have no quarrel with people who carry positive activities to the extreme. Exercise would be a good example. There has been much written about exercise addictions and their negative aspects. As with all things, one can find people whose lives have been harmed by an exercise addiction, but they are few and far between. No reasonable person need worry in the least that launching into an exercise program, aimed at becoming fit, will lead to a crippling addiction of any type. This kind of an academic dialogue is generally initiated by doomsayer personalities or attention-seeking individuals and, of course, the media would never avoid an attention-getting expose. Remember, you only pass this way once. This isn't a dress rehearsal. If

you're enjoying whatever you're doing, do it to whatever extent you desire as long as it's not interfering with the lives of those around you or hurting you in any obvious way.

Morton's neuromo: A moderately common pain occurring beneath the balls of one's foot due to a pinching of nerves in the foot by the metacarpyl bones at the base of the toes. It occurs between the third and fourth toes, causing swelling, numbness, and pain which can make running impossible. It can be treated in three ways: by wearing a shoe insert with a lump under the toes in question, which tends to spread the metacarpyl bones, relieving pressure on the nerve; a variety of medicinal drugs can be injected into the foot to reduce the swelling for long periods of time; or the condition can be eliminated by out-patient surgical procedures. The best prevention of the problem is to wear shoes that are very wide across the toes so that compression is minimized.

Motivation: Motivation should not be difficult when you realize that achieving excellence among your peers, as these peers age, gets easier and easier. The vast majority give in to the cries of "give up;" only a few ignore those exhortations and carry forward. The recognition that you are one of those places you in the thin air of aging athletes. This is satisfaction in itself which can begin a self-motivating momentum that makes all your training sheer enjoyment instead of drudgery. One doesn't have to become an egotistical bore in the company of more normal peers to enjoy one's prowess. One can simply smile inwardly and look around the room at a social gathering with the knowledge that he or she is in better shape and can run farther, swim faster, and cycle better than anyone in the vicinity. Sometimes we feel guilty that achieving a relative level of excellence among one's peers is so easy, but then we challenge ourselves to match those a few years younger.

It has been many years now that people have recognized that there is value in exercise, and at the very least, people would bet that while exercise may not add years to your life, it most assuredly adds life to your years. Medical studies are now beginning to show that there may be a distinct link between exercise and the improvement of one's immune system to a variety of diseases. This may increase longevity or, at the very least, reduce the chances of a lengthy uncomfortable period of true, old age. Thus, the built-in motivations are all around us. It's getting easier to be a participant in our later years because our particular peer group is increasing, and our odd-ball conduct is becoming more normal. While that makes little difference to us, being odd-balls is not commonly desirable to the normal social animal.

There is one additional area of motivation of which we think few of us take advantage — the sheer satisfaction of how we look in the mirror.

Mountain bikes: An extremely popular bike on the market today is the retooling of the 10- and 12-speed into a mountain bike with nubby tires that can travel effortlessly on all terrains at high speeds. If you live in a rural or country area lacking adequate paved roads, mountain bikes are a great investment and a good way to get exercise. The exercise will be quite different than simply logging miles at a particular speed, but is rather calculated in terms of the time spent tackling challenging hills and valleys and even rigorous creviced and bumpy paths in flatlands.

Muscle cramps: Painful contractions of muscle fibers that can last anywhere from a few seconds to a few hours. They may occur during or after exercise and are most commonly the result of reduced levels of potassium, resulting from the loss of potassium via sweat during exercise. They become more severe with age; thus all mature individuals should consider potassium supplements in some form. If you are concerned about the toxicity of large doses of potassium, consult your sports medicine physician to analyze your personal needs. Reasonably healthy individuals can handle supplements between 100 and 300 mg of potassium per day, depending upon their exercising regimen, without any concern for negative health impacts.

Muscle imbalance: A common occurrence wherein opposing muscles are not equal in strength. Every muscle movement has an opposing muscle movement, for example, the movement of the quadricep on the top of the thigh and the hamstring muscle below the thigh. If the muscle above is stronger than the muscle below, there is a muscle imbalance. The stronger muscle can, therefore, cause damage to the fibers in the weaker muscle. It is important, therefore, to balance all strength training programs. Any good book on strength training from your local fitness equipment store will assist you in achieving this goal.

Muscle pull: This refers to the tearing

of muscle fibers, resulting in sudden and localized pain. It can result from overuse, insufficient warmup, or muscle imbalance. Muscles heal slowly, so initial damage is best avoided by proper warmup and avoiding sudden, over-strenuous movements.

Music and the birds: The vast majority of fitness enthusiasts learn that exercising to music is very helpful. Thus we are seeing a proliferation of small headset radios and tape players, so much so that some communities have outlawed them for runners whose safety is threatened because of the inability to hear oncoming vehicles. We strongly recommend music accompanying any form of exercise, where it is feasible. However, one should never lose "sight" of the interesting sounds of nature itself. A run or bike ride in the country already has a built-in soundtrack of various birds, animals, and insects that frequently play a very pleasant concerto.

We claim to be the first to have ever run with a self-contained headset radio made by Panasonic, and it was ten times heavier than today's version. Observers laughed at us then. Running and biking brings forth both those who want to hear the sounds of nature and those who want to lose themselves in the commercial sounds they favor. We like to do both at times and thus find the lightweight headset radio to be a good accompaniment on all long jaunts into the hitherlands, whether on foot or bicycle tires. Every type of background music to fit the mood is available on FM stations today. Music can quicken your pace if you so desire or make a long leisurely sojourn much more enjoyable.

Neck: We tend to overlook the work of the neck as a result of the weight of the head and don't exercise the neck as much as we should. There are many neck exercises that can be done with special Nautilus-type equipment, as well as simple resistance exercises of an isometric (non-movement) variety in which one pushes the head against one's hand in all four directions. thus increasing strength in the neck.

Negative work: When we lift a weight, we say we are doing positive work. When we put down a weight, we say we are doing negative work. Both movements strengthen the muscle. Too often, negative work is overlooked, but it can actually more efficiently increase muscle strength. Look at every movement as having a positive and negative aspect. Positive movements can always be done rapidly, because gravity is working against you. Negative movements must always be done slowly; otherwise, gravity assists you far too much.

Nutrients: Most nutritionists tell us that if you eat a balanced diet, you don't need any vitamin supplements. We're still looking for the first individual who truly eats a perfectly balanced diet. We try very hard, but in this busy world very commonly fail. We have found through experimentation that a certain limited number of supplemental nutrients can overcome those bad eating days. You can start in a health food store where a well-meaning salesclerk will try to make several nutrient supplements a part of your life. You can go to a nutritionist, who might advise somewhere between nothing and a single multi-vitamin tablet a day, or you may take our advice, for what it's worth. We recommend any reputable vitamin manufacturers' multi-purpose, all in one, one-a-day vitamin supplement. Additionally, years of experience have proven to us that additional quantities of vitamin C taken daily will promote good health. 3000 mg of "C" a day has proved most effective for us. Any excess vitamin C simply flushes out of the system, but has a tendency to take vitamin B with it; thus if you take "C," a single multi-complex vitamin B is a good daily addition. Finally, the best-kept secret in the vitamin world for the older generation is potassium supplements. Without exception, we have found that people prone to stiffness, sore muscles, cramps, and chronic backache benefit from potassium supplements. Experiment with quantities between 100 and 300 mg of potassium a day and see what works for you.

Oat bran (see also *Health claims*): Perhaps the single most overrated, exploited factor in the human diet during the 80s. Hopefully, it will be put in its place in the 90s as a perfectly good, healthful, tasty cereal which will have no significant impact on your longevity or daily health in normal, reasonable, available quantities.

Orienteering: An activity involving the following of a trail through a wilderness-type area which requires both physical and mental acuity. It might be considered the fitness buffs' version of an automobile car rally. It's an activity that dates far back in history but has become popular in recent times with the increased focus on the outdoor environment of physical fitness and emotional stability.

Orthotic: A word for either a rigid or flexible support placed in a shoe to offer greater balance and stabilization of the foot when walking or running. It is normally made from a plaster cast of the foot, which an expert can read to determine problems in foot placement, arch, or posture which can result in excessive stress on the body. Orthopedists and podiatrists most commonly prescribe orthotics. For individuals experiencing constant discomfort in ankle, knee, and hip joints as a result of jogging or fast-walking, orthotics can be a heaven-sent solution.

Osteoporosis: A disease involving loss of calcium in the skeletal bones, making them considerably more brittle. It is common among women of advancing years. Some success has been achieved by the regular intake of calcium supplements. Dramatic improvement and reduction of bone loss can result from weight-lifting-type exercises.

Over-do (see *Extreme*)

Over-the-hill: Primarily a state of mind which need never be reached until, of course, you finally expire. We all know that at one point or another we have become "over the hill" with regard to one or another activity in which we had some degree of expertise and excellence in our youth. However, there are always additional mountains to climb that will keep us on this side of the hill mentally and physically as we attempt to reach higher ground at the top of another hill. Through one form of activity or another, we can always re-position ourselves on the right side of the hill.

Over-sleep: Scientists have proven that excessive sleep in the morning makes one groggy rather than more rested. Even though at times we may feel tired getting out of bed at our normal rising hour, it is better to do so than to over-sleep (see *Sleeping*).

Oxygen debt: Excess requirement of oxygen during exercise which the body is incapable of providing. It causes the muscles to sieze up, becoming all but immobile. This may result from excessive bursts of speed in a particular activity, which should be avoided for a variety of reasons in addition to the discomfort of oxygen debt.

Pain: Pain is a negative feeling with which we have great difficulty coexisting. It is different from aches (see *Aches*) as most of us are able to accommodate a certain amount of aches in our life. While aches are commonly a result of the soreness from activity following extended inactivity, pain is the result of a serious malfunction or damaged area within the body. While, like beauty, pain is in the feeling of the beholder, most of us can tell the difference between an ache and a pain. An exception is those individuals considered to be serious hypochondriacs to whom nearly any physical feeling can be experienced as discomfort. A good way to differentiate between aches and pains is to recognize the one with which you can continue activity and the one with which you cannot. If you can continue activity, you are probably not in pain unless you are a true stoic. We normally say with regard to injuries and continued physical activity, let pain be your guide. It is not a good idea to exercise through pain. See your doctor or physical therapist before continuing an exercise program if you are in pain.

Participant: Be one.

Pedals, toe clips, and locking devices: If you observe cyclists today, you will note that most have their foot clamped onto the pedal with some type of wire cage and leather strap clamping device or their foot is locked onto the pedal by a ski-binding-type device. Few regular riders use the bare pedal any longer. These advances allow for proper pedalling technique which involves a circular 360 degree stroke where pressure is applied in all four quadrants of the circle — pulling, pushing, pressing, and lifting. This, of course, cannot be done with the bare foot on a plain pedal. New systems allow for greater exercise benefit from bicycling, the utilization of more leg muscles, and the attainment of increased speed. They have the disadvantage of requiring a certain amount of time to become acclamated during which riders are a safety hazard. Obviously, one cannot escape as easily from toe clips or pedal-locking devices as one can by simply lifting the foot off a bare pedal. If one is to use contemporary locking devices (and we strongly recommend you do), one needs to ride for a time in empty parking areas where maneuvering can be practiced, as well as quick stops with rapid release of the feet from the clips or bindings. Toe clips require a very quick upward movement of the foot and then rear movement to remove the foot from the clips. Pedal bindings require a rapid twisting of the foot out of the binding. Expertise can be acquired quickly, but no attempt should be made to ride on the open road until that expertise is obtained.

Pepsi (see *Soft drinks*)

Performance: A word used to define how well or poorly you perform an activity. We would like to emphasize the fact that one should avoid severely grading one's activities in the area of fitness because the primary achievement we seek is simply the act of doing, not the act of doing well. We recognize that this concept may be considered heresy in the minds of the "reach-for-the-stars" people, but it's more suitable to real people.

There is, however, tremendous satisfaction in seeing one's performance improve with time. If the increments against which you make your measurement are long enough, your performances will indeed improve and yield satisfaction. The point is that you must focus more on quantity and not measure yourself against too rigid a standard. While this book was not written for the handicapped, we can learn many lessons from this group in the area of achievement. The expansion and attention given the Special Olympics athletic programs throughout the country today provide an outstanding example of achievement that can be gained at any level of capability and expertise. While the concept that everyone who finishes a marathon is a winner has been overused, it is, nevertheless, quite true.

Persistence: The old story of the turtle and the hare says it all. Then there's the "journey of a thousand miles begins with the first step". And of course, "the race belongs not to the swift but to those who keep on running." And then there's the song about "Oops, there goes another rubber tree plant," reflecting what an ant can accomplish. We'll take an average person with persistence any day over a superstar without it. In short, persistence coupled with attitude is the whole ball game.

Personal best: An individual's personal record for any particular athletic endeavor. It can be fun to keep track of one's best performances, but not if you are the kind of individual that gets discouraged when you can't frequently best your earlier performance. Competition with oneself can be stimulating and rewarding, but it can just as often be frustrating and demoralizing. Be cautious about keeping such records, depending on your personality. Activity, exercise, and fitness are the point of all of this, not performance excellence or records. We are always happy with our performance. We're just happy to be healthy and alive.

Philosophy: People are not fit by accident. Fitness cannot be purchased at the supermarket. It must be part of your philosophy of life, not unlike a religion. What comes casually, without thinking about it, is being overweight and out of shape. That doesn't require any thought or preplanning — fitness does. If you care about having your mind in order and having precise goals for your spiritual life, you may be impressed by the fact that a healthly body promotes a healthy mind. Build it into your philosophy, whether its humanistic or deistic. Have you ever seen an overweight portrait of Jesus Christ?

Physics: In essence, the science of motion, which is obviously involved in all fitness activities. Physics relating to the body is called kinesiology.

Students have studied this subject to better understand the mechanics of all motions involved in athletic activities. Its study can be a fun hobby for individuals interested in fitness, but the accomplishment of physical fitness can be achieved with no knowledge of it at all.

Physiology: A branch of biology that deals with the functions and activities of life or living matter (as organs, tissues, and cells) and the physical and chemical phenomena involved.

Pinch test: A test of body fat performed by measuring the thickness of fat-folds held between the thumb and forefinger at different points on the body. It is surprisingly accurate, but is age dependent. Special manual, mechanical and electronic calipers have been developed for the test. All sports-therapy clinics can perform it. It can be a good periodic measure of progress for dietary and fitness programs. Don't measure it very often, because reduction of fat, indicated by the pinch test, is a relatively slow process. If you are pursuing an ultra-dedicated program, you might try it every three months, but every six months might be more realistic to see results.

Pit stop: A slang term used to describe the necessity for stopping to urinate or defecate during an athletic event. It comes, of course, from car racing — a vernacular where drivers stop for fuel and mechanical repairs.

During exercise, the vibration will require bladder emptying more frequently than during non-exercise. Similarly, the ability to resist a bowel movement will decline. Make every effort to go to the bathroom prior to long periods of exercise, or know the location of a bathroom that can be visited during extended periods away from home. If such does not exist, work on reducing your pride by carrying toilet paper in a small plastic baggy tucked inside your running shorts. There are, normally, wooded areas enclosed enough for the runner to use. Though initially it will be very difficult for those not used to spending long periods in the woods, once you get the hang of it, the fear of long-distance running will diminish. Remember, the key is an adequate length of toilet paper carried in a small plastic bag.

Pleasure (see *Enjoyment*)

Polo: If you don't already play now, forget it. If you do, enjoy it and keep at it. Congratulations! Very possibly, you're already fit.

Positive addiction: A term applied to people who exercise compulsively. Unlike drug or alcohol addiction, there are positive benefits as a dividend. It is possible to be addicted to exercise without exhibiting a negative, compulsive behavior.

Positive attitudes (see also *Mental attitude*): Everyone has heard the expression, "We are what we eat;" a more appropriate one is "we are what we think." If we think negatively, we will act and respond negatively. If we think positively, we will become positive role models. We learned our positive attitude 40 years ago from a popular song: "You Gotta Accentuate the Positive, Eliminate the Negative, and Don't Mess with Mr. In Between." A tip that will help accomplish this, which is difficult but important to follow, is to avoid negative people. They steal your energy and your resolve. Nothing you do or say is going to change them. Your positive attitude will likely suffer in their company.

Posture: The manner in which you hold your body erect. Correct posture minimizes debilitating physical stress on the body in an erect position. Poor posture is not just poor because it looks bad, but because it is an unnecessary strain on one's spine, neck, lower back, and sometimes knees and ankles. Standing "smartly" erect is not simply a macho military matter but a matter of fitness.

Power: There are many connotations to this word as it relates to fitness. A positive aspect is the power you feel when you are fit, healthy, and exhibiting a positive attitude. It is a powerful feeling, especially at an advanced age, when your peers appear to be losing their mental and physical powers. In the area of strength, however, power relates in little or no way to fitness. One can be fit, firm, sturdy, resilient, and capable of tremendous endurance and yet not have the power that is synonymous with significant strength. Power, as it relates to strength, is achieved through special exercises focused directly on gaining that attribute. For example, body builders and power lifters utilize distinctly different weight-training regimens. One builds significant muscle fiber for the sake of looks, and the other focuses more on instantaneous power that does not require the voluminous muscle fiber. One can be fit without being strong; thus, we should never be intimidated by another's greater strength or by our lack of that particular attribute.

Practice: It may not make perfect,

as the old saying goes, but it certainly moves one closer to any goal, be it mental or physical. Thus, practice relates to the concept of just doing it. The simple repetition of any fitness or exercise function moves one closer and closer toward any objective. When we're young, however, we practice, practice, practice to get somewhere in the near term. We may be readying for a game this week, or the next sports season, or a place on a team next year. Now there is no pressure for us because our goal, really, is fitness for life. As long as we are moving on that positive path and practicing some worthwhile regimen, we will get where we want to go. It really doesn't matter when as long as we keep moving on that path toward fitness and away from the less healthy situation that many of us begin to experience in middle age.

Procrastinate: It means to put something off until later; commonly done by individuals attempting to avoid a workout. Be very aware of this tendency in yourself when beginning an exercise program. Giving in to procrastination will ultimately destroy the possibility of making exercise a permanent part of your lifestyle.

Productivity: Something that will increase in every phase of your life when you're fit. A clear head improves thought processing, improves physical energy, extends the time you can apply to any activity, increases enthusiasm, and enhances the quality of your effort. The net result is significantly increased productivity.

Proficient: A level of expertise that need never be achieved to become fit. We do not have to become excellent

runners, bikers, swimmers, or rowers to gain fitness benefits from these
activities. The greater our level of
proficiency, the more efficient our
bodies move and perhaps the more
we will get out of each hour we put
into the activity. But it's not crucial
and you should not give up an activity
you enjoy just because you have not
achieved proficiency. Remember,
you are doing this for yourself, not to
impress others.

Progress: Toward ultimate fitness is
slow; toward road sign indicators of
fitness advancement, it is very quick.
In a few weeks of a fitness program,
you'll know you are moving in the
right direction and you'll feel a lot
better. The visual results may take a
lot longer.

Progressive, resistance exercise:
Gradually increasing a resistance
against which you exercise a particular muscle or muscle group. Gradually increasing resistance will continue to lengthen the muscle fibers,
increasing the strength of any particular muscle or group of muscles.

Pronation: A small flaw in a a jogger's
stride which tends to cause the inside
of the foot to rotate forward and incur
undue stress at the joints of the ankle
and knee. Certain running shoes are
built to reduce pronation. Serious
pronation can be treated by the insertion of orthotics into the running shoe
(see *Orthotic*).

Protein: The primary dietary building block for human muscle and tissue. It should comprise approximately 20 percent of one's diet. It is
primarily found in fish, fowl, or animal meat, but can be derived from
carefully blended amino acids in
vegetable products. If the body does
not get an adequate quantity of protein daily, generally considered to be
around 75 grams, it will absorb it
from its own internal organs, which
can lead to serious physical deficien-
cies. It, thus, requires very special
regimentation to be successfully
healthy as a vegetarian.

Proud: What you'll be when you
achieve fitness. We have never
understood why pride is a sin, because pride in one's physical capability is the very incentive required to
maintain the quality of life we all
desire in our later years.

Psychoanalysis: A common hobby of
many people of advanced years.
While many of our problems are,
indeed, emotional and mental, many
relate to our lack of physical fitness.
The old saying, "healthy body,
healthy mind," is as true today as it
ever was.

Pull: A stretching of muscle fiber beyond its natural flexibility commonly
caused by an off-balance movement
and/or the lifting of an excessive
weight.

Quadriceps: The major muscle on top
of the thigh. What we call a "charley
horse" is a pulled quadricep. Its development is crucial to running and
cycling. Nautilus-style leg-lift machines develop it better than anything else. It's one of the strongest
muscles in the body and, thus, great
advances in its fitness can be
achieved on weight-lifting equipment. Its development can be a
source of tremendous satisfaction for
mature people for whom gains in
muscle strength normally come
slowly.

Quality years: Each one lived in a fit
condition.

Race walking: The act of walking
very rapidly in the style that makes

the hips swivel and the feet touch tangentially on either side of a line on the ground projected down the middle of the body, rather than in a normal walking stride where the feet might land with a horizontal separation of a foot or more. In order to walk in this manner, the arms must swing rhythmically like the connecting rods on the wheels of locomotives. It can be nearly as fast as slow jogging. At no time do both feet lift simultaneously off the ground as is commonly the case in running or jogging. Race walking utilizes 10 percent more calories than running because of the somewhat jerky motion required. Race walking entails far less stress on knee joints and thus can be an excellent alternate method of aerobic exercise.

Racing flats: Two words describing extremely lightweight running shoes used primarily for racing rather than training. Because of their light weight, they do not offer adequate protective cushioning. Use of this lightweight shoe for events of short distance will increase speed. We do not recommend their use for extended wear, but there are times when a very lightweight running shoe is exhilirating for periodic bouts of exercise.

Racquet ball: A game that probably offers more exercise benefit than most others: a lot of running, a lot of arm movement, and very little wasted time. It was the rage in the 70s when everyone found out how easy it was to play. It died out quickly when people found out how hard it was to become good at. Find someone equally as incompetent as you and enjoy a great game and a lot of exercise. Avoid playing with people who can hit the ball within a few inches of the floor. They eliminate the opportunity for exercise in the game. Racquet ball would be a far better exercise game and might still be more popular if it were made illegal to hit the ball lower than one foot off the bottom of the floor, which is the case in squash.

Range of motion (see *Flexibility*)

Recommended Dietary Allowances (RDA): The U.S. Government provides guidelines for proper nutrition by listing a prescribed level of a variety of vitamins and minerals which are beneficial as daily supplements. With few exceptions, these recommended allowances are incredibly low and most health food fanatics believe in dramatically increased quantities of a variety of vitamins and supplements to maintain an advanced level of good health. We tend to agree that RDAs are so conservative as to be ludicrous, but we'll draw no conclusions on multiple claims of health food fadists. We are convinced, and have so stated, that increased quantities of vitamin C and potassium have significant importance to individuals intending to maintain vigorous exercise programs.

Recovery heart rate: Following the cessation of strenuous exercise, the heart rate will slow to 60 to 80 percent of the maximum heart rate at which exercise is normally performed back to within 20 beats of the normal resting heart rate in 5 to 15 minutes. The shorter the recovery time, the greater the indication of advanced fitness. An extremely well-conditioned athlete will fall to within 20 beats of the resting heart rate within 2 minutes or less. This is another interesting self-measurement one can take to calibrate his path toward fitness. The pulse should be taken by the first two fingers, on an artery on the neck just below the chin or on the opposing wrist. Never use your thumb to measure your pulse because the thumb itself has a pulse and you can confuse the pulse rates.

Recreational sports: Such as bowling and golf do not provide adequate aerobic conditioning to be of significant value to a physical fitness program.

Reflex: The response of an organ to a stimulus. Our reflexes decline significantly with aging and bounce back quickly when fitness is achieved.

Relax: In his book, *Health and Fitness Excellence,* Robert Cooper describes an instant calming sequence worthy of note to anybody prone to excessive stressful situations. His instant calming sequence (ICS) contains five parts that, in a matter of seconds, can relieve stress.

1. Think about continued breathing. Stress tends to shorten or eliminate normal breathing patterns.

2. Smile — at least in a limited way. This alters facial tension and, believe it or not, has a positive impact as a brain stimulant.

3. Check your posture and be sure it is proper, allowing for maximal breathing capacity and oxygen transmission.

4. Quickly focus on all the muscles in your body from head to foot as though a wave were washing over you triggering all your muscles to relax.

5. Quickly alter negative thoughts to give a positive accent to your mental focus.

It takes a little practice, but once you master it the entire process can take but a matter of seconds and will eliminate stress. Stress, very definitely, works against our efforts to be physically fit. This is a valuable technique to learn.

Repetitions: Referring to the number of times you continuously perform an exercise such as a weight lift. A single group of continuous repetitions is called a "set."

Resist: the efforts of others to dissuade you from separating yourself from the unfit crowd by following a healthier than normal lifestyle.

Resolve: to begin a program this week.

Rest: Something you probably already get too much of.

Resting heart rate: This normally refers to what we commonly call our pulse. It is measured when you are not performing strenuous exercise. The average pulse or resting heart rate is between 68 and 76. Excessively fit individuals will approach 60 or lower, while overweight, out-of-shape individuals have a resting heart rate in excess of 80, which is another outstanding calibration to measure your approach toward fitness.

Rolfing: A rigorous form of massage which concentrates on applying heavy pressure to places on the body with elbows and fists. It can be effective, but is painful.

Roller blades: An innovation in roller skates which places 4 wheels in a straight line such that skating action is identical to ice skating except that stopping quickly is all but impossible. It is an excellent form of aerobic training if you are already an expert ice skater.

Roman chair: A Roman chair is an advanced fitness device, better than any other, to strengthen back and abdominal muscles. Excellent back exercises can be found in a variety of exercise books in any athletic or bookstore. Once you have achieved a moderate level of strength in the abdominal muscles and lower back, you may wish to buy the Roman chair. It is also called a hyperextension device. It consists of two elevated pads parallel to each other separated by a foot or more on which you can support your upper body or mid-section while locking your legs under the second pad so that you can allow your upper body to bend at the waist, either forward to exercise the back muscles or in a backward position, then lifting to exercise the abdominal muscles. When exercising the abdominal muscles, the face is to the ceiling, the body begins in a horizontal position, and the upper body lifts up 10 or 15 degrees toward the vertical. When exercising the lower back, the face is looking at the floor, and the upper body bends in a vertical position and then lifts up toward the horizontal position.

Rope skipping: This is an excellent exercise traditionally performed by young children and boxers. In recent years, it has become a popular form of adult exercise. It was once thought that a few minutes of jumping rope was the equivalent of many minutes of jogging or running. This, however, has been disproved. Rope jumping continues to be a popular exercise but should be undertaken cautiously by those with sensitive knees. It is not an exercise commonly recommended for older individuals but one which you should not hesitate to try because of the benefits of being able to perform indoors. It makes an especially agreeable alternative to running in excessively inclement weather.

Rowing: An outstanding alternative aerobic activity that can be readily substituted for cycling, running, or swimming. It should be performed vigorously, which represents a greater challenge than the aforementioned activities. Rowing takes many weeks to adjust to because the rear end must be broken in slowly. Initially, rowing will literally create a pain in the butt after just a few minutes. Eventually you, not your rear, can determine how long you choose to row; this juncture will not occur for many weeks into a rowing program.

Form is important with rowing. One's back should remain relatively straight (not too much lean — perhaps 30° during the forward reach). Hands should pull directly into the midsection while concentrating on flexing the abdominal muscles for greatest benefits.

There exist a wide variety of rowing machines for less than $200 all the way up to thousands of dollars. The most efficient machines range between $250 and $700. The machine provides an outstanding exercise which works a wide variety of muscles while offering excellent aerobic training effects. Machines which offer too many bells and whistles add very little to the aerobic benefits. One way or another, you should be able to time the period during which you utilize a rowing machine and be able to calculate the number of strokes per minute so as to measure your efficiency against a particular resistance. More expensive machines have built-in computer systems that do this. If your machine does not have such a system, you can periodically count your strokes for a minute on your watch and keep track, close enough, to recognize your progress. For the person who wants to know what he/she is accomplishing through every moment of a workout, we strongly recommend the more advanced machines that give automated readouts for a few hundred dollars more.

Runners' bra: As the advent of running among women increased, it became quite obvious that conventional bras were severely lacking in adequate support for athletic women. Bras have now been designed by female runners which decrease, if not eliminate, the stress placed upon women's breasts as the result of irregular vertical and horizontal movements required by jogging. When considering embarking on an exercise program that includes rapid ambulatory movement, you should check with a good running store or some of the better running magazines to select a good running bra.

Runners' high: The euphoric condition commonly experienced by runners at some time or another during an exhilarating run; not, however, to be expected frequently (see *Beta-endorphin*).

Runners' knee: One of the most common running injuries occurring when the kneecap wears excessively on the long bone of the thigh, creating irritation. It generally results from the pronation of the foot (see *Pronation*) and can be treated quite successfully by the insertion of an orthotic in your running shoe (see *Orthotic*).

Runners' nipple: A now common irritation occurring in both men and women running in loose fitting garments which can rub excessively over a nipple. It can be alleviated with the application of a little bit of Vaseline or, in extreme conditions, with the application of a Band-aid.

Runners' toe: Few runners, at one time or another, have failed to experience a black-and-blue toenail produced by constant jamming of the toenail into the end of the running shoe. This is the result of short shoes or long toenails. Be sure your shoes are adequately sized and that your toenails are closely clipped. Another important preventive measure for runners' toe is to make sure that your shoes are properly laced around the arch of the foot so that the foot is prevented from sliding forward in an exaggerated fashion toward the end of the shoe, bringing the toenail into contact with an immovable surface.

Running and remembering: One of the enjoyable and productive things to do on a long run is to think out some work or family-related problem. You will be amazed at how clear your mind is and how effective one can be during these periods. At the same time, it can be frustrating to forget the details of the solution you might work out to a problem while running. This can be overcome by developing some type of pneumonic memory device that will enable you to retain the details of some of the things you thought about. We use two such devices. First, we use the fingers of our hands to store imaginary rings — each ring standing for some idea or word that triggers our memory to fill in the details of whatever problem we had been dealing with on the run. Second, we use car appurtenances to hang ideas on such as the door handle, the hood ornament, the windshield wipers, the rear-view mirror, etc. This is a fairly standard memory device. The stranger the things you hang on these parts of the automobile, with key words related such that you can recall the thought processes, the more effective the memory device. Get a good book or pamphlet on memory devices to aid in developing your own techniques.

Running/pacing/distance: If running is a part of your fitness program, and well it should be, you always have the problem of determining how fast and how far to run, jog, or walk briskly. The worst way to figure out a program is to combine distance with time. That is to say, do not decide to go a certain distance in a fixed time. This puts too much pressure on you. Decide either to go for a certain time or to go a certain distance. Thus a run, jog, or fast walk can be done for a set period of time by moving out for half that time away from your starting point and then returning to your starting point. If you know the distances between things or around things, you can easily calculate how far to go or how many times around to meet that distance requirement. It's best not to start a run without having in mind either the time or distance. It's too easy otherwise to just quit at a point where little is accomplished. Adjust your energy level entirely by the speed or pace you put forth in covering the distance. There's noth-

ing wrong with starting out slowly and tapering off. There's something very wrong with starting off slowly and stopping altogether. Thus, it doesn't matter how you do it as long as you do it. If you prefer the confines of your home, running on treadmills is an excellent and affordable substitute to the great outdoors.

Running shoes: The wearing life of the running shoe brings us to the next point. We all periodically look at the bottom of our shoes and see one quadrant or another of the sole worn down. We say to ourselves, "I guess I'm going to have to get a new pair of shoes pretty soon." Of course, we've already made a mistake. We should have purchased a new pair of shoes some time ago. As running shoes get more and more expensive, our tendency to over-use a single pair is strengthened. But if your feet are striking the ground hundreds of thousands of times a month, as mine are, it doesn't take much of an imbalance in your stride to show up as a major pain in a joint, muscle, tendon, or bone. Figure out something else you can give up in order to buy shoes more often. Believe me, it's money well spent. If you think about the mental cost of your running injuries, I think you'll agree it's worth the extra cost.

Furthermore, you should buy new shoes well in advance of putting your current shoes to rest. If you haven't learned by now not to run in a new pair of shoes, you either have a high pain tolerance or your shoes are too large. To avoid unnecessary sore feet, the shoe needs to become molded to your foot and this can only be accomplished in comfort while walking. Buy your next pair of shoes at least a month before you're going to need to press them into service. Walk in them everywhere you can get away with, and that includes at work.

Sailing: An outstanding athletic event for people who want to combine the skill of a chess game with the relaxation of a summer breeze. The sport will certainly keep you hopping at one moment and tranquilly relaxed at another. It is a terrific mental escape from the normal pressures of the work day. Its bottom line contribution to fitness is far more mental than physical. This description, however, would not apply to the crew of an America's Cup ship who are engaged in what could well be called a continuous 100-yard sprint for the period of an entire race. These people have to be incredibly fit to sail, and sailing returns something to them in the form of fitness; for the average sailor, however, one can be less fit and, in turn, gains less fitness benefit from it.

Salt tablets: Eating sodium chloride in tablet form was once recommended to replace salt losses, but is now recognized to produce little more than stomach irritation. If you've been using salt tablets following exercise, now is a good time to stop.

Sauna: A dry heat often produced by heating rocks. It has a relaxing effect for most people, but is not of any special value from a fitness standpoint.

Sauna belts: These are wide rubber belts that fit tightly around one's waist, generally advertised as having benefits of spot-reducing: they do not. On the other hand, since they are worn around the lower back as well as the waist, some people find that they have the effect of warming the lower back muscles which can become sore from exercise. Thus, you might try them for that purpose but ignore them as an aid in weight reduction.

Scar tissue: A dense layer of tissue that commonly forms over a wound. It is often lumpy in feel because it forms in a matted and inelastic manner. When you damage muscles internally and allow them to heal without exercise, the same type of inflexible scar tissue will form. It is for this reason that it is best to at least gently exercise damaged muscles so that the new fibers will form in an orderly matrix that will allow you to maintain muscle, ligament, and tendon elasticity.

Sciatica: A common lower back ailment occurring as a result of damage to the sciatic nerve, which passes through the lower back. It controls the pain running all the way down the right or left leg, depending on whether the damage is to the right or left sciatic nerve. It is common with age and inactivity to find the sciatic nerve under pressure resulting in pain. Exercise and stretching of the lower back will usually reduce the inflammation and resulting trauma to this area.

Sciatic nerve (see *Sciatica*)

Scuba diving: Scuba stands for self-contained, underwater breathing apparatus — a wonderful hobby for people of all ages. It helps to be fit to enjoy it but it isn't necessary. Many out-of-shape people do it. The more fit you are, the more you enjoy it. Though tiring, it does not count as an aerobic activity that will contribute to fitness.

Seasonal rest: Most of us will have different energy levels in different seasons of the year and thus will tend to work more on our fitness programs at some times and less at others. It's probably best to try to smooth out these highs and lows and stay relatively constant over the year. We all tend to want to be more fit in the summer, when we are likely to wear less clothes and show more of our bodies, while in the winter we are all covered up and less concerned. To a certain extent, these attitudes cannot be avoided but they should be minimized when possible. Because all training can be done indoors with the advent of stationary bikes, running machines, rowing machines, and the like, there is no need for seasonal weather variations having any dramatic effect on training programs. If you're among the small percentage of readers who enjoy age-group races of some sort or other you will, of course, work a little harder prior to the racing season than at the conclusion. But, generally, you are trying to stay fit for life and a level year-round program will work the best. Again, though, if it isn't fun, don't do it. So if there are times of the year in which you want to reduce your intensity, you shouldn't feel guilty about it. While you can feel free to reduce the intensity at any time, do not go below a minimum time input for either aerobic training or muscle development programs. The bare minimums for these should remain 7 hours of aerobic exercise per week and 1 $\frac{1}{2}$ hours of muscle toning weight training.

Second wind: A common phenomenon during aerobic exercise, in which there is a transition from a feeling of tiredness or fatigue to a feeling of reinvigoration, allowing activity to proceed with greater ease. It is a real, not an imagined, phenomenon that is a result of improvement in the body's capacity to transmit blood and oxygen as well as the likely removal of lactic acid that accumulates in the initial phases of exercise or that is left over from past exercise. Depending upon the level of one's fitness, one may experience a second wind more or less frequently.

Self-fulfilling prophecies: In earlier entries in this encyclopedia, we have discussed things such as attitude and philosophy, all of which relate to self-fulfilling prophecies. The point is that whatever you think you can do, you can do, or whatever you think is likely to happen is going to happen. If you think negatively, negative things are likely to happen because you will subconsciously cause them to happen. If you think positively, positive things will tend to happen because you will engineer them in that manner. Obviously, circumstances beyond your control alter these cause-and-effect relationships. But in every area of human endeavor, we have gained a great deal of appreciation for and recognition of the fact that the mind controls a great deal of the outcome of our lives. If you want to be fit, and you say you're going to be fit, the likelihood is that you will be fit. You can be whatever you want to be. Admittedly, there are many real obstacles to the achievement of lofty and positive goals. For this reason, elsewhere we have argued against setting goals unrealistically high. Thus there are limits to what positive prophecies can achieve. Conversely, however, there are no limits to what negative prophecies will achieve. If you foretell that you are going to win your state's lottery, the odds are you're going to be wrong. But if you are sure you're not going to win the lottery and thus do not buy a ticket, rest assured you will not win. So, it is always easier to make certain of a negative outcome, and it is amazing how many people shoot themselves in the foot by prophesying negative outcomes. If you believe you'll always be overweight, out-of-shape, and lethargic, you can count on being just that.

Senile: This adjective pertains to the loss of mental faculties with advancing age and is now recognized to be a direct result of poor circulation of oxygen to the brain, which is a result of poor circulation in general. Doctors are becoming more and more confident that senility can be almost entirely avoided by maintaining a physically fit population of elderly people. It is probable that one does not need to be a conditioned athlete to achieve the level of fitness that will ward off what we so commonly saw in the past as the senility of the aged. This happy circumstance is a result of a dramatic change in philosophy. Where previously we told old people to slow down and sit down and rest, at which time their circulatory system declined dramatically, bringing on early senility, nowadays, we are recommending more strenuous activity throughout life which will have dramatically positive results on our aging population in the future.

Sew-ups" vs. "clinchers" (see *Bicycle tires*)

Sex: Few will argue that all aspects of a mature person's sexual life will improve with physical fitness. This includes both desire and performance.

Sex appeal: It almost goes without saying that people who are physically fit are more appealing to the opposite sex. Of course, a difference in taste is what makes horse racing and so people of all sizes and shapes are, fortunately for the human race, found to be attractive to other people of different sizes and shapes. Few, however, debate the fact that the universal model of an attractive person is one who appears physically fit, and most people are sexually attracted to those same people. We have met individuals who are so attractive that they have purposely gained weight so as to be less attractive to people of the opposite sex who tend to make passes at them, but few of us have this problem. Sex appeal is considered by most to be a positive attribute and a very distinct bonus for becoming physically fit at any age. While our younger friends may think such things don't matter so much to us older folks, we know they don't know what they're talking about.

Shape: A word commonly used to describe your condition or well-being. You're in good shape, bad shape, or moderate shape. Most people, frankly, are in bad shape. Hopefully, this book will generate the interest, energy, and enthusiasm to get into good shape.

Shiatsu: A type of muscle massage that utilizes pressure points. It can be painful, but is considered effective by some in relieving tension in the muscles.

Shin splints: This expression describes very fine tears in muscles commonly residing along the front of the leg on the shinbone between the knee and ankle. They may also occur in the back of the leg between the lower calf and the ankle. They are extremely painful and may require a certain amount of rest from active running. Our experience, however, has shown that the discomfort can be dramatically relieved by the placement of heel pads into running shoes to slightly lift the heel, reducing the stretch required of the muscles along the shin and thereby reducing trauma.

Shoe goo: This is a material that can be purchased to build up worn down soles of running shoes to make them flat and whole once again. We strongly recommend against it, because it is difficult to do a very precise job and the net result might be creation of further imbalance in the stride of a runner. The cost of your shoes is small in comparison with the importance of your feet, ankles, and knees.

Shoulder: The joint connecting the arm and body. It is one of the most problematic joints in the body for the mature individual. Shoulder flexibility is commonly lost in the aging population, partly as a result of disuse and partly as a result of a certain amount of calcification or arthritic condition in the joint. Loose and limber shoulders are one of the joys of being fit and can be obtained by a variety of flexibility exercises. Older people should regularly rotate their arms at a high speed in a windmilling fashion in order to maintain movement in their shoulder joints, moving the arm clockwise and counter-clockwise at different angles to the body. If you have ever attended a college swimming meet, this is an exercise you will invariably see the swimmers performing just prior to entering the water in order to ensure that their shoulder joints are loose enough to facilitate an efficient swimming stroke. You will additionally see them try to bring their elbow behind their neck by pulling their hand across the back of their head to the opposite side of the body. This is another useful way of keeping your shoulder loose and flexible.

Simple: A good word to describe how uncomplicated it can be to be physcially fit. In fact, if you don't keep it simple, you won't do it. Eventually, in some form or another, you must work toward an hour a day of aerobic activity broken up into two or three segments if you wish. You must do resistance exercises with weights or machines and/or certain calisthenics three times a week. The results are no mystery and no miracle, just good, common sense. There are even some who believe you can attain fitness with considerably less time input. One author we have read subscribes to a total of 30 minutes a week. While we find that absurd, it's not impossible. The problem is that as the time input goes down, the precision of the activity required goes up, thus increasing the complication of what you need to do. Keep it simple and realize that an hour a day of physical activity is not too great an investment to ensure a significantly increased quality of life.

Singing: An excellent exercise for the lungs because it requires disciplined breath control.

Singlet: A running shirt that has no sleeves; it makes arm movement very easy in warm weather but can create the opportunity for chafing between the bicep muscle on the arm and the trapezius muscle on the side of the body. We generally prefer T-shirts with relatively long sleeves approaching at least half-way to the elbow for maximum comfort, but everyone should experiment with clothing in different weather.

Sitting: A position which can contribute to skeleton problems if posture is not correct; a comfortable position during which many weight-lifting exercises can be performed with dumbbells.

Skate: Ice skating or roller skating can be excellent aerobic activities if you are proficient enough to move at a high enough rate of speed to increase your pulse to a conditioning level.

Skiing — downhill (see also *Cross-country skiing*): A sport which, to do well, requires a great amount of fitness. Only the very best skiers ski as a form of exercise. In turn, the very best skiers exercise in a wide variety of ways to be fit so they can ski rapidly and with great endurance. Downhill skiing, under rigorous conditions, can require large amounts of energy which are magnified by the high altitudes at which it is normally practiced and the consequent reduction in oxygen content of the air. When a skier achieves a high level of skill, skiing can clearly be used as an outstanding aerobic activity that will help maintain a very high level of fitness. The average recreational skier, however, is not extremely fit and skis at a pace and at intervals which do not allow skiing to contribute significantly to a fitness program. That is to say, the average skier rests so often on the hill that no aerobic benefit is achieved and skis too slowly to get the working heart rate up to a level that positively stresses the heart. Clearly, downhill skiing is a wonderful activity that, under all circumstances, has benefits, but the benefits are over-rated for all but the truly fit, highly skilled

skier who attacks the mountains with a certain degree of abandonment. Poor skiers will appear to exhaust themselves in the effort and thus assume they are gaining tremendous fitness advantages from the sport when, in fact, it is their fear of the activity that creates a great deal of fatigue. The soreness that develops is more from the use of unused muscles in very strange positions for short periods of time rather than from excessive use of muscles and aerobic capacity which bring on a true fitness effect.

Skill: An attribute that one may be totally devoid of while still attaining a high level of fitness.

Skin: The largest organ of the human body. It ages as does any organ. It thins and loses its elasticity and thus sags and wrinkles with age. This is also a direct result of a decline in the capacity of the body to adequately circulate blood and oxygen. Skin tone dramatically improves with physical fitness. Many older people who seek a variety of cosmetic solutions to improve their skin would get more efficient and economic results by investing their time and money into physical fitness effort rather than cosmetic care. That is not to say cosmetic care is not important, because it is, at least to the extent of affording your skin good moisturizers to counteract the negative aspects of the environment around us such as wind or dry air.

Skin care: There's little question that as we age, one of the organs of our body that deteriorates is our skin. We also know that there is some truth to the adage "healthy body, healthy mind," and there's also truth to a newer adage, "healthy body, healthy skin." The skin will improve up to a point, with the overall aerobic or vascular fitness achieved from exercise. Obviously, a certain amount of cosmetic skin care is also required. It is probable, however, that women use far more cream on their skin than is necessary, and men use far less. Nowadays people are afraid of the sun because of all the health scares relating to skin cancer. As with all environmental terror movements, there is little doubt that we have over-reacted to the negative aspects of the sun. Obviously, we can overdo it and skin cancers are a real concern. Moderate exposure to the sun and the acquisition of a healthy tan, however, has many positive benefits to both physical fitness and mental health.

If you are determined to become physically fit, you are going to exercise more and you are going to need more showers; thus your skin is going to lose more of its natural oils. You will definitely have to compensate by applying moisturizers to your skin.

Skinfold measurements: They can determine the body-fat content of an individual. By measuring the thickness of a pinch of skin usually taken on the thigh, the back, or the side of the waist, one can get a reasonably accurate measurement of body fat. The most accurate measurements are made using age-related tables. Skinfold calipers can be obtained to allow an individual to make the measurement on himself. This can also be done simply with the fingers. The most accurate body-fat measurements are generally performed by weighing the body in and out of a tank of water with air fully expelled before the submerged water weight

is taken. Such measurements are not readily obtainable but are worth the effort from time to time to gain insight into one's fitness, as body fat content is certainly a useful measure.

Sky: The limiting factor in what we can achieve toward physical fitness at any age.

Sleeping: The average adult requires $6\frac{1}{2}$ hours of sleep per night. Many get by very well on 6 hours and a few can do with even less. If you were to survey the population of unfit people, however, you would find that the vast majority gets 7 to 8 hours of sleep per night, with many getting as much as 9 hours. There is some evidence that too much sleep can have a negative impact on the human body, but we will not argue that 7 to 8 hours is too much sleep. We will argue, however, that the extra 30 to 90 minutes of sleep (over 7 to 8 hours) that many people get could be more productively spent in aerobic exercise than in rest. If you are an unfit individual claiming not to have time to exercise, the first place to look for time to exercise is in your sleep pattern. If you're sleeping over seven hours a night, that is a reservoir of time that can be tapped and used for exercise. Simply get up earlier than you are used to, and begin your exercise program in whatever form you choose. We don't care if you're jumping rope, jogging, running in place on a mini-trampolene, bicycling outdoors or in, swimming, or taking an aerobic class. If you can get to it at the crack of dawn, you can use those last minutes of sleep more productively to get your blood flowing, jump-starting your day, and getting on the road to physical fitness. We do want to emphasize again that the most convenient, relaxed, and easy way to start an exercise program in the morning is on a stationary bicycle.

Slowly: A word that creates comfort, good feeling, and well-being in all exercise programs. Go slowly. Start slowly. Slow down, but just be sure that you GO. When speed is not a concern, the mind and body will be relaxed. It might even go surprisingly fast. But who cares as long as it's going. We like to recommend that people start slowly and then taper off. Obviously, we're kidding but we think you get the message.

Slow twitch fibers: These are red muscle fibers that act more slowly than fast twitch fibers. They have a low anaerobic capacity; that is, they do not perform well in the absence of oxygen but perform very well with a continuous supply of oxygen. They are, therefore, most suited for low-power output activities such as endurance events like marathons. People who are successful at short, fast activities invariably are found to have a super abundance of fast twitch fibers, and it is the former that enable the mature individual to sustain a considerable exercise program.

Smoking: There aren't many people left on the planet who haven't heard that smoking is bad for you. Clearly, it is the leading cause of cancer. Smoking has no redeeming qualities, and all people who do smoke should endeavor to stop. Heavy smokers are most assuredly certain of a shorter life span than they would have otherwise achieved. In addition, along the way, they may suffer a wide variety of lung and heart problems. Most people who want to achieve physical fitness have the will to give up smok-

ing. Some do not. For those, there is heartening news that, at least for the present, there appears to be very little evidence of a strong, negative impact upon health as a result of smoking less than five cigarettes a day. It appears that the body may be capable of processing three or four cigarettes without the dramatic negative impacts that we know to be the result of heavy smoking. One can argue, however, that if you have the willpower to cut back to three or four cigarettes a day, you should have the willpower to cut to zero. Note, however, that the studies on individuals who smoke a very small number of cigarettes a day are not extensive, because there aren't many subjects to study.

Anecdotal evidence does exist indicating that as individuals become more fit, their dependency on nicotine for their highs will decline. Thus, serious exercise programs will aid in the kicking of the cigarette habit.

Snacks: A between-meal repast. The vast majority of popular edible items are unhealthy because of incredibly high fat and sugar content, which is why they are instantly satisfying and good tasting. Healthful substitutes for what you probably eat include pretzels, air-blown pop corn, fruits, carrots, celery, radishes, and other raw salad ingredients.

Snorkling: A delightful sport in which swimmers wear goggles or face masks, a surface breathing apparatus, and swim fins to propel oneself along the surface and look at fish below. A lot of fun, but no significant exercise.

Soccer: An outstanding game requiring a great deal of aerobic effort. Nowadays, there are a large number of adult soccer leagues throughout the United States, both indoor and outdoor. Most teams consist of individuals with a great deal of experience in their younger days, but among them are quite a number of individuals beyond 50. If you have either a good deal of soccer experience or you are extremely fit, it's an outstanding way to get some of your weekly exercise and have a lot of fun doing it. If you have no skill and are not fit, the sport could be too challenging.

Soft drinks: Generally referring to carbonated beverages which in years past always contained a good deal of sugar. These are, at best, empty calories and, at worst, ingredients which materially fatigue the stomach. Today, diet drinks which contain artificial sweeteners command much of the market and are a distinct improvement over conventional soft drinks. Many health experts speak strongly against the diet drinks because of the variety of chemicals they contain. In moderation, however, we see no reason to eliminate them from your diet.

Soreness: The common feeling of light to moderate pain in muscles as a result of the strain of exercise which is actually caused by the slight tearing of muscle tissue. This tissue becomes stronger upon healing. It commonly disappears in 48 hours and can be effectively treated with ice for periods of 20 minutes per hour immediately following exercise, and this can reduce the period of soreness. Be fully aware that soreness comes with embarking on a fitness program, and do not let it dissuade you from fulfilling your plan.

Spasms: A sudden, involuntary contraction of a muscle or group of muscles normally occurring during, or immediately following, exercise. They are related to muscle cramps and are a result of lost electrolytes in the body, most commonly a reduction of potassium.

Specialist: One who is extremely good at some particular activity. It is surprisingly possible to be very good at a particular athletic activity without being fit. The reason is that a great deal of skill can mask a lack of fitness. For example, we have seen excellent age-group soccer players who are so deft with their feet and so knowledgeable of the strategy of the game that they can mask their inability to run rapidly for long or short periods of time. The same can be true in games like ice hockey, badminton, or, at times, tennis. Thus, don't always be assured that because someone is good at an athletic activity, he or she is in extremely good physical condition. It may not be true.

Specificity: This refers to the idea that exercise is very specific to the muscles utilized for a particular athletic event. Thus, one type of exercise does not contribute as much as we would like to our capacity to perform another type of exercise. Mixing exercises or cross-training, as it is commonly called, does build strength and very definitely aerobic capacity, but it is generally true that bicycling will not make you a better runner, nor will running make you a better bicyclist. Needless to say, the best way to become a good golfer is to swing a golf club, but strength gained from weight training will enable you to push the ball out further on the fairway if your hand/eye coordination is equal to the task.

Speed play (see *Fartlek*)

Spinning: A term describing bicycling at high revolutions per minute (rpm). It is a technique that should be used by most bicyclists and virtually all mature bicyclists. In order to turn bicycle cranks at high rpm, one must be pedalling against very low resistance. That, in fact, is the point. You should ride in very low gears. Those are the ones where the chain in front is on the small sprocket wheel, and the chain in back is on a large sprocket wheel, offering low mechanical resistance. This eliminates the aggravation of the knee while still exercising all of the leg muscles to a more moderate degree and the full aerobic capacity of the body to an acceptable degree. Bicycling should be easy and fun. Thus, spinning is a requisite to achieving this most satisfactory state.

Sports medicine: Sports medicine has become a major field of the medical profession. Our nation's emphasis and delight in athletics has produced a great deal of research and knowledge about the medical problems resulting from athletic endeavors. Numerous research journals now exist covering this field, as well as professional societies catering to the needs of doctors who specialize in sports medicine. Ultimately, the object is to cure a problem through some type of therapeutic procedure. Sports therapy and sports medicine clinics have sprouted up in every major metropolitan area of the country. If you have a sport, recreation, exercise-related injury, disease, or discomfort, you'd be well served to visit a sports medicine doctor or therapist. They simply have more experience and knowledge about such problems than doctors who see problems that develop in the general population, as related to their particular specialty or body part.

Don't be afraid to ask your own family doctor for a recommendation to a sports medicine specialist — though you may hear that your family doctor is sure he or she can treat you adequately. That may or may not be the case. We have had very positive results the past decade with sports medicine specialists, and we highly recommend them. Perhaps one of the greatest benefits they offer is that they recognize your goal of continuing your exercise program as quickly as possible. Normal medical practitioners have no concern for this goal and are likely to recommend long periods of rest as part of the cure, with little concern for the impact that rest will have on your overall state of physical fitness.

Sports therapy (see *Sports medicine*)

Spot reducing: If it were possible, people who chew gum would have thin faces. They don't and it isn't. Fat is normally stored and eliminated more or less evenly throughout the body. Women are most commonly taken in by claims of spot-reducing possibilities. Sadly, there is no substitute for reduction of fat in the body and overall exercise of the entire body. Some people, unfortunately, have a slower metabolism, which make reduction of body fat a slow and tedious process. But with patience anyone can come close to achieving the body shape they desire. Sadly, exercise has a smaller impact on fat reduction than we would like. By far, the most important way to eliminate fat from the body is to eliminate it from the diet. Then, slowly but surely, the body will consume any stored fat.

Sprain: Over-straining the muscles of a joint. We sprain, most commonly, our ankles, our knees, our shoulders, and our elbows. We do this because we do not strengthen the little muscles that hold the joints together. If we make a special effort to exercise our ankles, our knees, our elbows, and our shoulders, we could reduce common sprains by 80 percent. Any book on calisthenics will show a number of ways to exercise these joints very simply, without great effort or complication. Free weights and exercise machines can also be geared to strengthen the same muscles that protect against sprain.

Sprint: To move one's body at a high rate of speed for a short period of time. A common training technique for people desiring to win races, but neither necessary nor advisable for one seeking fitness. On the other hand, sprinting can be fun on occasion when you are physically and psychologically prepared for it. There will be days where your zest for life is at such a high peak that moving short distances at high speeds will feel wonderful. More often than not, they are the dread of most athletes on most days.

Squash: A game similar to racquet ball but played with a smaller, deader ball and a lighter, long-handled racquet that can be used considerably more as a weapon. Because the ball is deader than in racquet ball, the game requires a considerably greater amount of speed than racquet ball and is not recommended for novices of advanced age. It does, however, have one wonderful advantage: it is not legal to hit balls lower than approximately sixteen inches from the floor. A hollow, metal embankment placed against the bottom of the front wall precludes the possibility of not recognizing a low shot. Play the game if you must, but be sure to wear eye protectors because, on occasion, you will be hit in the head by your opponent's racket.

Stair climbing: One of the most popular exercise machines today is the stair-climbing machine. There are several different makes on the market. One of the more popular is called the "Stairmaster." There are many inexpensive imitations, all of which are very worthwhile. If you enjoy the activity of climbing stairs, it is an excellent alternative to running, biking, rowing, cross-country skiing, walking, etc. Some people find it quite boring and difficult and, thus, it is another personal opinion alternative. It's best to do it watching TV to get your mind off the repetitive factor involved in the muscles of the legs. It must be done at a great enough pace to have an aerobic effect so that you are not simply getting exercise for the muscles of the leg, including the calf, quadricep, and hamstring muscles. Just like walking, its primary benefit is achieved when done at a brisk pace. Stair-climbing devices can now be purchased for anywhere between $400 and $4000, and the benefits of the more expensive machines, as compared to the less expensive machines, are minimal.

Stationary bicycle: In our minds, the single most effective exercise device that can be placed in the arsenal of a mature fitness buff. See *Bicycling.*

Steak: Commonly recognized as a healthy slab of red meat. Cooked to perfection, a good steak is a meat lover's dream. While today's society has reduced its love affair with red meat, there's nothing wrong with a good steak every week or two. It's a great source of needed protein. And, a little fat, once in a while, won't hurt either. While the leaner the meat the more healthy it is, it is, in fact, the nicely marbeled fat that gives most steaks their exceptional flavor.

Steam baths: These were a favorite of the health clubs of old and are not uncommon today. Sitting in a steam room certainly has the impact of loosening one's body and opening one's pores; add a few eucalyptus leaves and you can clear your sinuses as well. They do improve circulation, as does all heat, but are primarily of aesthetic value and create mental relaxation rather than contributing significantly to fitness. They are one of the luxuries of the elegant health club and make the club worthwhile but do not contribute in any significant way to the effectiveness of a fitness program.

Steroids: Chemical substances which have been ingested by athletes and body builders to increase muscle growth by the activation of growth hormones and increased generation of testosterone. They have now been proved, beyond any doubt, to have widespread deleterious impacts on a variety of human organs, bringing them into the category of plain and simple poisons. Their use should be totally eliminated.

Stimulant: Anything that stimulates or excites. Most stimulants are illegal. The one that is definitely not illegal is caffine (see *Caffeine*).

Stomach: The organ which receives food from the esophagus for diges-

tion. It tends to get more sensitive with age, and thus we develop types of food allergies. This is partly psychological and partly a matter of over-indulgence. A healthy stomach should be able to tolerate a wide diversity of food, which is, in the long run, what is most healthful for all of us. The most common stomach ailment is the acid stomach. It results from a wide variety of over-eating or poor eating habits.

Strength: Do not confuse strength with fitness. Many overweight behemoths are strong but not fit. Some well-muscled body builders are not particularly strong. Some thin, sinewy people are very strong. Strength tends to increase with muscle size and muscle tone, but by no means in direct proportion. When we talk about fitness, we clearly talk about having the strength to fulfill one's normal, daily, and weekly chores without strain or fatigue, but we do not necessarily mean excessive strength to lift very heavy weights.

Stress fracture: A hairline crack in a bone along which there is no displacement. It can be a result of overuse or a specific traumatic injury. It can be very painful, and while difficult to diagnose, as always, ice is a good prescription. Reduction in exercise stress will assist healing, but full rest is not required. Support of the fractured area with an elastic bandage will commonly yield a reduction in discomfort. If in doubt and pain persists, x-rays should be requested of sport physicians.

Stretching the old body: While a modicum of stretching before a workout is okay, its importance pales in comparison to the critical need to stretch when you complete a workout. The older athlete should always begin any workout slowly, so as to build in the "stretch" through relaxed performance of the early segment of his or her run, cycle, swim, or other activity. Old, cold muscles demand this. A little stretching before a workout is okay, but the downside of overstretching "cold" muscles is considerable. At the end of a workout, however, when the body is warm, virtually every tendon used in the preceding activity will have been drawn taut and will remain that way, bringing on considerable discomfort unless a few minutes is set aside to restretch those old, but now warm, tendons and fibers.

Correct stretching exercises are the secret to injury-free training. I propose that if you are putting in much more than five minutes stretching before running, you're doing more than is necessary. Let me describe for you what I consider to be the three most important stretching exercises that can be performed in two minutes prior to a run and should be carried out, to a limited extent, during and after the run.

I have found three primary areas which require stretching in order to avoid limited or extensive discomfort. These include the hamstring tendons, running from the buttocks down the back of the thighs, behind the knee joint into the calf muscle; the groin muscle tendons, connecting the thighs to the pelvic area; and the lower back muscles. In my half century of ambulation, discomfort in these areas has accounted for 80 percent of my athletic injuries. I have at last found what appears to be a near foolproof solution to the problem.

I have solved part of the lower back problem and all of the back-of-the-leg tendon problems with a simple 20- to 25-second stretch prior to exercising. It consists of leaning over with your knees locked and allowing the weight of your upper body to carry your hands down to the floor, first reaching with your fingertips, then slowly feeling your knuckles reach the floor. With practice, over a matter of months, this exercise will lead you to a palm-to-floor extension when standing in your bare feet. This gravity stretch does wonders in extending the muscles of the lower back, ultimately reducing or eliminating lower back problems while at the same time stretching the tendons behind your leg. These tendons draw tight from extensive running, cause your stride to shorten, and create the soreness frequently felt following long runs.

This particular exercise has such wondrous results that I strongly recommend it be done during long runs. If you're going to run over an hour, I suggest you stop and do this for 20 to 30 seconds somewhere between the 40- and 60-minute mark. You will be amazed when you first lean over how far your fingertips are from the ground, but how soon, with your knees locked, your upper body weight will carry your hands down to the ground, stretching tendons behind your leg that you didn't realize had tightened so severely. Twenty seconds of this will set you up for an amazingly loose get-away. Your gait will be rejuvenated to the point that you will feel as good as you did much earlier in your run. From that point on, I recommend you take this 20- to 30-second break every 20 to 30 minutes. At the end of the run do this same stretch again, extending it to 45 seconds, attempting in stages to get your fingertips, then knuckles, and finally one day your palms to the ground.

Two other stretching exercises that should be performed prior to a run, cycle or even swim include a leg split and a set of half push-ups. The leg split will stretch the groin muscles and reduce the tightness felt there by many runners. This should be done by facing forward and slowly spreading your legs into the widest split possible, easing your feet out until you can comfortably balance yourself by touching your hands to the ground in front of you. Once you have reached the greatest expansion of your split with your knees locked and your toes extended outward to either side, hold this position for 30 seconds and you have completed the second phase of the two-minute stretching procedure.

Half push-ups are performed lying face down prone on the ground, placing your hands beside your shoulders, holding your pelvis to the floor, and pushing your upper body up as high as you can without raising your pelvis off the ground. This exercise will maintain the important arch in the lower part of your spine and strengthen the area in which sciatic nerve problems frequently develop among athletes. Do 10 to 12 of these half push-ups, holding at the top of the push-up for one second and then letting yourself down slowly each time. I recommend all three of these exercises before and after all workouts, as much to assist you in your workout as to strengthen these important areas of the body.

Sugar: Sugar has no redeeming qualities regarding fitness. It is, of course, a simple carbohydrate that can translate into energy production. However, it burns too fast, giving you a high-energy-level perception, and then plunging you down to a low, lethargic level. Actually, sugar by the teaspoonful doesn't have many calories — about 18 — and thus poses no problem in your coffee, on your cereal, etc. In desserts such as cakes, pies, pastries, and candy, however, the levels add up to big calorie totals which have no nutritional value. Total abstinence from sweets is not necessary if one eats a balanced diet, and the reward of small quantities of dessert-type food can offer psychological benefits. Therefore, we don't recommend going cold turkey; we simply point out that desserts are wasted calories, have no redeeming qualities, and the lower your consumption the better off you are. Enough said!

Sun (see *Sunglasses*)

Sunglasses: Exercise out-of-doors will always subject your eyes to excessive amounts of sunlight, wind, and dust. We strongly recommend the wearing of a good, pale-colored sunglasses which filter out all the ultraviolet radiation. Many people only wear glasses when it is excessively bright or excessively windy, but long-term protection of the eyes is gained by wearing glasses at all times. It is better, however, to wear no glasses than to wear cheap sunglasses that do a poor, if not insignificant, job of filtering ultraviolet light while possibly even distorting one's vision. There are numerous brands of excellent athletic glasses that are extremely light and amazingly comfortable, which will do the job and increase the enjoyment of all outdoor exercise activities.

Surfboard: A wonderful toy for young people.

Sweatband: An absorbent cloth which wraps around either the wrists and/or forehead to prevent sweat from dripping onto the face and hands. Such headbands are advisable in hot weather to keep salty perspiration out of the eyes, which can cause considerable discomfort. They also give one a generally "macho" look and feel. It can be a nice touch for senior exercisers.

Sweets (see *Sugar*)

Swimming: Swimming is clearly one of the three most popular aerobic exercises, which also include running and biking. Some statistics indicate that swimming is actually the most popular sport. While that may be true, it is likely that not a very large percentage of swimmers achieve optimal exercise value from the activity. The reason for this is that they swim neither far enough nor fast enough. Unlike running and cycling, where virtually any speed attained offers significant value as a caloric burner, swimming at a very slow speed can utilize the buoyancy of the water to such an extent that very little exercise value is achieved. Each individual can easily determine if he or she is swimming at a speed which creates enough physical stress to obtain beneficial exercise. At that speed (as with all aerobic activities) a minimum time of 20 minutes should be expended to optimize the value of the workout. While the most efficient stroke is the crawl on one's stomach, utilizing one arm at a time, individuals can obtain good workouts doing the breast stroke, back stroke, or even side stroke.

Swimming has the advantage of working virtually all the muscles in the body, which is less true of running and biking. It also places less stress on the skeletal muscles, though it can, at times, cause discomfort in the shoulders which are not commonly moved in the rotation required by both the crawl and the back stroke. As with all other exercises, the mature person should not set speed alone as a goal once the lower critical speed previously discussed is reached. At that point, the individual should decide to swim so many laps in a pool, a certain distance in the open water, or, even better, swim for a particular length of time. In a pool, we strongly prefer time, as it does not require the counting of laps, which can be so terribly boring. If you swim for a prescribed amount of time, you can allow your mind to wander, dealing with the solution of problems in your personal or business life or just musings on beautiful places or interesting narratives. Because the authors are inclined to swim extensive distances and are constantly asked by observers how far we swam, we always find it charming to respond that we have no idea, but we enjoyed "X" minutes of recreation and exercise.

Avoid swimming in cold water (72°F), as it tends to be unpleasant. Always wear eye goggles to protect your eyes from chlorine in pools or grease and dirt in most open bodies of water or ocean saltwater. After swimming, be sure to carefully clean your ears so as not to leave any water, which can support the growth of bacteria; also, wash your hair so as not to leave any chlorine, which can destroy its body over time. Conditioning shampoos are very beneficial.

Swimming on land: There are available, in some exercise equipment stores and catalogs, swimming benches for use indoors. For people who enjoy swimming but can't get to a pool frequently, the swim bench provides an excellent workout. It consists of a bench on which you lie horizontally, then reach forward and place your hands in paddle assemblages attached to ropes and pulleys which extend from a resistance box. The arms are pulled back against the resistance and strokes identical to those used in the swimming crawl can be achieved in an amazingly representative manner that offers both good exercise and training for improving one's swimming. Unfortunately, the devices are quite expensive. Lower cost benches are entirely mechanical, and higher cost benches offer you computerized resistances and readouts. The range is between $800 and $2000. The leading company providing the Biokinetic Swim Bench is Counsilman Co., Inc., P.O. Box 6397, Berkeley, CA 94706.

Talent: None required for fitness.

Talking about exercise: It is not uncommon to ridicule people who spend more time talking about what they are doing than actually doing it. While we cannot quarrel with that, we find that talking about exercise serves as an incentive to performing exercise, just as it is for somebody on a strict diet to talk about the diet because it helps them to stay focused. It is also valuable to openly discuss the exercise program you are involved in with others. While some may see it as a form of bragging, others will be interested in the subject and the interchange will serve to secure the permanence of an exercise program into your daily and weekly regimen.

There's an additional satisfaction in talking about exercise because of the information you frequently impart to others who may be on the verge of developing a program and only need a little extra impetus, which you might provide. Additionally, interchanging ideas with others in your age group who are also engaged in fitness programs will have a tremendous educational value. While we try to cover all the bases in a superficial manner in this text, you'll never reach a point where you can't learn more about fitness and exercise. Every person is different and has different requirements to satisfy their needs, both physically and psychologically. Ideas derived from others are always helpful in defining our own approach to fitness.

Teddy Roosevelt used to say, "Walk softly and carry a big stick." We don't think you have to walk so softly.

Target heart rate (see *Training effect*)

Team sports: A great way to combine aerobic activity with social comraderie, but as we get older, there are very few team sports we are capable of playing that offer significant aerobic exercise. Softball and bowling do not; tennis and basketball do. There now are masters' teams in track and swimming which are excellent, but they don't qualify in the strict sense of team sports. Soccer is great if you can find a senior team matching your skill level, but that may not be easy. If you're lucky enough to find an aerobic team sport, don't hesitate to go for it. And if you like softball, don't hesitate to play, but don't fool yourself into thinking it has fitness value. On the other hand, if you get fit, you will most definitely play better softball.

Tear: The actual separation of muscle fibers resulting from too strenuous or too extensive a movement. With few exceptions, an entire muscle or tendon does not separate or tear — only a portion of the many fibers which make up a muscle will normally tear at any given time.

Tedious: When exercise becomes tedious, it becomes history for most people. You have got to make it pleasant and fun. It can be pleasant because it feels so good when you stop, and it can be pleasant because you visualize the good it's doing for you. Music, educational tapes, attractive scenery, or challenging thoughts can turn any period of exercise from tedium to delight.

Tendons: Since so few of us laymen really understand what tendons are or do and because so many of us suffer from their damage, let's go into some detail here.

A tendon is comparable to a cable that connects a muscle to a bone. When a muscle is exercised, tremendous force is applied to the tendon at both its junctions with the muscle and bone and in its main body. The tendon is made up of collagen fibers that are parallel to one another. Their significant tensile strength is capable of withstanding large forces. However, there is a limit that each tendon fiber can endure before breaking. They are bonded so firmly into the bone that it is rare for the tendon to rip out.

The tendon is separated from surrounding tissue by a tube or sheath. This sheath allows the tendon to move without interference and produces fluid for lubricating its motion.

What causes painful tendons? This is caused by the forceful repetitive movement of the tendon within the sheath. Eventually a few of the fibers of the tendon rupture. If pain along a tendon does not ease up after a couple of days of rest, see your sports medicine physician.

When a few fibers break, nature tries to bridge the gap with scar tissue. Scar tissue is weak and does not have adequate strength to allow full use. It takes several weeks, or even months, after a tendon is injured for the scar tissue to form mature collagen in which the fibers are aligned in a parallel and linear manner so as to return the tendon to adequate strength.

Prevention of these injuries can be achieved by stretching and warming up slowly, thus less strain will be applied to the tendon.

Tennis: Tennis is an outstanding game with tremendous benefits to physical fitness once you achieve a level of expertise that allows you to run continuously and vigorously in pursuit of a point. Individuals whose expertise at the game is not very advanced will obtain very little exercise. For most people, in order to play tennis, they must become fit through an exercise program. Then, and only then, can they achieve optimum benefits from the enjoyment of the game. Once an individual achieves a certain level of excellence in the game, tennis can be used as part of a fitness program. You'll know when you achieve that level of excellence because you will recognize a level of stress throughout your tennis game as a result of continued, rigorous activity rather than the very common swing, miss, and walk that prevails in the game of the novice.

Tennis elbow: Inflammation of tendons connecting muscle to the elbow joint; a common problem connecting all muscles to all joints. It most commonly occurs in tennis players, as a result of the change in speed and motion as the arm swings and then is radically slowed upon contact with the ball. Discomfort lessens with activity and can be minimized by heating the elbow prior to activity and cooling it with ice immediately following the conclusion of the activity. This elbow condition is also very common to weight lifters. If you engage in a free-weight program and notice discomfort in the elbows, consider the warm-up, cool-down program just described.

Thin: It will always be "in."

Time: There is never enough of it, although you always have time to be sick, have an accident, and recuperate. Make time for your exercise, and you'll need less time for the aforementioned three activities.

Time to exercise: We can glibly say that the time to exercise is any time, but more productively we like to stress that working up to a 30-minute aerobic exercise program when arising in the morning is optimum. It gets your blood moving through your body, loosens you up, and gives a vigorous jump-start to your day. A similar 30-minute program of exercise in the evening washes away the stress of the work day, and sharpens all of your faculties, virtually extending the effectiveness and enjoyment of your evening hours. Exercise in the evening is best done before dinner but better done after dinner than not at all. Thirty minutes of rest after dinner, before exercise, is recommended but not necessarily essential if the meal was light. Many people enjoy exercising during their lunch hour, at their job, and this can be a very satisfactory program. The critical factor, however, is to attempt to maintain a schedule of one total hour of aerobic activity each day. There is no need to schedule days off. With most people, days off will be forced with the press of personal and work responsibilities. As we've stated time and time again, we cannot accept the argument of an individual who says that he or she has no time to exercise. The time can be borrowed from sleep, if your sleep exceeds seven hours per night; it can be borrowed from TV watching or extended meal hours. If scheduling pressures short you five weekday hours in any given week, make an effort to make up the time with additional aerobic exercise on weekends when, for most people, a greater amount of time is available. Attempt to consider seven hours of aerobic exercise a week as your basic minimum for fitness. You may include time spent playing games only when the game is very vigorous and your level of excellence is beyond doubt. Time spent lifting weights which we recommend in three half-hour sessions per week, should not be included in your seven aerobic hours.

Many people inquire about exercising before bedtime, because they are aware that exercise wakes you up and may make it difficult to sleep. This is quite true — late night exercise will have that effect on some people. However, if you are fit, you will not have any trouble sleeping whether or not you exercised shortly before retiring for the night.

Time to train: You must decide the time that is most compatible with your schedule.

Don't turn yourself inside out trying to get the time in and become filled with guilt when you can't. To begin with, if you're sleeping more than seven hours each night, ask yourself if you really need that much rest. Some people do, but most physically fit people need no more than six and one half hours of sleep a night. Once you've established the amount of time you need to sleep, you can determine the best time to get up in the morning.

I've always believed the easiest and quickest way to log some training time is an indoor bike when you're still half asleep. If you sleep from 11:30 p.m. to 6:00 a.m., you can be on that bike a few minutes after 6 and cycle for a half-hour or more. The rest of the day is a real high built on this early morning accomplishment. I do my running in the evening — right before dinner. I try to get home a little earlier in the winter when it gets dark early; in the summer, there's no rush. It may require a little negotiating with your family about dinner time, but this can be resolved.

Timid: Timidity discourages many people from leading a more active, athletic life. People are afraid to expose themselves in physical activity. Fitness is a personal thing that is wonderful to share with others but need not be. If you are timid and desire to become fit, you have to insulate yourself from any negative feedback you think may occur from those around you. Remember, any nega-

tive feedback may be a result of jealousy.

Tiredness: The normal feeling resulting from either the expension of more energy than the body can sustain from its stores or inadequate circulation of oxygen and nutrients to parts of the body. A portion of tiredness can be attributed to the mind's perception rather than the body's reality. With virtually no exception, chronic tiredness is reduced significantly with increased fitness, which may be the supreme reason for becoming fit.

Tobacco: A plant leaf containing the addictive drug nicotine, which has the parallel capacity of exciting the brain and destroying the lungs while inhibiting the vascular system. The government subsidizes its agricultural production, then rails against its only economic use, namely the manufacturing of smoking products. This is one of the greatest dichotomies in society today. It is likely that the sale of tobacco will become illegal within two decades.

Toes: Some of us experience toe discomfort from regular walking shoes; all of us at one time or another experince toe discomfort in running shoes or biking shoes. Because of the constant forward movement, pressure almost always exists between the toes and the front of an athletic shoe. For this reason, much greater care must be given to selecting running and biking shoes that are long enough to provide a little extra room for the toes.

Secondarily, the width of the shoe across the balls of the feet, commonly referred to as the toe box, needs to be generous enough so as not to provide excessive pressure across the shoe. The shoe must be properly laced so that the foot is held in the proper position in the shoe and not allowed to glide too easily forward against the front of the shoe. A narrow toe box will also cause squeezing of the nerves leading into the toes, which can readily cause numbness at the bottom of the foot just behind the toes, which can lead to excruciating pain making exercise difficult or impossible. Most of these problems stem, initially, from shoes with too small a toe box. Perhaps of greatest importance for all athletes is the necessity to keep toenails closely clipped at all times, as pressure on the nail accounts for more than 50 percent of the discomfort felt by runners and cyclists.

Tomorrow: Never as good a day to exercise as today.

Too old: You are never!

Topography: The detailed account of the surface features of the land around us. While we prefer running and cycling on flat land, we recognize the benefits of running and cycling up and down hills, as well as the aesthetic enjoyment the hills provide. Thus, make the best of what nature has provided in your community.

Toxin: A poison of animal, vegetable, or bacterial origin. From a fitness perspective, it's anything you put into your body that detracts from, rather than adds to, your well-being.

Train, don't strain: A phrase made popular by former University of Oregon track coach William Bower. It is the underlying philosophy of the authors of this book and a fact that fitness can be achieved without pain.

Training: The process of preparing oneself for an event. In the context of this book, the event of which we speak is life. All we have to say does, indeed, deal with training to improve our capacity to live. The training regimen is largely your option. But, if you're serious and you wish to live while you're alive, it will require some form of aerobic activity for an average of one hour a day and resistance activity three times a week for one-half hour. Of course you can get by with much less, but you will most assuredly lose the contest, which is to get the most out of life in the relatively short stay we have on this planet.

Training effect: This refers to the capacity of the body to undergo increasing stress and become stronger. It allows for continued improvement at nearly any age and is largely dependent on your ability to function at an elevated pulse or heart rate. The maximum heart rate that a person can attain is normally equivalent to the number resulting from the subtraction of one's age from 225. Thus, the maximum heart rate of a person 50 years of age would be 225 minus 50 or 175. The range to which the pulse must be raised to achieve a cardiovascular training effect from exercise is normally thought to be between 60 and 85 percent of the maximum rate or, in the case of a 50-year-old, between 104 and 149. Our own personal experience indicates that it is worthwhile trying for 65 percent to ensure efficient training and not to exceed 80 percent, so as to avoid the discomfort that accompanies that level of stress. Thus, we like the 114 to 140 heart beat range for training a 50-year-old person. Most people desiring to engage in aerobic exercise "briskly" will raise their heart rate into this range and thus need not measure it regularly.

Travel and exercise: Those of us who travel extensively in our work can find it difficult to maintain a regular exercise schedule. This need not and should not be the case in this day and age. Clearly, travel is fatiguing and there may be an initial tendency not to exercise when one is on the road working. This is exactly the opposite of what you should do. Exercising on the road is critical to eliminating the common fatigue that stems from traveling. Today, many hotels are aware of this and provide exercise rooms and recommend running courses for joggers. Additionally, many hotels have swimming pools of an acceptable length for lap swimming. When out of town, morning exercise should be maintained at all costs. Runs can be substituted for sessions on exercise bicycles in hotel facilities. Some hotels won't have an exercise bike for your use. Others will likely not have bikes of the quality of your own, but they will do for a short stay. If you think clearly about your work schedule on the road, you might actually recognize that you have more free time available than you have at home without the normal family responsibilities. If this is the case, focus on this extra time and make it work for you as a way of getting in extra exercise rather than, as too often is the case, using travel as an excuse not to exercise. If you travel through multiple time zones, there is nothing better to minimize the impact of jet lag than a rigorous exercise program. If you are into weight lifting and exercise machines and your hotel does not have an exercise room with adequate equipment,

they will be happy to tell you the location of a nearby gym which accepts travelers on a day-rate basis.

Traveling: Valuable exercise can actually be done while you are traveling. If you don't have to hit the ground running on your average business trip, get in the habit of traveling in workout clothes, saving the wrinkling of your business suit. Then you can use dead times in airports, or at rest stops when traveling by auto, to do valuable stretching exercises. Even on airplanes and trains there's usually a wide place where you can do a little beneficial stretching. When you're traveling in workout clothes, you won't look too odd to passersby, and most of them will envy you rather than ridicule you. Either way, you shouldn't care.

Triathlon: Any athletic competition consisting of three sporting events held one right after the other. Most commonly, it refers to swim, bike, run races popularized by the Hawaiian Ironman. The latter is a 2.4-mile swim, 112-mile bicycle ride, followed by a full 26.2-mile marathon. More common triathlon distances today consist of a 1.5-kilometer swim, a 40-kilometer bicycle ride, and a 10-kilometer run. They have become popular because of the enjoyable benefits of cross-training between three sports, which is less boring, more forgiving on the body, and generally fun.

Twenty-minute workouts: We recommend beginning aerobic exercise programs with 5-minute sessions and building up to 30-minute sessions. However, once you have achieved the ability to perform for a significant length of time, you should realize that 20 minutes is the minimal aerobic period to experience beneficial results. Conversely or consequently, you can make valuable use of a period as short as 20 minutes — a point you should keep actively aware of when time constraints make exercise difficult.

Unset agendas: We like to stress the advantage of not being rigorous in following a prescribed exercise regimen. While we want to achieve a minimum of 1 hour of aerobic activity a day, when we reach our stride as active, fit individuals, we need not be regimented in how we achieve it. Most of us will tend to do the same thing day after day and this is fine. But it is important to realize that you can awaken on any given day and decide to achieve your aerobic fitness goal in any manner that appears attractive to you on that day. We believe that we have been able to maintain rigorous fitness programs for many years because we have never suffered the burn-out of boredom. We go with the flow and the dictates of our body on a daily basis. On a given day, we might have a general idea of what we are going to do the next day, but we are ready to change that plan at a moment's notice to fit our psychological mood and our physical feelings. The only hard-and-fast rule is that we don't give in to laziness because we know too well the benefits of exercise — no matter how much at times we may wish to remain sedentary throughout the day.

Variety: An important ingredient in a physical fitness program. Avoid regimentation or sameness if it becomes boring to you. Feel free to vary the time and place of any aerobic activity; vary the aerobic activity itself. Regimentation is good for some people to ensure they get the job done, and that is fine. For those who don't like regimentation, variety is the answer in maintaining enthusiasm toward achieving fitness and staying fit.

Vegetarian: There are two types of vegetarians: those who eat no animal products whatsoever and those who will eat eggs, milk, and perhaps even poultry. The latter type who simply avoid red meat have very little problem with their diet or their health. Those who avoid all animal by-products and eat truly only vegetables can, at times, find it difficult to maintain a high energy level and, in fact, what may be considered good health. While it can be done, in order to obtain the proper protein for muscle and tissue growth, one has to combine certain vegetables to form the needed proteins. Strangely, while animals such as cows grow to be robust on grasses alone, there are few human vegetarians who one would consider robust. While avoidance of large quantities of red meat is admirable, and a desire not to eat living things can also be looked on as a reasonable philosophy, one wants to be sure not to limit one's health by being overly radical in these views. Dietary moderation in all things, in the long run, will lead to the best fitness and health.

Vicarious: Experiencing the emotions of another, which is an attribute of or even a way of life for many unfit people. When you lack the energy or physical capacity to participate in a variety of exciting activities and human endeavors, you tend to live them vicariously through others. No one will argue that that's never as good as the real thing. Fit people tend to live far more through themselves than vicariously through others.

Videotapes: Videotapes are a marvelous way to develop exercise and fitness programs. Your video rental store, today, has a wealth of different exercise tapes from a variety of instructors. Rent a few. Watch them and see what strikes your fancy. For many people, exercising along with an instructor on television is a great way to get started in a program that might suit your fancy. Remember you have to like what you see and enjoy what you're doing. If you do, then purchase the tape. If you don't, give it back and try others. While we recommend cycling in the morning and running in the evening, this can be replaced by a wide variety of aerobic activities such as rowing, cross-country skiing machines, stairmasters, as well as some excellent aerobic programs. If you find a program that suits you, that's great, as long as you end up doing aerobic activity at least one hour a day. Also please note that this hour can be divided up into two, 30-minute periods or three 20-minute periods if you wish.

Visualization: Any activity you do in the area of exercise can be significantly improved by visualizing the activity during periods of non-activity. Divers and gymnasts have benefited dramatically by performing their routines in their minds over and over. They've found that by virtue of that mind exercise, their actual physical performance improves. You can similarly benefit in the efficiency of your performance in any physical activity by thinking about it during your quiet, non-active periods. This practice can also have the effect of

reducing any fear or concern about the activity and its difficulty, which may tend to create a resistance on your part to continue performing it. This is true of all activities whether they be running, rowing, cycling, or climbing stairs. The act of visualizing or imagining your performance will make that performance easier and more comfortable. It will not, however, burn up a single calorie, so eventually, as the saying goes, you gotta do it.

Vitamins: Complex organic substances essential to the human metabolic process. We believe that people who are fit should probably take certain vitamin supplements. A single multi-vitamin tablet taken daily may be all that is required to obtain the necessary vitamin A, B, C, D, and E combinations. The vitamin controversy rages on, with many in the medical profession feeling that a balanced diet is all one needs. Unfortunately, a balanced diet is sometimes difficult to obtain, making vitamin supplements a reasonable and conservative approach. We are strong believers in megadoses of vitamin C, such as 3 grams per day, to reduce the potential for the common cold and stronger advocates, with doses as much as 1 gram per waking hour, when a cold is perceived to be coming on. The proof of the efficacy of vitamin C when battling a cold can be seen by the crystal-clear color of the urine in spite of heavy doses of vitamin C. When vitamin C is not being utilized by the body, such as normally would be the case when not fighting a cold, the urine will be canary yellow.

Vitamins and supplements (see *Nutrients*)

VO₂ max (see *Maximum oxygen uptake*)

Walking: Walking cannot be faulted as an excellent exercise, although it requires a brisk pace in order to realize its maximum benefits. Sauntering or casual walking is enjoyable and beats being a couch potato, but with the same amount of time input and a little more effort, the advantages that can be achieved in walking can be doubled or tripled by learning to walk at a brisk pace. Race walking, now sometimes termed power walking for non-competitive individuals, requires tremendous coordination, agility, and technique, but also burns 10 percent more calories than jogging an equivalent distance. Normal exercise walkers need not do either race walking or power walking to achieve tremendous benefits. But they must walk at a pace that approaches 15 minutes per mile or 4 miles per hour to get maximum benefit from their effort. With practice, 14-minute miles can be achieved and comfortable conditions still experienced. Exceptionally fast walkers can approach 12-minute miles without having to adopt the form of the race walker.

Although a brisk pace is required to optimize walking benefits, walkers should not worry once they have achieved reasonable paces for the distance they cover in a set period of time. Again, it's best to walk a set distance or a set period of time and not worry about achieving a particular pace. Practice, of course, is required to be able to walk efficiently and effectively, but once achieved one shouldn't worry about dramatic improvements in terms of walking speed. With time it may come, but it's

no longer important once one is comfortable with a sub-15-minute mile.

Walking fast: Determined by a heartbeat elevated to 60 percent of your maximum, which is 225 less your age. If you're 55, you need to reach 108. This is easily accomplished at a 14-minute mile pace, but as you get fit, you may have to walk faster to achieve it. You should experience a slight shortness of breath when walking fast. It should feel both brisk and exhilarating because of the increase in oxygen coursing through your body. Your stride should be of moderate length and each step quick enough that you have the feeling of falling forward and catching yourself on each stride.

Walking tall: Keeping your back erect and shoulders straight rather than round will contribute to more efficient bearing load on your joints and easier oxygen intake.

Wall: An imaginary obstacle all athletes and exercisers feel that they hit on occasion when they expend a maximum effort for a greater period than their body can continue to support with adequate oxygen and nutrients. It is the feeling of total system shutdown, where all movement is difficult. It happens to all competitive runners, swimmers, rowers, and cyclists who go all out. It is also a point where one is thought to go into oxygen debt, where the body is working anaerobically or in the absence of oxygen. The wall can be a pleasant masochistic experience, because it feels so good once you recover. A normal person pursuing fitness need never experience hitting the wall.

Warm hands and short socks: If you choose to walk or jog outdoors in the winter, cold hands can be your enemy. Gloves and mittens may be suitable but can also be awkward and heavy for a long distance or time period. A wonderful trick of experienced winter runners is the use of short socks as mittens. They are always at hand, easily interchangeable, can be washed regularly, weigh almost nothing, and keep your hands extremely warm at virtually any outdoor temperature.

Water, water: Water for fitness could be the subject of an essay all by itself. Few people drink enough water. We need water to cool our entire physical system. We need water to flush toxins from our body. We need water to control our body temperature. An absolute requirement of a fitness program which consists of a considerable number of aerobic activity hours per week is to drink an adequate quantity of water. Eight 8-ounce glasses a day is commonly recommended by most experts, but if you are exercising vigorously, you might actually need more. The best way to be sure that lack of water does not inhibit your physical progress is to drink copious quantities prior to your aerobic activities. This is especially true if you are going to be riding, running, or walking outdoors, where water is not readily available. A few glasses of water prior to going outdoors will normally set you up for your exercise program. If you are going to be running or biking in the heat, carry water on your bike or carry a water bottle with you on your walk or run. If you're going to be running around a circular course, leave some water in a bottle somewhere along the course that you can revisit on each circuit. While the health requirements of water previ-

ously mentioned are generally well recognized, what many individuals don't realize is that they simply perform and feel better when hydrated. It's not uncommon to get down on ourselves for not feeling up to par or not performing well when our primary problem is simply a slight amount of dehydration. Athletes and endurance racers know that being dehydrated by as little as 1 percent of body requirements will reduce optimal performance by as much as 15 percent. Increases in dehydration beyond that point cause exponential declines in performance and eventually illness. Get into the habit of drinking a lot of water before exercise, during exercise, and after exercise.

Weak: Lack of strength is normally an attribute of unfit individuals. Sometimes, it is a measure of fitness, though always inaccurately so. While it is true that most unfit people are weak, it is possible to be fit without being very strong (see *Strength*). We tend to think of weakness or strength in terms of our capacity to lift weights. It is probably more realistically thought of as our capacity to carry our own bodies physically through a strenuous day of work or play. The inability to fill very many hours of a day with human activity is the most accurate measure of human weakness and very definitely a most precise measure of lack of fitness.

Weather: Weather frequently interferes with exercise. This need not be the case for two reasons. First, an indoor stationary bicycle can always replace outdoor activities when the weather is totally inclement. Second, walking, jogging, or running out of doors can be performed in weather which is less than optimal. People tend to be dissuaded by the lightest drizzle or the least bit of cold or heat. While initiating a walk, run, or jog in such weather may be difficult, a properly dressed body quickly adjusts. The key, of course, is to be properly dressed at all times. Clothing which protects from wind and mild rain but is light in weight is a requirement for outdoor exercise.

Bicycling outdoors in bad weather can be another story altogether. Bicycling in the rain is totally unacceptable because the increased speed of the cycle makes the apparent velocity of the rain very distressing. High winds are dangerous for bicycles. Excessive cold is not readily accommodated on a bike because all body parts are not moving and the increased wind-chill factor due to the movement of the bike can make temperatures which are acceptable for running unbearable for biking. The bottom line for most people, however, is to reconsider decisions to stay indoors if outdoors is where you want to be. You will find you can enjoy a lot more exercise outdoors in moderately inclement weather than you ever thought possible, if you will only try it.

Weekends: A time when you can make up for exercise time lost during the week. A clever way to treat your weekend is to arise earlier and get in a large dose of exercise in the morning, still leaving your entire day for other activities with family and friends. If you're guilty of cheating yourself of your hour per day of aerobic exercising during the week, make it up on weekends. If you find that excessive, perhaps you would be less likely to eliminate the simple hour if you normally broke it up into two 30-minute segments during the week. Weekends are also the perfect time to involve others, who are less dedicated, in your exercise program. Relatives or friends can be coerced into short bike rides, moderate-length walks, or even a few laps in a pool. It's a time when you can have a positive impact on others by being persuasive about their accompanying you, but extremely patient about doing it at an acceptable pace and distance. If you enjoy a companion in exercise activity, you have got to cultivate one by moving at his or her speed, making it fun, not intimidating. So many men could find exercise partners in their wives if they would only be willing to invest the time in going along at their pace until they have learned to enjoy it. Eventually, their pace will improve. You can or bike with anyone and still get exercise out of it (see the entries under *Bounding* and *Spinning*).

Weight lifting: Most senior athletes never consider using free weights for exercise or body building so reading that it's a "must" will come as a surprise to most. The fact remains that free weights are a must. As an athlete ages, he or she will begin to lose serious amounts of lean muscle mass that either disappears or converts to fatty tissue. It's simply part of the genetic clock. You can undoubtedly remember the few senior athletes you have seen with well-muscled bodies because there are so few. While seniors are achieving remarkable performances in running, cycling, and swimming, and their bodies remain trim, they are not generally well-muscled and, thus, do not perform up to their potential even though their performances are excellent.

It's no surprise that lifting free weights and body building have been the sole domain of young athletes, although it can be shown to be less critical to these athletes who will retain lean muscle mass through aerobic exercise alone. While there is the rare body builder who maintains his regimen from youth to senior status, there has been no significant number of senior athletes who initiated a free-weight body-building program past 45 or 50 years of age. This situation must be corrected if senior athletes are going to reach or maintain their potential, as they can and should, through their 50s and 60s and very possibly their 70s.

The neat thing about free weights is the amazingly rapid results that we can achieve in shaping a muscle or adding muscle mass. While this can be done on weight-lifting machines, it is considerably more difficult because of the fixed motion position they demand. Of course, that is what has made them safe and popular. Free weights demand more muscle fiber, but definitely require greater care in manipulation.

By now many readers have a vision of barbell-thumping muscle men doing things well out of the range of their own capabilities. You can put that image out of your head, as free weights for seniors can, and perhaps should, omit the use of barbells entirely. While barbells obviously can be of great value in body building, they offer the disadvantage of less flexibility of movement and the need for a second person spotting for safe manipulation of heavy weights.

Everything that can be achieved with barbells can be achieved with dumbbells, safely and more flexibly. So it is a dumbbell program on which we wish to focus. Dumbbells are individual, hand-held weights which can be built to any weight level with plate weights on a short bar or in fixed configurations. Most gyms have the latter starting at 5 pounds and proceeding, in 5-pound increments, to 65 or 70 pounds. But the neatest thing about dumbbells is that you can purchase your own set, inexpensively, with a double-deck rack to hold them and thus create a weight gym in the corner of your basement or even your living room, where watching TV and weight lifting are amazingly compatible. We think of ourselves as real couch potatoes, but our couch is a weight-lifting bench, and instead of keeping our hands busy moving a munchy from dish to mouth, we move dumbbells from place to place to work every muscle group in our upper body.

Our dumbbells are chrome and are attractive enough to be allowed in the living room. However, 50 cents a pound will buy you adequate dumbbells.

Now, if we have semi-convinced you that we know of what we speak when it comes to being an old body builder, let's draw some word pictures of how you may use your dumbbells. We learned from the best, Frank Zane, Mr. Olympia 1977, 1978, and 1979. He did it all almost exclusively with dumbbells, so it stands to reason that you can expect at least moderate gains the same way. Exercise for the upper body includes dumbbell presses both flat and on an inclined bench using essentially the same motion as one would with a barbell.

Also, flat on a bench, one performs an exercise called a "fly," which brings the weights together above your chest in the back-to-bench position as though you were trying to hug a tree. All of these work the large chest muscles such as the pectorals, deltoids, and latimus dorsi. In the sitting position, bent over, one can extend the weights outward to work the shoulder muscles as well as do wrist curls for the wrists and forearms. In the standing position, there are a series of side raises that work the lats, shoulders, and arms and of course the well-known curls which work the biceps in a number of different positions. A variety of kick backs and pull-over motions work the triceps and round out the upper body.

All exercises with dumbbells should be performed in three sets. The first set is done with the heaviest dumbbells that you can lift for 15 repetitions of the exercise. The second set is done with heavier dumbbells (either a 2-, 3-, or 5-pound weight increase) performing 12 repetitions, and the final set with still heavier dumbbells performing 8 repetitions. Rest between sets can be anywhere from 30 seconds to 2 minutes, depending on the time it takes for your breathing to return to normal. With time, you will graduate to heavier dumbbell weights at 15 repetitions when the first set becomes too easy for you.

One of the neatest and unexpected side effects of weight lifting is the fact that it rapidly increases the incentive to remain slim and not overeat. The reason for this is that as new muscle texture develops, few in their right minds want to cover up the new

found gains with fatty tissue resulting from the injection of sugar and fat.

While we don't expect everyone to properly visualize the exercises we have discussed, every barbell store sells a myriad of body-building books with an abundance of pictures illustrating most of what we have described.

We have a videotape we give to all our friends who get interested in free weights. It shows us going through a workout, and we would be happy to copy it for anyone who would like to send a blank 30-minute tape and return postage. Before you run down to your local barbell store (there are no dumbbell stores), let me tell you about something else to pick up — amino acids. They are not a must, but they will yield about a 30 percent improvement in muscle development over what you achieve without them. A brand of pharmaceutical-quality formulated (there are about 17 different amino acids the body does not synthesize) capsules will do. You can take up to 1 gram per 25 pounds of body weight per day quite safely as a food supplement before meals. They tend to promote growth hormone releases in older bodies, which doesn't commonly occur without them. Here again, the proprietor of any good local barbell store or weight gym can fill you in on the whole book on amino acids. They do work, and safely.

Well, if you have gotten through this, you should be dizzy with dreams of a body you long ago thought was left behind in your youth. Not so. Clearly, the body's genetic code does work against us, but it is now proven that we can resist by heightening our physical activity instead of giving in to the naysayers and slowing down all those activities that we really need to be speeding up. It's not too late. It may never be too late. Go for it.

Where and when to train: Let's now look at some of the specifics that can help training be more fun. The first item on our list is convenience. We hate to waste time going places to exercise, so we recommend finding running courses that start and end at our front door. Occasionally, we have the desire to go elsewhere — perhaps work out on a high school track — but easy access maintains optimum enthusiasm.

Windsurfing: An exciting new sport not intended for a mature audience. Windsurfing is both great exercise and great frustration for those who aren't very good at it. Most of the time is spent climbing onto a surfboard and falling off of it. It requires incredible coordination, strength and determination. When you really get good at it and can stand on the board and hold onto the sail, the primary exercise is one of dynamic tension — simply holding onto a heavy weight. It's really great fun, but will never be a significant contributor to man's physical fitness.

Winning: Feeling good about yourself.

Wrinkle: What tends to happen to the skin of all mature and aging individuals. While some of us are blessed with just the right skin tone and moisture content to reduce wrinkles to a bare minimum, the vast majority of people over 50 have wrinkles to show for it. There is a great deal that one can specifically do for the skin to minimize wrinkles, though probably not eliminate them. Overall physical fitness is one contributor to that minimization but, by no means, is a significant answer to the problem. We know many individuals of advanced age that have bodies of 25- or 30-year-olds, but the wrinkles on their face will give away the fact that they are decades older than that.

Yawn: An indication of drowziness that can be observed in all people at one time or another. It is more commonly an indicator of people who are chronically tired and unfit.

Youth: It is said that it is wasted on the young. That may be so, but the capacity to enjoy life and live an active life, which we think of as being lost on the young, can be recaptured in our advancing years when we re-achieve a high level of fitness and a concurrent, youthful mental attitude that allows us to strip away the baggage of age and recognize that life offers largely the same opportunities for enjoyment and fulfillment to all ages.

Zilch: The amount of exercise done daily by the average adult over 50 years of age.

BIBLIOGRAPHY

Fit, Firm & 50 focuses on the mental aspects of physical fitness for people over 40. It is oriented toward athletics and uses the A-to-Z encyclopedic concept to convey most information. The purpose is to overcome the mental barriers of self-motivated people, thereby helping them perform enjoyable physical exercises that lead to improved health and quality of life.

Once interest and motivation have been established, the subject of improved health and fitness can be pursued in depth via a large number of published books. Most fitness books deal with exercise and nutrition; some focus on selected age groups and some are oriented to athletes. In additon, many positive-thinking books are available to help develop and maintain the right attitude. Although mental aspects of physical conditioning are often included in fitness books and the A-to-Z concept has been used in various ways, neither has been found to exist in book form such as *Fit, Firm & 50*.

Following is a brief bibliography of books dealing with health and fitness for people over 40.

Aerobics by Kenneth H. Cooper, M.D. (1968, M. Evans and Company, New York). Dr. Cooper's research identified the form and amount of exercise needed to improve health and longevity, and his book marks a turning point in America's outlook toward fitness. *Aerobics* provides "a scientific program of exercise aimed at the overall *fitness and health* of your body with a unique point system for measuring your progress towards maximal health."

315

Ageless Athletes — *The Scientific Approach to Achieving High-Level Fitness and Counteracting the Effects of Aging* by Richard A. Winett, Ph.D. (1988, Contemporary Books, Chicago). Dr. Winett is a health psychologist and fitness expert, a bodybuilder and former runner, and a writer. Using his research studies in psychology to form a focus for the book, Winett analyzes the programs, routines, and strategies of 17 superbly conditioned middle-aged athletes, and he presents training techniques for achieving health and fitness.

Endurance — *The Events, The Athletes, The Attitude* by Albert C. Gross (1986, Dodd, Mead & Company, New York). Gross reviews the history of endurance sport, positive and negative effects of training, and the astounding results of many athletes.

Fitness After 50 — *An Exercise Prescription for Lifelong Health* by Herbert A. de Vries, Ph.D. with Dianne Hales (1982, Charles Scribner's Sons, New York). This book provides an exercise regimen for people over 50, including those who have been out of shape for years.

Fitness for Life — *Exercises for People Over 50* by Theodore Berland (an AARP book published by the American Association of Retired Persons, Washington, D.C.; Scott, Foresman and Company, Glenview, Illinois). This book features 97 exercises and direction on designing a fitness program. Also included are chapters to assess current fitness levels, select equipment, and choose sports.

Fitness Through Pleasure — *A Guide to Superior Health for People who Like to Have a Good Time* by Porter Shimer (1982, Rodale Press, Emmaus, Pennsylvania). The goal of this book is to help the reader to improved health without forsaking happiness derived from the pleasure of bad habits. It's a "how to" book on habits: how to keep bad habits from killing you and how to keep good habits from boring you. Since pleasure provides rewards, relaxation, and a means for coping, the book acknowledges its place in a total health program.

Forever Fit — *The Exercise Program for Staying Young* by Morton D. Bogdonoff, M.D. (1983, Little, Brown and Company, Boston). Dr. Bogdonoff developed the exercise program presented in this book for men and women who want to improve their fitness. The program features a series of stretching, walking, jogging, swimming, and biking workouts that begin at an easy pace and gradually escalate.

Golf Begins at 50 — *Playing the Lifetime Game Better than Ever* by Gary Player with Desmond Tolhurst (1988, Simon and Schuster, New York). Gary Player, who is one of the best-conditioned golfers on the PGA Tour, reviews his positive viewpoint toward life and, in particular, physical health and fitness. He describes his diet and exercises, and he recommends ways for mature golfers to improve their games by improving their fitness.

Health & Fitness Excellence — The Scientific Action Plan by Robert K. Cooper, Ph.D. (1989, Houghton Mifflin Company, Boston). Cooper presents in a seven-step approach the latest information on health and fitness to dispute popular myths, fads, and fallacies. The seven steps are stress strategies, exercise options, nutritional wellness, body fat control, postural vitality, rejuvenation and living environments design, and unlimited mind and life unity.

Inside Running: Basics of Sports Physiology by David L. Costill, Ph.D. (1986, Benchmark Press, Indianapolis). Written by an authority in the field of running, this book provides information on the problems and questions facing runners and other athletes. It addresses the athlete's body, demands placed on the body, nutrition, training, and peaking for performance.

Jim Palmer's Way to Fitness by Jim Palmer with Jack Clary (1985, by Mountain Lion, Inc. and James A. Palmer Enterprises, Inc., Harper & Row, New York). "Jim Palmer — award-winning pitcher, sportscaster and jockey model — now offers his complete, lifetime program for staying in great shape, dressing smart, and being well-groomed."

Marathoning by Bill Rodgers with Joe Concannon (1980, Simon and Schuster, New York). Rodgers won the three major marathon races — Boston, New York, and Fukuoka — between the fall of 1977 and the spring of 1978. He then went on to repeat his New York win in 1978 and 1979 and his Boston win in 1979. He ran ten marathons in less than 2 hours and 12 minutes, which is the time that represents a 5-minute-per-mile pace. This is an inspirational autobiography.

Medical and Health Guide for People Over Fifty — A Program for Managing Your Health (1986, an AARP book published by the American Association of Retired Persons, Washington, D.C.; Scott, Foresman and Company, Glenview, Illinois). This is a "how-to" guide for older people to manage their health and lives.

Orienteering for Sport and Pleasure by Hans Bengtsson and George Atkinson (1977, The Stephen Greene Press, Brattleboro, Vermont.) This is a "how-to" book on orienteering, which the authors define as "the art of navigation through an unknown area using a map and compass as guide."

Perfect Parts — A World Champion's Guide to "Spot" Slimming,

Shaping, and Strengthening Your Body by Rachel Maclish and Joyce L. Vedral, Ph.D. (1987, Warner Books). Bodybuilders McLish and Vedral present a program to help women reshape specific parts of their bodies "for a sleeker, sexier, fitter you!" Each prospective reader is challenged to "discover how beautiful you can be — in only 30 minutes per week!"

Prime Time Tennis *—Tennis for Players Over 40* by Vic Seixas with Joel Cohen (1983, Charles Scribner's Sons, New York). Vic Seixas, a Wimbledon and U.S. Open champion and a U.S. Davis Cup veteran, shares his knowledge and enjoyment of tennis. Written for the mature player, Vic suggests cures to many problems experienced by amateur players. His good nature and humor make this a delightful book to read and a helpful ally to tennis players.

Staying with It *— On Becoming an Athlete* by John Jerome (1984, The Viking Press, New York). Jerome ties his experiences as an athlete and master swimmer to the essence of athletics — muscle and nerve endings, physiology, concentration, and obsession. He also relates aging to athletics in the sense that both deal with muscles and nerves. This book has been dubbed a "classic."

Superpump: Hardcore Women Body Building by Ben Weider and Robert Kennedy (1989, Sterling Publishing, New York City). Don't be fooled by the gross title. This book features a variety of beautiful women of all ages and careers dedicated to body building ,who share their diets and exercise routines.

The Athlete Within *— A Personal Guide to Total Fitness* by Harvey B. Simon, M.D., and Steven R. Levisohn, M.D. (1987, Little, Brown and Company, Boston). This book, which is based on the author's belief that we are all athletes, is loaded with information on exercise, nutrition, and stress management. Common injuries and practical instructions for constructing a balanced program are included in this hands-on guide.

The Complete Book of Walking *— The Way to Total Fitness— Step-by-Step* by Charles T. Kuntzleman and the Editors of *Consumer Guide* (1979, Simon and Schuster, New York). This book presents "the easiest and most efficient way yet devised to get fit and stay fit."

Walking for the Health of It *— The Easy & Effective Exercise for People Over 50* by Jeannie Ralston (1986, an AARP book published by the American Association of Retired People, Washington, D.C.; Scott, Foresman and Company, Glenview, Illinois). This is a "how-to" book on walking, which is described as the "best exercise" because "it uses more of the body's muscles than many other types of exercises, improves cardiovascular efficiency, and is virtually injury-free."